Sudden Deaths in Sports

# Sudden Deaths in Sports

*75 Athletes Lost Without Warning*

Douglas Putnam

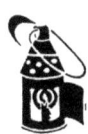

McFarland & Company, Inc., Publishers
*Jefferson, North Carolina*

Library of Congress Cataloging-in-Publication Data

Names: Putnam, Douglas T., 1953– author.
Title: Sudden deaths in sports : 75 athletes lost without warning / Douglas Putnam.
Other titles: Seventy-five athletes lost without warning
Description: Jefferson, North Carolina : McFarland & Company, Inc., Publishers, 2024 | Includes bibliographical references and index.
Identifiers: LCCN 2024006483 | ISBN 9781476694443 (paperback : acid free paper) ♾
ISBN 9781476652412 (ebook)
Subjects: LCSH: Sudden death—Popular works. | Athletes—Health and hygiene—Popular works. | Athletes—Health and hygiene—Miscellanea. | Athletes—Diseases—Popular works.
Classification: LCC RB150.S84 P88 2024 | DDC 617.1/027—dc23/eng/20240319
LC record available at https://lccn.loc.gov/2024006483

British Library cataloguing data are available
ISBN (print) 978-1-4766-9444-3
ISBN (ebook) 978-1-4766-5241-2

© 2024 Douglas Putnam. All rights reserved

*No part of this book may be reproduced or transmitted in any form or by any means, electronic or mechanical, including photocopying or recording, or by any information storage and retrieval system, without permission in writing from the publisher.*

Front cover: (left to right) Dale Earnhardt (Darryl Moran), Ray Chapman (Library of Congress), Flo Hyman (Texas Sports Hall of Fame)

Printed in the United States of America

*McFarland & Company, Inc., Publishers
Box 611, Jefferson, North Carolina 28640
www.mcfarlandpub.com*

# Contents

*Introduction*  1

## 1. In the Arena  5

- Harold Moore: Gladiator
  *College Football 1905*  5
- Francisco Lázaro: No Sweat
  *Olympic Marathon 1912*  9
- Ray Chapman: Beanball
  *MLB 1920*  10
- Bill Masterton:
  The Unforgiving Ice
  *NHL 1968*  13
- Chuck Hughes:
  A Moment's Notice
  *NFL 1971*  15
- Duk Koo Kim: Live or Die
  *Boxing 1982*  18
- Sergei Shalibashvili:
  Kiss the Tower
  *Platform Diving 1983*  22
- Lane Frost: Born to Ride
  *Bull Riding 1989*  23

## 2. Spilled Blood  27

- David Berger: All Gone
  *Olympic Weightlifting 1972*  27
- Lyman Bostock:
  Pure Happenstance
  *MLB 1978*  29
- Ron Settles: Jailhouse Shock
  *College Football 1981*  31
- Andrés Escobar:
  Brave to the End
  *World Cup Soccer 1994*  33
- Dave Schultz:
  Pinned by a Madman
  *Wrestling 1996*  35
- Greg Halman: Brothers for Life
  *Baseball 2011*  38
- Celia Barquín Arozamena:
  Broad Daylight
  *Golf 2018*  41
- Mike Ryan: Covid Rage
  *Hockey 2021*  44

## 3. Dark Waters  47

- Ed Delahanty: Swept Away
  *MLB 1903*  47
- Joe Delaney:
  Great with a Capital G
  *NFL 1983*  49
- Craig Arfons:
  Last Run on Lake Jackson
  *Speed Racing 1989*  50
- Tim Crews and Steve Olin:
  They Never Saw the Dock
  *MLB 1993*  52
- Shannon Smith: Paradise Lost
  *College Football 1997*  55
- Marquis Cooper and Corey
  Smith: Engulfed
  *NFL 2009*  57

## 4. Sound of Impact  61

- Knute Rockne: Dreadful News
  *College Football 1931*  61
- Thurman Munson:
  Out of His League
  *MLB 1979*  65

- Davey Allison: Chopper Down
  *NASCAR 1993* … 68
- Rodney Culver: Nosedive
  *NFL 1996* … 70
- Payne Stewart: Flight of Doom
  *Golf 1999* … 73
- Cory Lidle: Manhattan Fireball
  *MLB 2006* … 75

## 5. Accidents Will Happen … 79

- Terry Sawchuk: Senseless
  *NHL 1970* … 79
- Don Wilson: Beyond Strange
  *MLB 1975* … 82
- Richard Wertheim: Lethal Ace
  *Tennis 1983* … 84
- Owen Hart: Real as Can Be
  *World Wrestling Federation 1999* … 85
- Matīss Kivlenieks: Fiasco
  *NHL 2021* … 88

## 6. Demons and Disease … 92

- Flo Hyman: No Warning
  *Volleyball 1986* … 92
- Len Bias: Shock to the Systems
  *Basketball 1986* … 94
- Reggie Lewis:
  Too Young, Too Soon
  *Basketball 1993* … 98
- Sergei Grinkov: Shattered Dream
  *Pairs Figure Skating 1995* … 100
- Andreas Munzer: Hunger Pains
  *Bodybuilding 1997* … 103
- Korey Stringer:
  Water Is for Cowards
  *NFL 2001* … 106
- Tyler Skaggs: Black Cloud
  *MLB 2019* … 109

## 7. In the Arena Redux … 113

- Hank Gathers: Heart of a Lion
  *Basketball 1990* … 113
- Ulrike Maier: No Chance
  *Skiing 1994* … 116
- Fabio Casartelli: Deadly Descent
  *Tour de France 1995* … 117
- John McSherry: Last Call
  *MLB 1996* … 119
- Caleb Moore: Fatal Obsession
  *Snowmobile, X-Games 2013* … 121
- Oshi: Breaking Point
  *Iditarod 2019* … 124
- Yellow River Stone Forest:
  21 Gone
  *Ultramarathon 2021* … 128

## 8. Win, Place or Die … 131

- Frank Hayes:
  First Win, Only Win
  *Steeplechase 1923* … 131
- Ruffian: She Reigns
  *Match Race 1975* … 134
- Billy Haughton: Breaking Gait
  *Harness Racing 1986* … 138
- Mary Bacon: Riding Is Living
  *Off Track 1991* … 140
- Santa Anita Meltdown:
  How Many More Have to Die?
  *Thoroughbreds 2019* … 142

## 9. Motorsport Mishaps … 147

- Bill Vukovich: The Fearless One
  *Indy 500 1955* … 147
- The Dakar Rally: Desert Storm
  *Off Road Racing 1988* … 149
- Ayrton Senna: Collision Course
  *Formula One 1994* … 153
- Dale Earnhardt:
  Long Live the King
  *NASCAR 2001* … 155
- Jessi Combs: Speed Kills
  *Speed Racing 2019* … 158
- IMTT: Full Throttle
  *Motorcycle 2022* … 160

## 10. Team Tragedy … 164

- Spokane Indians: Such Hell
  *Baseball 1946* … 164

- Duluth Dukes:
    North Country Inferno
    *Baseball 1948* ............ 166
- Cal Poly Mustangs:
    Lost in the Fog
    *College Football 1960* ............ 167
- USA Figure Skating:
    Total Eclipse
    *Figure Skating 1961* ............ 170
- Wichita State Shockers:
    Gold Flight
    *College Football 1970* ............ 172
- Marshall Thundering Herd:
    The Worst
    *College Football 1970* ............ 174
- Evansville Purple Aces:
    Basketball's Darkest Night
    *Basketball 1977* ............ 176
- USA Boxing: KO'd by Fate
    *Boxing 1980* ............ 178

**11. Red Highways** ............ 179
- Steve Prefontaine: Bell Lap
    *Running 1975* ............ 179
- Pelle Lindbergh:
    A Man and His Porsche
    *NHL 1985* ............ 181
- Jackson State Tigers:
    Blue Bengal Curse?
    *College Football 1988–1990* ............ 184
- John Rodolph: Pure Soul
    *Wheelchair Racing 1995* ............ 186
- Judith Flannery: End of the Road
    *Triathlon 1997* ............ 187
- Dwayne Haskins:
    Running on Empty
    *NFL 2022* ............ 189

**12. The Savage God** ............ 191
- Rick Carter: No Goodbyes
    *College Football 1986* ............ 191
- Jeff Alm: Very Close
    *NFL 1993* ............ 194
- Erica Blasberg: Final Breath
    *Golf 2010* ............ 197

*Chapter Notes* ............ 203
*Bibliography* ............ 207
*Index* ............ 213

# Introduction

This book chronicles the lives and deaths of athletes who departed our world suddenly, unexpectedly and without warning during their playing careers.

For many the end came early, cruelly robbing them of the chance to keep competing. For others it arrived in their hour of greatest glory. And for some it came at the end of the road as they struggled to survive in the sports they loved and lived for. All of them faced the same merciless truth—there would be no next year.

My interest in the subject began in my college years when I watched mesmerized as three events unfolded on the television screen—the on-field collapse of NFL wide receiver Chuck Hughes at Tiger Stadium in 1971, the kidnapping and murder of 11 Israeli athletes and coaches at the Munich Olympics in 1972 and the breakdown of Ruffian on the track at Belmont Park during her match race with Foolish Pleasure in 1975.

They captivated and upset me, and I was far from the only one who felt that way. Athletes dying young attract widespread attention. The shock of premature death stirs up deep feelings in millions of fans.

In the 1990s I began collecting source material in earnest, starting with contemporaneous newspaper accounts provided by more than 40 public and private libraries. From there I proceeded to longer retrospectives and books that offered insights into the tragedies and the contexts in which they occurred. By the time I began writing early versions of this work I had files on nearly 150 incidents.

The book is not an exercise in celebrity reportage, featuring only the famous. Nor is it a master scroll that attempts to record every sudden death in every era in every sport. If a story contained an element that aroused my interest I dug deeper. I was drawn in by the tortuous brotherly bond that led to the passing of Greg Halman and the ain't-afraid-to-die bedlam of the Isle of Man motorcycle races and the unspeakable horror of Payne Stewart's flight of doom from Florida to a farm pasture in North Dakota. The coverage ranges from 1903 to 2022. Time, space and endurance constraints led me to forgo many compelling stories, particularly from earlier times with source material that is often sparse and difficult to access.

Most of the 75 accounts take place in America, but 20 other countries factor into the narratives. The highlighted realms are football, baseball, basketball, hockey, motorsports and horse racing. Overall more than 25 sports are included. While writing the main draft I expanded my scope and added eight accounts centered on coaches, game officials, racehorses and sled dogs.

A third of the stories focus on "in the arena" deaths, arising from injuries sustained while competing in games, races, matches, bouts, runs and rallies. The rest of the deaths cover the waterfront. Cold-blooded murder at the hands of a perfect stranger, a disgruntled fan, and a deranged tycoon. Accidents in jets, prop planes, buses, fishing boats and sports cars. By drug overdose. By drowning in bodies of water large and small. By way of disease and genetic defects. In freak accidents in a backyard hot tub and a barbecue pit and the rafters high above a wrestling ring. Grimmest of all, in four cases, and maybe a fifth, by suicide.

There are no perfect human beings in our world, and you will not find any here, although a few come close. Furthermore, many of the fallen contributed to their own demise through arrogant, reckless and downright stupid behavior. I'm not condemning them. Nor am I mourning them less than I otherwise would. At the same time, I don't sweep their actions under the rug or absolve them of deserved blame.

During the course of the project several recurring themes emerged. One is the squabbling about protective headgear that persisted in football, hockey, baseball, motorsports and biking for decades and continues today with the mandated use of Guardian Caps in NFL training camps.

Another is the ongoing, pervasive presence of illicit drugs in the sports world. Whether they're classified as performance-enhancing like steroids and amphetamines or as drugs of abuse like cocaine and non-prescribed opioids, they've been around for a very long time. Then of course there are the legal substances—alcohol and tobacco. They've been around even longer. There are also repeated instances of accusation and protracted legal action by the families of the departed, directed at the parties they held responsible for their loss.

Another takeaway is that sudden death can lead to constructive change. When tragedy strikes, the powers that be often respond. After Tyler Skaggs died of a fentanyl overdose in 2019, MLB revamped its drug violation policies to emphasize rehabilitation and treatment instead of monetary fines and suspensions. The brutal pounding from Ray Mancini that killed Duk Koo Kim on the Las Vegas Strip in 1982 led boxing to adopt the standing eight count and require extensive pre-fight medical exams. There has not been a heat stroke fatality in the NFL since Korey Stringer collapsed and died in training camp in 2001. Dale Earnhardt's death in the same year prompted NASCAR to require use of the HANS (head and neck support) device for all drivers in its top three series. And the deaths of 30 horses during the 2019 racing season at Santa Anita Park in California led Congress to mandate uniform anti-doping regulations at tracks nationwide.

A book that explores personal tragedy and the darker aspects of human existence can be challenging for both writer and reader. But by delving deeper into death and all it signifies we can reach a greater understanding of life. I didn't allow all the grim morbidity to overshadow the accomplishments of these magnificent athletes and I hope you won't either. Their drive to excel was surpassed only by their desire to compete. Each and every one of them was a warrior.

# 1

## In the Arena

### Harold Moore: Gladiator
*College Football 1905*

The game was played in the Bronx on November 25, 1905, at a place called Ohio Field on a bluff overlooking the Harlem River. It was quirky that the home of the New York University Violets football team shared a name with the home of the Ohio State Buckeyes way out in the flatlands, 560 miles to the west.

Perhaps it was a sign of college football's way of connecting people all across America. As the new century unfolded, the sport was surging in popularity, fueled by rabid fans drawn to the robust action on autumn afternoons in every region of the country.

The NFL would not exist for another 16 years. MLB—the American and National Leagues—reigned supreme. But as squads like Harvard, Chicago, LSU, Michigan and Stanford gained renown, football was getting as much coverage in newspapers and magazines as horse racing, boxing and golf.

NYU would see some glory years down the road but in 1905 they were hardly a power. Neither was their opponent that day, Union College out of Schenectady. NYU came into the contest at 2-3-1. Union was 3-5. Their schedules included Lehigh, Trinity, Hobart and Wesleyan. It was the last outing of the season for both.

The game they played was in many ways vastly different from the one we see today. The field was 110 yards long. The goalposts were on the goal line, not at the back of the end zone. There was no passing, no neutral zone along the line of scrimmage and no protective equipment, except scattered nose guards and goofy looking padded hats. Leather helmets wouldn't be widely used until the 1920s.

Games were usually 70 minutes long, divided into two halves with no quarters. The starting elevens played both offense and defense. If a player left the game, he could not return. Only five yards, not ten, were needed for a first down, so there was little incentive to run around the end. Straight up the middle was the way to go. Three yards and a cloud of dust was the order of the day.

The preferred way for the offense to operate was the flying wedge. With their hands wrapped tightly around each other's "wedge belts," the unit formed a chevron-like shield in front of the ball carrier. The job of the defense was to smash through the shield as it rumbled down the field and tackle him. Each side could accomplish its goal by just about any means necessary. Though they existed, "rules" were not much of a factor.

The entire exercise was an inch or two above the level of street thuggery, and the results were predictable. Broken arms, legs, ribs, shoulders, jaws and noses. Ruptured spinal cords. Fractured skulls. Mangled knees. Bruised buttocks. Dislocated hips. And ample helpings of blood.

The brutality on the field was so extreme that the game was getting a bad reputation. Not everybody loved it, and a lot of those who didn't were very outspoken.

Many were college professors, mortified that their esteemed institutions of higher learning had gotten tangled up in something as sordid as football. The dean of the University of Chicago divinity school called it a "boy killing, education-prostituting, gladiatorial sport."[1]

Some were activists who viewed football reform as an agenda item in the Progressive movement that peaked during the presidency of Theodore Roosevelt. Progressives are best remembered for fighting trusts and big business and securing the right to vote for women. But they also strived to promote moral improvement, and curtailing the Saturday afternoon bloodshed fit in well under that rubric. There were also a few muckraking journalists following the lead of Nelly Bly, always on the prowl for scandals that exposed the shortcomings of society's elites.

Notably absent among the critics were Bible thumpers, evangelical Christians who wanted to rid the world of John Barleycorn, dice games, houses of ill repute and loose morals of every shape and stripe. They didn't have much of a beef with football. That's not surprising because religion—at least one version of it—played a vital role in the birth of the game. Football bloomed in the decades after the Civil War, during the era of Muscular Christianity. For members of the sect, sports had spiritual value. The male body was something to be cultivated, improved and celebrated. Playing football was a godly pursuit. The Heavenly Father approved. Churches and YMCAs sponsored many teams before the focus shifted to schools, colleges and universities. Players often took the field holding hands in a circle, singing the Doxology or reciting the Lord's Prayer.

The naysayers did have a point about violence. If only because the deaths that year were widely recorded, 1905 was a notably lethal season. Sources differ on exactly how many young people perished—13, 18, 19, 21. And it was often hard to determine if the injury suffered on the field was the primary cause of death.

One case in which it clearly was occurred on November 3, with the demise of Bernadette Decker, 18, a member of the girls' team in Eckhart Mines, Maryland. In medical language, the injury she suffered "resembled malignant peritonitis."[2] In other words, somebody's knee or head or foot rammed her in the gut so hard that it blew her stomach apart.

Another occurred on the day before the NYU-Union game when Carl Osborne, 18, died playing for Bellmore High School in Indiana. He got slammed in the chest by a charging opponent and one of his broken ribs ripped through his heart.

The *Chicago Tribune* called the parade of bodies that fall "a death harvest."[3] The situation had grown gruesome enough to draw the concern of Roosevelt. Raised as a Muscular Christian, TR loved the game even though he'd been barred from playing at Harvard because of poor eyesight. On October 9, he hosted a small, clubby gathering at the White House. Present were the football men from Harvard, Princeton and Yale—all superpowers. Also in the room was Walter Camp, the grand old man of the gridiron who'd gone 79–5–3 in eight years as coach at Yale and Stanford from 1888 to 1895.

The Rough Rider delivered his message in a soft voice. My eyes are on you. Adhere to the codified rules of the game. If the roughhousing and anarchy on the field doesn't abate, I am going to swing my big stick and insist on some serious changes. Consider your sport to be on probation.

Roosevelt's role in the controversy likely has been exaggerated. He was joining a chorus of criticism that was loud and in tune well before he jumped on stage. But his involvement was key. It wasn't every day that a president thrust himself into the inner workings of colleges and universities.

That was the situation as November 25 arrived seven weeks later. One of the players on Ohio Field was Harold Moore, 19, an engineering student and two-year starter at halfback for Union. His father made the 390-mile trip from Ogdensburg on the banks of the St. Lawrence River to watch him play.

Early in the game, Moore busted through the NYU flying wedge. The ball carrier's head crunched right under his chin. Or maybe Moore was kicked in the head. Or his head smacked down flush on somebody's knee. Maybe all three happened. He collapsed to the turf, blacked out and went into convulsions. He was hauled to the sideline and transported to Fordham Hospital where he died of a cerebral hemorrhage some six hours later, his father at his bedside. On November 28, he was buried in Ogdensburg. Shaken by the tragedy, Union cancelled its entire 1906 season.

Because it happened in New York City and received extensive national publicity, Moore's death became the catalyst for change. In December, college presidents from all regions met and formed the Intercollegiate Athletic Association, the forerunner of the NCAA.

The group enacted a slew of rule changes. They shortened the game to 60 minutes, legalized the forward pass, created the neutral zone, changed the distance needed for a first down from five to ten yards and added a penalty for unnecessary roughness. Projecting nails on the soles of shoes were prohibited, as were iron insets. Knee and thigh pads for all players were encouraged.

Within the tribe of old school jocks that ruled the domain, there was fear that the radical revamping would make their game too effeminate. Walter Camp did not approve. Neither did Amos Alonzo Stagg, the coach of the Chicago Maroons juggernaut that had just finished an 11–0 campaign. The tribe also feared that fan interest would wane.

Instead just the opposite happened. At first an incomplete pass resulted in a turnover, so very few were attempted. But after that rule was scrapped the aerial game soon proved to be electrifying. In the Roaring 20s, with the rise of radio and the emergence of major conferences and rivalries, college football stood second only to baseball in the breadth and depth and intensity of its fan base. The seeds were planted for a sport that after World War II would tie its fortunes to television and mushroom into a multi-billion-dollar entertainment enterprise.

More than a century has passed since the pioneer era. How much has really changed about the game? In some ways virtually nothing. Football has never been simply a contact sport. It's also a *collision* sport. That's the essence of it. Woody Hayes said that football was about two things—blocking and tackling. And the point of both of those endeavors is the same as ever—knock some guy across the line from you in a different color jersey on his butt.

But some things are different. Rules for rough play are strictly enforced, protective equipment is far more effective, and medical treatment is extraordinary. What we have today instead of death on the field by blunt force trauma is an insidious disease called chronic traumatic encephalopathy (CTE). It's caused by repeated blows to the head and also afflicts boxers and soccer and hockey players.

The blows don't have to be strong enough to spawn concussions. A sizable number of CTE victims never suffered a concussion in their lives. It's a matter of quantity. The more slaps and punches and jolts to the head, the greater the damage inflicted by an overload of a protein called tau that strangles cells in various parts of the brain and impairs its ability to function.

CTE can only be diagnosed after death. The brains of some 315 NFL players—including Hall of Famers Frank Gifford and Ken Stabler—have been found to contain evidence of CTE. Symptoms can show up quickly or lay dormant for years before they erupt. Violent rage, paranoia, aggression and memory loss head the list, and they're sometimes accompanied by suicidal impulses. Junior Seau, Jovan Belcher, Aaron Hernandez, Andre Waters and Phillip Adams are among the NFL's CTE-induced suicides.

So here's a thought. The Grim Reaper is probably claiming just about as many football players as he ever did. These days, he's just practicing his craft more patiently.

But this volume is about swift, unexpected, unforeseen death, with an emphasis on those that spring from competition. Let's move on from Ohio Field to more places where stars have fallen in the arena—the streets of Stockholm, the Polo Grounds, an ice rink in Minnesota, Tiger Stadium, a boxing ring on the Las Vegas Strip and the Frontier Days Rodeo in Wyoming.

## Francisco Lázaro: No Sweat
*Olympic Marathon 1912*

Francisco Lázaro arrived in Stockholm, Sweden, for the 1912 Summer Olympics as a confident, accomplished long distance runner. He'd won three marathons in his native Portugal, 1,800 miles to the south, with a personal best of 2:52:08. Sporting thick black hair, a brick house body and a handlebar moustache, the bowlegged carpenter who worked in an automobile factory in Lisbon was the proud flag bearer of his country's first Olympic team.

You could even call him a bit cocky. Asked for his thoughts on the upcoming race, he responded "either I win or I die."[4]

That quote might be accurate. Or it might have been dreamed up by other people after the fact because it fit the story line so well. The sad truth is that his prediction was spot on. He didn't win the race. The gold medal went to Ken McArthur of South Africa. And Lázaro left Stockholm in a coffin, the first athlete to die in the modern Olympics from an injury suffered in competition. There has only been one since.

Lázaro concocted a borderline crazy scheme to boost his performance in the 26-mile, 385-yard race. A few hours before the start, he slathered a substance called suet all over his body. Suet is the hard white fat surrounding the kidneys of cattle, sheep and horses. It's the base material in tallow, used in cooking and for making candles, soap and lubricants.

He applied the suet to his skin for two reasons. First, he wanted to reduce frictional drag and resistance to air flow in order to increase his speed. It sounds nutty but it works. Many swimmers shave their body hair for the same reason. Second, he wanted to prevent painful, blistering sunburn. He no doubt was successful to some degree on both counts.

But the suet also had a huge downside. The thick waxy gunk clogged the pores of his skin so tightly that it prevented him from sweating. Did he know that sealing up his skin with the organic version of Saran Wrap was dangerous? It's hard to believe he didn't. But we can't be certain. The state of medical science in 1912 was primitive—shockingly so by today's standards. Diseased limbs were amputated with hacksaws and the flu was treated by bloodletting and forced consumption of 100 proof alcohol. If Lázaro was aware of the risk, it was one he'd decided was worth taking.

The gun sounded at 1:48 on Sunday afternoon, July 14, in Stockholm's new Olympiastadion. The temperature was 89 degrees Fahrenheit. Of the 68 runners from 19 nations who started only 35 finished, the rest forced to the sidelines by the brutal heat. Lázaro wore a painter's cap to protect his head from the sun. He was used to running in hot conditions and he believed that would give him yet another competitive edge.

His strategy worked for 90 minutes or so. Then halfway through the race, just past the turnaround point, he went down hard. He bounced up and soldiered on, staggering badly time and time again, until he collapsed for good climbing a hill at the 30-kilometer marker. Boy Scouts patrolling the course found him prostrate on the dirt road.

At a modern hospital nearby he turned delirious, and his body temperature rose to 106.7 degrees. Cramping and convulsing, he spent the night in an intensive care bed and died at six o'clock Monday morning. Spurred by a lack of perspiration, a severe electrolyte imbalance in his body fluids sealed his fate. He was 21.

Might Lázaro have lived if officials had moved the race to the cooler morning hours? Or if an enlightened medical professional had gotten wind of his scheme and convinced him to back off? Those questions must remain unanswered.

Lázaro's death is largely forgotten now, lost in the foggy mists of time. A simple monument stands in the Stockholm suburb of Sollentuna near the point where he first fell. The novel *The Piano Cemetery* by Portuguese writer José Luís Peixoto is based on his life.

The only other athlete to die from an injury suffered in Olympic competition is Knud Enemark Jensen, a 23-year-old Danish biker. During the 100-kilometer team time trial at the 1960 Summer Games in Rome, Jensen collapsed on the course and fractured his skull on the concrete pavement. The official cause of death was heatstroke.

But during his autopsy traces of Roniacol were discovered in his body. It's a liquid substance that widens vessels to improve blood flow. Another find was amphetamines, known today under a variety of names—speed, beans, bennies, black beauties, speckled birds, uppers, pep pills. Whatever it's called, the stuff is used solely for the purpose of enhancing performance by increasing energy and endurance. Like Lázaro, Jensen was simply trying to move faster toward the finish line. His death is viewed today as a seminal event in the relentless rise of doping in the sports world.

## Ray Chapman: Beanball
*MLB 1920*

It was a Monday afternoon game in front of a big noisy crowd of 21,000, with the teams in the thick of a pennant fight. The temperature was 88 degrees, the air was damp and drizzly, and the sky was very dark.

In the top of the fifth the shortstop led off for the visitors, who were leading 3–0. He hunched over the plate as if preparing to bunt. The third pitch whistled right at his head straight and hard. He never budged. It was as if he didn't see the ball coming. It smashed into his left temple with a loud smack and rolled all the way back to the mound. The pitcher flipped the ball to first base because he thought it had hit the handle of the bat.

# 1. In the Arena

With blood gushing from his left ear, the batter sank to the dirt and blacked out. He came to, stood up, and collapsed again on the way to the dugout. His teammates carried him to the clubhouse, where he blacked out again. But he came to and seemed to be on the upswing until later that evening when he was rushed to the hospital.

His skull was cracked wide open, and a piece of his brain was crushed. He died early the next morning at age 29 after doctors failed in a desperate attempt to save his life. He left behind a pregnant wife who gave birth to their daughter six months later.

Since the founding of the National League in 1876, there have been 147 seasons of MLB through 2023. Cleveland Indian Ray Chapman remains the only player in that long span to die after being hit in the head by a pitch. His beaning at the hands of Yankee pitcher Carl Mays at the Polo Grounds in New York City on August 16, 1920, remains one of the game's most notorious moments.

The submarine delivery of a doctored-up ball was the pitch that killed that day. But many other pitches at all levels of play have also killed. While it is impossible to determine the true mindsets of human beings, the vast majority of beanballs are thought to be accidental. After an inquiry by the New York district attorney, Mays was found not to have acted with intentional malice. He reached that conclusion even though Mays had a longstanding reputation as a nasty SOB who liked to throw at batters. Whatever the motivations of the pitchers, the beanball has been a dangerous staple of the game for a very long time.

Robert Gorman and David Weeks compiled accounts of fatal beanings in their exhaustive book *Death at the Ballpark* (2015). They documented 11 in professional minor leagues between 1906 and 1951, two in Black pro leagues in 1908 and 1929, and nearly 300 on school, college and amateur teams, starting with a 24-year-old shortstop for the Red Bluff (CA) Athletics in 1880 and ending with a 13-year-old Babe Ruth League player from Gillette, New York, in 2011. There were three deaths in 1920, including one in Silver Creek, Michigan, the day before Chapman's beaning and another that killed a 14-year-old Boy Scout in Corning, New York.

Those numbers do not include fatalities from thrown or batted balls or from pitched balls that hit batters somewhere other than their heads. Gorman and Weeks consider all of those to be separate categories.

As your eyes roll through page after page of the memorial scroll, something stands out. It's downright amazing that there hasn't been a beaning death in MLB since Chapman's more than a century ago.

The zero out is largely due to blind dumb luck—and the now mandatory use of batting helmets. Ray Chapman was a talented nine-year veteran, a popular, affable player on a good team, one that would rally from the depths of grief to defeat the Brooklyn Dodgers in the World Series six weeks after the tragedy. His death received extensive publicity. You might think that all that would have led to the swift advent of helmets in MLB.

You would be wrong.

The campaign for helmet use inched forward at a glacial pace, held back primarily by opposition from players. In the 1920s some started wearing tight-fitting leather headgear similar to the football helmets of the day. There was another contraption lined with cork and another that resembled a large pair of earmuffs. None of them caught on, and today the reasons offered by players for shunning protection just sound kind of silly. Helmets obscured vision and slowed them down on the basepaths. Their inner linings accumulated sweat that dropped down into their eyes during the course of a game. The fans would razz them. Worst of all, helmets would make them look and feel like sissies and wimps and pantywaists. Could there be anything worse than that?

In 1940, Pee Wee Reese and Joe (Ducky) Medwick of the Dodgers were both beaned within a span of three weeks. That prompted GM Larry McPhail to mandate headgear for the team the next year. The prototype for the modern helmet was introduced in 1952 by Pirates GM Branch Rickey. Four years later the NL mandated protective headgear. The AL followed in 1958. Plastic or cork liners that fit underneath cloth caps passed muster. Helmets themselves were not required until 1971, and after their use became standard procedure in MLB and other leagues, the number of beaning fatalities and injuries declined dramatically.

So today beanings are virtually extinct and helmets are worn everywhere. But there's another aspect of Chapman's story in which very little progress has been made.

The fatal pitch that Carl Mays threw at Chapman was widely viewed at the time to be a spitball. That's a generic term used to describe a ball that has been altered by the application of a foreign substance. It doesn't have to be pure saliva. Most of the time it is saliva mixed with something else—resin, talcum, licorice, dirt, mud, petroleum jelly, pine tar.

In the case of Mays it was likely mud and dirt, perhaps with a squirt or two of tobacco juice added in. He was throwing a "rough" ball to begin with, one that had been nicked and dirtied up in the regular course of play. In 1920 umpires didn't replace balls nearly as frequently as they do today, and they took a real beating. That just made doctoring them up all the more tempting.

Whatever the substance applied, the point of the exercise was always the same—to make the ball harder to hit. If a pitcher loaded up a ball with gunk and goo it gave him a firmer grip. A firmer grip led to a faster spin rate that in turn created more ball movement. The pill might go over, under, sideways or down, confusing and confounding hitters.

Goo and gunk also made the ball harder to see. The most plausible explanation of Chapman's death is that the rough ball was further darkened by mud and dirt and tobacco juice to the point that it blended in perfectly with the infield turf. The sunless, overcast day reduced visibility even more. It all explains why the shortstop stood in the batter's box like a frozen statue as the ball smashed into his temple.

Citing Chapman's death, safety concerns, and the fact that spitters gave pitchers an unfair advantage over hitters, both major leagues imposed a partial ban on spitballs before the 1921 season. Under a bizarre "grandfather" clause, each of the 16 teams could name two pitchers who would be allowed to throw them legally until they retired. Carl Mays was not on the Yankees designated spitters list. But he continued to throw them anyway because enforcement was lax, and he knew he could get away with it. Dozens of other pitchers through the years have done the same. The spitter may technically be illegal, but the pitch has not merely survived on the diamond. It has thrived.

Preacher Roe was a master ball doctor with the Dodgers in the 1950s. Don Drysdale continued the practice into the 1960s, and Gaylord Perry, the Ancient Mariner who played 22 seasons in MLB, threw it steadily until his retirement in 1983. He was so fond of the pitch that he titled his autobiography *Me and the Spitter.*

Fast forward to 2021 and the abrupt rise of the "sticky stuff scandal." With the number of strikeouts skyrocketing and offenses in the doldrums, parties well-versed in physics and statistics documented an alarming rise in spin rates throughout MLB. Their conclusion was that ball doctoring was rampant. The substances being applied were a bit more exotic—sunscreen, glue, hair gel, fir tree sap—but the results were the same. Pitchers win, hitters lose. There were nine no-hitters in the 2021 season. One observer brashly stated the deluge of sticky stuff was the biggest scandal in the entire sports world.

That summer rules were enacted to allow umpires to check pitchers for the presence of foreign substances during games. The crackdown met with some resistance. White Sox hurler Lance Lynn was ejected from a game after he threw a hissy fit and flung his belt at an umpire during a check. Sergio Romo of the A's dropped his pants on the mound in protest. In 2023, Mets ace Max Scherzer and Yankee right-hander Domingo German served 10-game suspensions for doctoring their pitches.

What the future holds in terms of enforcement is uncertain. But for now here's the gist. Pitchers of the modern era—at least until 2021—have been throwing doctored balls at batters just like the doctored ball Carl Mays threw at the Polo Grounds on that dark, drizzly afternoon in 1920. That's the most overlooked aspect of Ray Chapman's death.

## Bill Masterton: The Unforgiving Ice
### *NHL 1968*

Bill Masterton was keenly aware of the many risks that confronted those playing the fast, rough game of ice hockey. He had been on skates most of his life. In junior leagues in his native Winnipeg, Manitoba. At the University of Denver, a hockey powerhouse, where he earned All-America honors and led the Pioneers to NCAA titles in 1960 and 1961. And in the minor leagues with teams in Hull-Ottawa and Cleveland in the Montreal Canadiens organization. Every time he took the ice he faced brutal body checks, sharply-honed skates, airborne pucks, flying sticks and opponents' fists, all in a game played on the most unforgiving of surfaces.

Masterton left pro hockey after two seasons. He felt he'd gone as far up the ladder as he could. He married, adopted two children with his wife Carol and went to work for the Honeywell Corporation in Minneapolis as a contract administrator. But he never let go of his dream of playing in the NHL. In 1967, when he was offered a chance to try out for the Minnesota North Stars, he jumped on it. He knew it would be a tough go, but he was confident he could catch on with the expansion team.

He did. The 6–0, 186-pounder earned a roster spot as a center and scored the first goal in North Star history against the St. Louis Blues on October 11.

The tragic end of his comeback story came just four months later. Four minutes into a game against the Oakland Seals on January 13, 1968, Masterton had just slid a pass to right wing Wayne Connelly when he was checked harshly from the back and side in a crowd of high-sticking players in the Oakland zone. He flew backward and landed on his head. By all accounts they were powerful, even vicious hits. But in the eyes of the referees they were clean. No penalty was called.

Masterton's eyes were loose, and he'd swallowed his tongue. Bleeding from the nose and ears, he was taken from the Metropolitan Sports Arena to Fairview-Southdale Hospital seven miles away. Neurosurgeons were unable to operate on him because of the extreme gravity of his injuries. He died without regaining consciousness at 1:55 a.m. on January 15, 30 hours after his fall. He was 29.

There have been many near fatalities in the NHL, most notably Gordie Howe's skull fracture in a 1950 playoff game. And way back in 1907, Owen (Bud) McCourt of Cornwall died after brawling with opponents in a game against Ottawa in the Federal Amateur Hockey League, a forerunner of the NHL. But after 105 seasons through 2023, Masterton remains the only player to die from an injury sustained in an NHL game.

A new take on his death has arisen in recent years and gained considerable credence. The theory is that Masterton did not die solely from the blow he took in the Seals game. He'd been playing with heavy damage from an earlier concussion that was never diagnosed or treated and did not heal properly. Doctors call it second impact syndrome. It can cause rapid, severe swelling. The brain more or less explodes, and death quickly follows.

Several North Star players said later that Masterton seemed woozy and disoriented in the days leading up to January 13. He complained of headaches to his wife and a few close friends. But otherwise it was business as usual. Playing hurt was the order of the day in the warrior culture of the NHL. The protocol was to shake the pain off and get back in the rink, lest you be branded a yellowbelly by your teammates. An even greater threat was incurring the contempt of management and losing your roster spot.

The North Stars headed for Boston after the incident for a Sunday game with the Bruins. Coach and GM Wren Blair, who hadn't slept in three days, waited until Monday morning to break the news to his team. They did not take it well. They looked like zombies on the ice and proceeded to lose their next six games before rallying to stay in the playoff hunt. After finishing their inaugural season with a 27–32–15 record, they won their first-round playoff series against the Los Angeles Kings.

The Bill Masterton Trophy was established in 1968. Awarded by the Professional Hockey Writers Association, it recognizes the NHL player who best exemplifies the qualities of perseverance, sportsmanship and dedication to hockey. His number 19 jersey was retired. It hung from the rafters of the Metropolitan Sports Arena until the North Stars moved to Dallas in 1993. It is now in the United States Hockey Hall of Fame in Eveleth, Minnesota.

Masterton's greatest legacy is the universal use of helmets by NHL players today. He wore a helmet at every stage of his career until he reached the NHL. Carol said that if her husband had been wearing one on the night of his last game "he would have had a chance."[5]

But as in baseball, there was longstanding resistance to helmets among the league's players. Knitted woolen caps called tuques were common in the early years of the game, but they were used to keep the head warm, not protect it.

Even as players added other forms of protection through the years—shoulder and kidney pads, heavier gloves, shin, ankle and instep guards—helmets continued to be viewed with disdain. They were too confining, too hot, too uncomfortable. They impaired vision and reduced rink awareness. They were unpopular with fans and media as well because they concealed the faces and hair of the players. The aversion lingered despite the fact that many prominent players wore them, including Eddie Shore, Red Kelly, Maurice Richard and Ted Green.

Masterton's death was the watershed event in changing that outlook. It didn't happen overnight, but by the 1978–1979 season two-thirds of the players were wearing them. On June 1, 1979, the NHL enacted a rule requiring helmet use for anyone entering the league after that date. A grandfather clause allowed veterans to continue to play without them if they wished. A sizable number did. The helmetless era finally ended in 1997 with the retirement of St. Louis Blues center Craig MacTavish, the last holdout.

## Chuck Hughes: A Moment's Notice
### *NFL 1971*

The NFL is into its second century of existence and one player holds a grim distinction similar to Ray Chapman in MLB and Bill Masterton in the NHL.

Although several players have perished within hours or days after sustaining injuries in games, Chuck Hughes is the only man in the history of the league to die on the gridiron. Damar Hamlin of the Buffalo Bills nearly became the second in 2023 at Riverfront Stadium in Cincinnati, but he pulled through. Hughes was not as fortunate. He collapsed on the field at Tiger Stadium in Detroit on October 24, 1971, and never regained consciousness. The doctors who rushed to his aid at the stadium believed he died within minutes of his collapse, if not sooner. His wife Sharon, who burst out of the stands to be at his side, agreed.

The irony of his death is that he wasn't taken down by the violence of the game.

It wasn't like Harold Moore getting trounced in the tumult of a flying wedge or Chapman being smashed in the temple by a blazing spitball or Masterton's bare head meeting the unforgiving ice after a fierce body check.

Hughes had a degenerative disease that slowly but surely clogged his arteries and prevented his blood from circulating. His family had a history of heart problems, and the seeds of his demise were very likely imbedded in his genetic code. The medical name for the condition is atherosclerosis. It's common in people over 50 but is rarely found in anyone under that age. In many instances it goes undetected for years, and in the insidious manner of heart disease death can arrive on a moment's notice.

That moment arrived for Chuck Hughes in the last minutes of the Lions game against the Chicago Bears. He was in his second season with the team after playing three with the Philadelphia Eagles. One of 13 children, he grew up in Abilene in central Texas and starred at Texas Western College in El Paso as part of the "Flying Miners" aerial attack. Nicknamed Coyote by his Lion teammates, he lacked blazing speed and was small at 5–11, 175 pounds, but he ran crisp routes and possessed great hands.

On his first play in the offensive lineup that Sunday, Hughes caught a 32-yard pass from quarterback Greg Landry and was brutally sandwiched between two Bear defenders on the tackle. It was a brilliant reception, only the 15th of his NFL career. It would be his last. Two plays later, as he trotted back to the huddle after running a downfield post pattern, he grabbed his chest and faceplanted onto the field near the 20-yard line.

Nobody noticed him right away, but after he didn't get up Bears middle linebacker Dick Butkus knelt over him and screamed to the sidelines for help. As Hughes lay twitching on the ground in front of a silent crowd of 54,418, team doctors worked feverishly to revive him. Legs crossed, arms limp at his side, his hands turning blue, he was wheeled off the field on a stretcher and taken by ambulance to Henry Ford Hospital, where he was pronounced dead at 4:41 p.m.

A minute and two seconds remained on the clock. After a long delay play resumed, and the Bears intercepted a Landry pass and won the game 28–23.

At first it was thought that the force of the tackle after his pass reception

## 1. In the Arena

17

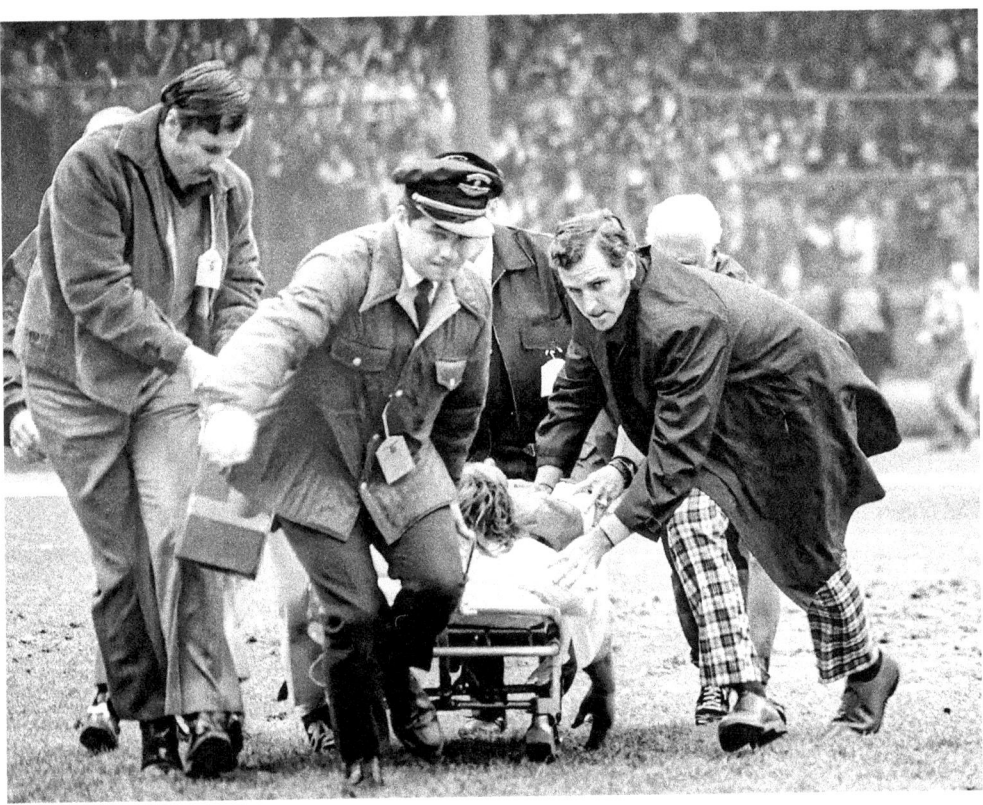

**Chuck Hughes is wheeled off the field at Tiger Stadium in Detroit on October 24, 1971. The Lions' wide receiver collapsed late in the fourth quarter of the game against the Chicago Bears and never regained consciousness. Doctors traced his death to a congenital heart defect that hardened his aorta and clogged his arteries. On the right is Dr. Gerald Boyle of Grosse Pointe Woods, Michigan, who bolted from the stands to assist (AP Images / Don Merrein).**

had burst a vital vessel in his abdomen, heart or brain. But an autopsy revealed no such damage. Nor did it indicate the presence of any type of stimulant that may have been a contributing factor. The culprit was a hardened, thickened aorta, the main trunk of the heart that pumps blood to all limbs and organs except the lungs. One doctor described his condition as "an old man's disease in a young man's arteries."[6]

The saddest aspect of the situation is that his death might well have been prevented—or at least delayed. Hughes had not been feeling right for a couple of months. He suffered sharp, severe chest and stomach pain after an exhibition game with Buffalo on September 4. After three days in the hospital and extensive testing, doctors found nothing abnormal. On September 26, before a home game with the Patriots, the pains returned and again doctors could not pinpoint any specific problem.

Despite those findings his condition existed, and playing football couldn't possibly have been a plus. The extreme physical stress of the game was undoubtedly a factor in the advance of the disease. If he'd been diagnosed that September or earlier, doctors might well have advised him to quit football, or at least recommended that he adopt a low-fat diet and use blood thinner or vascular dilators to stabilize his circulation.

Nor did Hughes have access to statins, the now ubiquitous drugs that fight high cholesterol, plaque in the arteries and blood clots.

Mevacor, the first statin, was not approved for medical use until 1987. Since then, the drugs have prevented and delayed millions of heart attacks and strokes. Some experts describe them as the greatest advance in the history of medicine. If they had been available to the public in 1971, they might well have prolonged his life.

But it wasn't to be. Charles Frederick Hughes was gone at age 28, leaving behind Sharon and 23-month-old son Brandon Shane. After funeral services in Detroit and San Antonio he was buried at Sunset Memorial Park in Bexar County, Texas.

## Duk Koo Kim: Live or Die
*Boxing 1982*

His birth name was Lee Deokgu. He grew up dirt poor in Gangwon Province, 60 miles east of Seoul, the fifth and youngest child of rice and ginseng farmers. His father died when he was two, his mother remarried three times, and at some point in that tumultuous journey, he became Duk Koo Kim.

He moved to Seoul when he was 14 and worked as a shoeshine boy and newspaper hawker. In 1976, at age 21, he took up boxing. Like thousands of other young men before him, he saw the sport as a way out of poverty and hardship. In 1978 he turned pro and joined Tong-a gymnasium.

The southpaw lightweight soon became the best fighter on the premises. He won the Orient and Pacific title and compiled a record of 17–1–1. That earned him a ranking as the World Boxing Association's (WBA) number one contender for the crown held by Ray "Boom Boom" Mancini. In 1982, he accepted a $20,000 offer from promoter Bob Arum to challenge Mancini in a 15-round matchup at Caesars Palace in Las Vegas.

It would be Kim's first—and last—fight in America.

Mancini was a golden boy, a friendly, devout Italian Catholic from Youngstown, Ohio, in the heart of the recession-ravaged Rust Belt. In a business dominated by Black, Mexican and Hispanic fighters the 21-year-old stood out. So did Kim. There were few Asians on boxing's main stages.

Kim arrived in Sin City hell bent on making the most of his moment in the sun.

On a lampshade in his hotel room he scrawled a cryptic phrase—*Live or Die.*

## 1. In the Arena

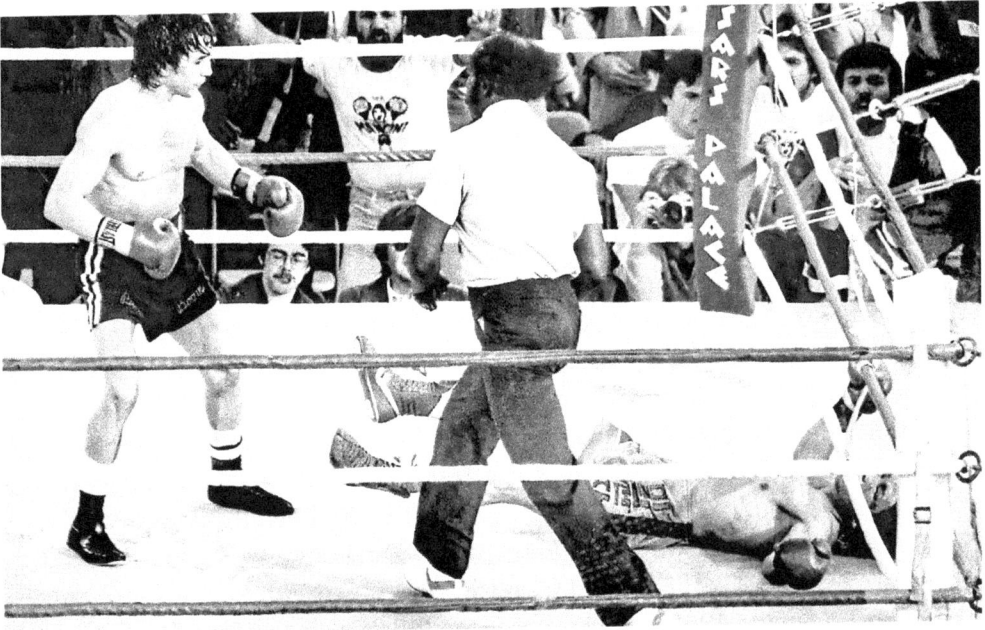

**Duk Koo Kim lies prostrate on the canvas after a potent punch from opponent Ray Mancini sent him flying into the ropes in the 14th round of their lightweight title bout in Las Vegas on November 13, 1982. He died five days later. Stepping in between the fighters is referee Richard Green (AP Images / Jeff Scheid).**

It was eerily similar to Francisco Lázaro's comment before his fatal marathon at the 1912 Olympics—*either I win or I die.* Did Kim view the fight as a death match in which the winner would survive and the loser would not? He never clarified exactly what he meant by his words. But that is certainly what it sounded like.

On Saturday night, November 13, some 10,000 spectators filled a temporary arena outside Caesars on the Strip. Along with a nationwide television audience on CBS, they witnessed one of the most savage fights in the history of boxing. Kim laid a bloody beating on Mancini, tearing an ear open, puffing up his left eye and swelling his left hand to twice its normal size.

The golden boy gave back as good as he got and gradually assumed control. In the first seconds of the 14th round he landed a roundhouse right flush on Kim's chin and sent him flying into the ropes. As he bounced off his head smacked onto the canvas. He managed to rise to his feet but at that point referee Richard Green stopped the action. Mancini was declared the winner by technical knockout.

Minutes later Kim blacked out and fell into a coma. He was carried from the arena on a stretcher and transported to Desert Spring Hospital in Paradise. Doctors discovered a fresh hemorrhage in his brain, caused in their view by a powerful single punch near the end of the fight. They performed emergency surgery in an attempt to save his life. Their efforts were in vain. After Kim's mother arrived from Korea with a squad of acupuncturists who failed to revive him, he was removed from life support. He died on November 18 at age 27.

Kim's death was yet another in a sport where death is as common as dry heat in the desert. Unlike any other form of competition, the entire point of the exercise is to render your opponent injured, defenseless, incapacitated, unconscious. Even in football, boxing's prime partner in the brutality business, there's a higher purpose—pushing the pigskin across the goal line or kicking it through the crossbars.

In boxing there is no higher purpose. And if every now and then human beings happen to get pummeled to the point of expiration—well, so be it. Nobody kills anybody on purpose, at least that we know of. Nobody can anticipate when it might happen, and nobody likes it when it does. But ring death comes with the territory.

Many prominent fighters have inflicted the ultimate punishment on their opponents. They saw the specter of death up close and personal between the ropes. Heavyweight Max Baer saw it with Frankie Campbell in 1930 in San Francisco. Sugar Ray Robinson saw it with Jimmy Doyle in a welterweight bout in Cleveland in 1946. Featherweight Sugar Ramos saw it twice—with Jose (Tiger) Blanco in Havana in 1958 and Davey Moore in Los Angeles in 1963. And Emile Griffith saw it in Madison Square Garden in 1962 with Benny (Kid) Paret, a man he despised with every fiber of his being.

There have been hundreds of more obscure incidents as well. When Kim died, *Ring* magazine reported that he was the 438th documented ring death since 1918. On October 15, 1995, flyweight Restituto Espinel in the Philippines and bantamweight James Murray in Scotland pulled off a macabre double by becoming the only ring death victims to die on the same day. Becky Zerlantes, 34, became the first female fatality on April 3, 2005. She was a contestant at the Colorado State Championships in Denver.

The deceased are not the only ones who suffer. Survivor remorse and guilt often set in. Robinson was so demoralized by Doyle's death that he almost quit boxing. Griffith, who fought 80 times after the Paret bout, was spooked for the rest of his life by the ghost of the man he hated. After super featherweight Gabriel Ruelas savaged Jimmy Garcia in 1995 in the same ring where Kim and Mancini fought, he visited his comatose opponent in the hospital and wanted to change places with him. Ruelas feared that after he died, God would think he killed Garcia intentionally and render His own brand of vengeful justice.

So it was with Mancini. Distraught after the fight, he fled Caesars with his parents and the family priest to an undisclosed location. From there he attended an impromptu Mass to pray for Kim's recovery. He then flew to Korea to attend Kim's funeral and burial in Kojin Village Cemetery. In a morbid coda to the tragedy, Kim's mother committed suicide three months later by drinking a bottle of pesticide. Then on July 1, 1983, referee Richard Green died of a self-inflicted gunshot wound in Las Vegas. The role that Kim's death played in their actions has never been fully determined.

There was speculation that Mancini would quit the sport, but he carried on at the urging of family, friends and fans. Sadly, his career fizzled out. He fought only six more times. In 1984 he lost his lightweight title to Livingston Bramble. He retired at age 24, saying that the thrill was gone. A comeback effort in 1992 against Greg Haugen ended with an ugly, embarrassing defeat.

Kim's death prompted a number of rules changes and new safety measures. There have been many boxing reforms through the centuries, starting with Broughton's Rule in 1743 that barred punches to the testicles. In 1838 came bans on head butting, eye gouging and kicking, and in 1866 the Marquis of Queensberry Rules mandated gloves and matched fighters by weight for the first time.

The Kim reforms eventually reduced the number of rounds in title fights from 15 to 12. The standing eight count was also created. It allows the referee, if warranted, to call a knockdown and pause the action even when a fighter is still standing. Pre-fight medical checkups were expanded to include electrocardiograms and brain and lung tests. Before Kim, doctors checked blood pressure and pulse rate and little else. More attention is also now paid to dehydration caused by extreme weight loss and pre-existing injuries and medical conditions that fighters bring into bouts.

Nearly everyone in the boxing hierarchy applauded the changes. But to the sport's many detractors they seemed feeble, a mere chipping away at the edges. They scoffed at the idea that boxing, when conducted "properly," can somehow be made safe. To them, the sport cannot be "reformed." They point out that the many changes through the years have done little to reduce the number of fatalities.

The NCAA discontinued boxing in 1961 after Wisconsin's Charlie Mohr died of an aneurysm after a bout. The American Medical Association has endorsed a total ban on pros and amateurs since 1984. Radio host and columnist Bonnie Erbe writes that the sport, for the benefit of a largely male audience, fixates on the basest and most deplorable aspects of human behavior. She speaks for many when she calls it "loathsome, nauseating, brutal, repulsive."[7]

Despite the strident objections of the critics, boxing endures. Crowds have gathered since before the time of Christ to take in the spectacle of two humans inflicting pain on each other in an enclosed ring. They still do. The biggest change in the 21st century is that the sport has spawned a number of variations that arouse all the same passions as boxing itself. Ultimate Fighting and Extreme Fighting combine elements of kick boxing, wrestling and judo in a discipline called Mixed Marital Arts (MMA). Toughman contests often take place in cages and feature amateurs with little or no experience or skill. The new variations have survived numerous bans by cities and states and continue to thrive in live, televised and pay-per-view formats.

So it seems that the people have rendered a mixed verdict. Yes, we despise this vile, vicious form of sporting entertainment. But please give us more.

## Sergei Shalibashvili: Kiss the Tower
*Platform Diving 1983*

As the diving competition got underway at the World University Games in Edmonton, Alberta, in July of 1983, a palpable sense of unease pervaded the Kinsman Aquatic Centre. Even the crowd was catching on to it.

The focus of concern was Sergei Shalibashvili, 21, the fourth ranked tower diver for the team from the Soviet Union. He was practicing a hugely demanding dive, a reverse 3½ somersault from the tuck position, known in the argot of the sport as a 307C. It had been authorized for less than a year and carried a degree of difficulty of 3.4, higher than any other dive. Only four men had ever attempted it in competition. One was Greg Louganis, the American superstar who was far and away the best diver in the world. Another was Shalibashvili himself. He'd successfully executed it at a meet in Minsk in his native country less than a year earlier.

But that was scant comfort to the onlookers in and around the pool. The dive was giving him fits. Everybody could see it. He took an eternity to prep himself on the platform. Ten to 15 seconds is the norm. He was taking 40 plus. And his efforts were ugly. He kept coming way too close to the platform as he lifted his body up and away from the tower and came tumbling back inward to complete the maneuver.

There's an exhortation often directed at a diver by coaches and fellow competitors—"Kiss the tower!" It means tighten your body up and bring the dive closer to the platform as you begin your descent. In Shalibashvili's case, nobody was doing any exhorting. The silence was deafening. He was coming so close to the tower on his own that he was scaring the daylights out of people. As the preliminaries began on the afternoon of July 6, the unspoken fear was that his 307C was a disaster waiting to happen.

As he climbed the steps for his eighth dive of the prelims, he was mired in sixth place in the standings and looking for the 307C to make up lost ground. Louganis was in the arena at the time. But he couldn't bear to watch. He closed his eyes and put his hands over his ears. When he felt the tower rumble and shake, he feared the worst. The loud, sickening screams confirmed it.

Shalibashvili had smacked his head on the platform and dropped feet first into the water, where he was floating in a thick mess of blood. He was eased from the pool by fellow divers and taken to the University of Alberta Hospital.

Information on his condition remained sketchy. Doctors performed a 48-minute operation to relieve extreme pressure on his brain, but he was soon placed on life support. He died a week after the operation on July 16 without regaining consciousness. His death was believed to be the first at an international diving meet. Four years later Australian diver Nathan Meade, 21, died after hitting his head on a concrete platform while practicing a 307C in Brisbane.

The finger-pointing erupted pronto. The question of the hour was this—if so many people knew the danger Shalibashvili was in, why didn't anybody step up and warn him off?

Provisions exist in the sport's bylaws that allow officials to bar divers from attempting dives viewed to be beyond their abilities. But that virtually never happens. Coaches bear that responsibility, and the athletes rely heavily on their judgment. So most of the fingers pointed at Vladimir Vasin, the head Soviet coach. The consensus was that Vasin *had* to have known of the risk his country's diver was taking.

Several Western coaches had in fact made tactful, discreet inquiries to some of their Soviet counterparts about Shalibashvili's safety. They were told, in effect, to shove it. The rude retort was rooted in the notion that coaches don't offer unsolicited advice to their colleagues. That was viewed as getting into somebody else's business. It also stemmed in part from the persistent Cold War mentality that continued to thrive in diving and other sports well into the 1980s. Relations between Soviet and Western coaches were far from cordial.

Another aspect of the situation was that Shalibashvili's personal coach was not present. That would be his widowed mother Thais Muntean. She'd remained home in Tbiliss, the capital of the Soviet republic of Georgia. If she'd been in Edmonton, she might have counseled her son to back off.

Half an hour after Shalibashvili was pulled from the bloody pool, Greg Louganis executed a splendid 307C. He told the media the next day that jet lag might have played a role in the tragedy. Shalibashvili's equilibrium was out of whack. The time zone shift was huge. He was disoriented and fatigued and not as strong as he needed to be.

Many dismissed his comments as nonsense, describing them as a case of a diver sticking up for a fallen comrade, trying to put the best light on the sad event. In their eyes the young man was in over his head, plain and simple. He died attempting a dive that was beyond his talent level. The fact that he had executed it in competition a year earlier, while compelling, apparently was not enough to change their viewpoint.

Two days after his death, Shalibashvili's body was embalmed and placed in a casket before being flown home to the Soviet Union for burial.

## Lane Frost: Born to Ride
*Bull Riding 1989*

Lane Frost started with rodeo early on in life. You can say that the bull riding legend he became was present at the creation.

As an infant he sleepwalked on all fours to his family barn clutching a bull rope, and as a toddler he starred in a home movie mounted joyously on the back of a small calf. His parents Clyde and Elsie tried to steer him away from bull riding into one of rodeo's less dangerous events like calf roping or bareback riding. But the young man had made up his mind.

At Atoka High School in Oklahoma, Frost won the national high school bull riding title. He also wrestled. In 1983 he began competing in Professional Rodeo Cowboys Association (PRCA) events. Two years later he marred Kellie Kyle, a barrel racer he met in 1980 at a high school competition.

In 1987 he won the "Big Buckle," the PRCA bull riding championship. And he did it his way, as a straight arrow who didn't succumb to the many temptations of the tour—bright lights, swelled heads, booze, drugs, buckle bunnies looking for hookups. He was praised not only for his marvelous skills but his modesty and infectious grin. His close friend and traveling partner Tuff Hedeman, a three-time world champion, said Frost just had a magic about him. He left everybody he met with a smile.

The young Sooner had reached the pinnacle of one of the world's most unusual sports. There are many other competitions in a classic rodeo—team roping, in which Frost also excelled, tie-down roping, steer wrestling, barrel racing, bareback bronc riding, and saddle bronc riding. But bull riding is the one that has magnetized a vast audience and broken out as a marquee, standalone event.

The goal of every competitor is to "ride" the bull. That means staying on it for at least eight seconds after the chute opens, with one hand on the saddle knob and the other hand and arm free and clear of both himself and the bull. If a rider falls or gets bucked off before eight seconds elapse, or if he touches himself or the bull with his free hand or arm, he scores zero. That happens frequently.

Four judges rate a rider's ability to match his movements to those of the bull while maintaining rhythm, balance, control and body position. Spurring the bull raises a rider's score. The spurs are dull and do not hurt the animal, whose hide is seven times thicker than human skin. The judging standards are highly subjective, perhaps too much so. As in diving and gymnastics and figure skating, appearance matters. The look test is real. Style points count.

The bulls themselves are also scored, even if a rider zeroes out. Judges rate the animal's overall agility and power, the speed of its moves and its spinning and kicking ability. Each of the four judges awards between zero and 25 points to both rider and bull. Those eight numbers are then combined and divided by two for the official score. A total score of 80 or higher is excellent and 90 or more is exceptional. For a rider to attain those marks the bull has to be performing at a high level—bucking hard, changing direction and rolling its body.

There have been any number of renowned bulls in the history of the sport—Dillinger, Tornado, Bushwacker, Mr. T., Voodoo Child, Smackdown. The year before his death Frost conquered Red Rock, becoming the first rider ever to stay on him for eight seconds. That hadn't been done in 308 previous attempts.

A pale yellow bull named Bodacious was so dangerous that he was banned from competition in 1996. At the MGM Grand Arena in Las Vegas in 1995, the animal Terry Bradshaw calls "the Michael Jordan of bulls"[8] headbutted Tuff Hedeman so fiercely that Hedeman broke every bone in his face. After 13 hours of surgery he somehow survived, but he lost his sense of smell and needed six titanium plates inserted into his face to allow him to function normally.

So like everyone else in bull riding, Frost lived with danger. It wasn't about if you got hurt. It was about how often and how badly. With most cowboys being true to their popular image—macho, hard-bitten, taciturn—there wasn't much chatter about it, and statistics showed that "wrecks" didn't occur all that often. But the possibility of severe injury—and death—was ever present.

It isn't just the riders who are at risk. In the ring with them are clowns, there to amuse the audience, and barrelmen and bull fighters whose job is to distract bulls after rides to allow cowboys to safely exit the arena. Any of them can get rammed or gored or trampled at any time by an angry beast weighing up to a ton. In 1987 a chuck wagon outrider was killed during a race at the Cheyenne Frontier Days Rodeo in Wyoming, the sport's biggest stage.

As 1989 began, Frost was looking to break out of a slump. At the Winter Olympics in Calgary, where bull riding was presented as a demonstration sport, he didn't think the judges were giving him a fair shake and he performed poorly. A few months later he got bucked off a bull and was unconscious for five minutes. Then in Fort Worth he lost his front teeth when his face slammed into the back of a bull's head.

The worst was yet to come. On July 30, the last afternoon of the Frontier Days Rodeo, Frost came out of the chute on a Brahman cross breed bull named MASO K Walsh. He was nicknamed Bad to the Bone because of his surly manner with riders. After scoring an 85-point ride, Frost was thrown off the back end of the animal. He landed on his hands and knees and tried to scramble away to safety. On its way to the escape chute Bad to the Bone knocked him down with his huge forehead, rammed his left side and back and stomped on him repeatedly with his feet. Frost bounced up after the attack, signaled for help, then collapsed face down on the ring floor.

"When he fell back down you knew he was hurt," said rider Cody Lambert. "When we rolled him over, you knew it was real bad. Looking back on it now, I think we all knew right then."[9]

Bad to the Bone had crushed several of Frost's ribs and one had pierced an artery in his chest. He was pronounced dead at 3:59 p.m. at Memorial Hospital in Cheyenne. Tuff Hedeman and Cody Lambert accompanied his body on the flight home to Oklahoma. Elsie Frost found a small degree of comfort in her son's last stand. "It's not much consolation, but he loved bull riding," she said. "So at least I know he died doing what he loved."[10]

Funeral services were held at First Baptist Church in Atoka on August 1. About 1,200 people gathered there, with many spilling onto the lawn to listen to the eulogies on loudspeakers. Lane Clay Frost is buried in Mount Olivet Cemetery in Hugo, 50 miles southeast of Atoka. He lies head to head with Warren "Freckles" Brown, a family friend and bull riding mentor who died in 1987.

A life-size bronze statue of Frost created by artist Chris Navarro was unveiled at the Cheyenne Frontier Days headquarters on July 24, 1993. The next year *8 Seconds*, a feature movie directed by John Avildsen of *Rocky* fame, debuted in theaters across America. The film starred Luke Perry as Frost and Stephen Baldwin as Tuff Hedeman.

There will be more accounts of in the arena deaths in Chapter 7 and elsewhere. Let's proceed now to a darker realm—murder and manslaughter, unlawful killings of one human being by another.

# 2

## Spilled Blood

### David Berger: All Gone
*Olympic Weightlifting 1972*

Unlike most athletes, David Berger didn't grow up in a house full of gloves, racquets, balls, bats, helmets and mountains of dirty laundry. He was surrounded by music, books and artwork in his home in Shaker Heights, Ohio.

So when he took up weightlifting at age 12 it was a bit of a shocker. He wasn't a big kid, and he didn't have a lot of muscles. Dorothy Davidson Berger didn't care for the way her son dented the basement floor when he slammed his barbells down during workouts. Benjamin Berger, an esteemed family physician, was puzzled that his passion didn't extend to other sports. Football, baseball and basketball didn't interest him. Neither did tennis or wrestling or swimming.

The young man was all in with the ancient tradition that started with cave dwellers in prehistoric tribes lifting huge rocks over their heads to find out who among them was the strongest. In the 19th century it flourished in circuses and theaters in Great Britain and Europe and was one of only nine sports in the first modern Olympics in Athens in 1896. In Berger's era and into the 1980s and 1990s it was dominated by lifters from the Soviet Union and Bulgaria. These days rampant accusations of bribery, cheating and doping have sullied the sport's reputation, and it's tentatively been booted out of the Olympics scheduled to held in Los Angeles in 2028.

Despite weightlifting's relentlessly macho image, it's not all about raw strength. Technique is just as vital. Focused, cerebral and disciplined, Berger was great at technique. He recorded notes on all his sessions in a handwritten log and he carried on. He carried on with academics too. High achievement in the classroom was an ingrained family value. Berger was about as far from the dumb jock stereotype as it was possible to be. As a psychology major and honors student at Tulane University in New Orleans, he won the NCAA title in the 148-pound class in 1965. While enrolled in the four-year joint MBA-law degree program at Columbia University, he trained at the storied McBurney Y.M.C.A. at 215 West 23rd Street in Manhattan. The vibrant community hub was once the residence of Al Pacino and Andy Warhol, and it was there that Charles Merrill and Edward

Lynch became friends in the swimming pool before opening up shop together in 1914. McBurney also inspired the 1978 smash disco hit "Y.M.C.A." by the Village People.

In 1968 Berger finished fourth at the Olympic trials for Mexico City, just missing a place on the team. It was a huge disappointment that stung hard. The next year he was on the U.S. team at the Maccabiah Games in Tel Aviv, the so-called Jewish Olympics first held in 1932. He won a gold medal in the middleweight (149–165 pounds) class.

The experience prompted him to make a fateful decision that would lead to his tragic end. Berger emigrated to Israel, in accordance with a doctrine that grants Jews living outside the country the right to leave their homes and reside there as citizens under Israeli law. The act is known in Jewish culture as "making aliyah" (AH-lee-uh).

After the country's swift, stunning victory in the Six-Day War in 1967, there was a surge of new arrivals. In the next seven years, some 60,000 North American Jews moved to Israel. More than half of them eventually returned to their home countries. We'll never know if Berger might have been among them.

Economic opportunity was largely a non-factor for the emigrants. Most moved for political, religious or ideological reasons. Berger had something different in mind for himself. At that point in his life his primary goal was to compete in the Olympics. And he knew he had a far better chance of doing that not as a citizen of the U.S. but of Israel, where the number of elite lifters was much smaller and the competition far less stiff.

So as he turned 26, he moved to Tel Aviv. He continued to train and compete, moved up to the light heavyweight (165–182 pounds) class and earned a place on the Israeli team for the 1972 games in Munich. Berger was one of 188 lifters from 54 countries. He competed on September 2 and was eliminated in an early round.

His brother Fred and sister Barbara were in Munich to support him. On the 4th, David bade his siblings farewell over an evening snack. They were leaving Munich early the next morning to go camping in the mountains of Austria. It was the last time he would see them.

Six hours later in the pre-dawn darkness of September 5, black-faced Palestinian commandos armed with rifles and submachine guns scaled the fences surrounding the Olympic Village. They were members of Black September, a militant splinter group of the Fatah movement. They stormed the apartment where Berger and five roommates were staying. Six team members were seized in another unit and brought there. One hostage escaped, two were shot to death as they tried to overpower the commandos, and in that hail of gunfire Berger was wounded in his left shoulder.

The rest of the day was a tortured descent into chaos and carnage, played out live in front of a worldwide television audience estimated at one billion. A tense standoff lasted for hours. Negotiations for the release of 200 Arabs imprisoned in

Israel ended in a stalemate. Then came a transfer of the hostages to Fürstenfeldbruck airbase west of Munich, where commandos thought they'd be boarding a Lufthansa 707 for a safe passage flight to Egypt.

But that promise was just a ruse to lure the commandos into an ambush. As German snipers opened fire on a runway illuminated by floodlights, Berger and three other hostages lay bound and gagged in a helicopter. With police closing in, a commando sprayed it with machine gun fire, killing the three others instantly and wounding Berger in the legs. When another commando tossed a hand grenade into the craft, Berger died of smoke inhalation in the ensuing explosion and fire. Five commandos and a German police officer also died.

At 3:24 a.m. Jim McKay of ABC Sports announced the deaths of the hostages to the television audience in America. "When I was a kid my father used to say 'our greatest hopes and worst fears are seldom realized.' Our worst fears have been realized tonight ... they're all gone."[1]

These are the other ten members of the Israeli team who died in the attack: Ze'ev Friedman, 28, weightlifter; Yossef Gutfreund, 40, wrestling referee; Eliezer Halfin, 24, wrestler; Yossef Romano, 32, weightlifter; Amitzur Shapira, 40, track coach; Kehat Schorr, 53, marksmanship coach; Mark Slavin, 18, wrestler; Andre Spitzer, 27, fencing coach; Yakov Springer, 51, weightlifting judge and coach; and Moshe Weinberg, 33, wrestling coach.

Berger's family wanted him to be buried in his hometown and President Richard Nixon ordered an Air Force jet to fly to Munich and return the body to Cleveland. After a memorial service at City Hall on September 11, he was buried in Mayfield Cemetery in Cleveland Heights. The David Berger National Memorial in Beachwood honors the memory of Berger and his teammates.

## Lyman Bostock: Pure Happenstance
### *MLB 1978*

On a sultry Saturday night, a Ford and a Buick Electra idled side by side at the intersection of Fifth Avenue and Jackson Street in Gary, Indiana.

As the light turned green, the driver of the Ford leaned out, thrust a .410-gauge shotgun up to a closed window of the Electra and blasted buckshot pellets into the back seat. They grazed a woman's neck and smashed into the right temple of the 27-year-old man sitting next to her, splattering blood, flesh and bone all over the four occupants of the vehicle.

At St. Mary Medical Center the damage inflicted on the wounded man was far too severe to mend. He had a three-inch hole in the side of his head. Emergency surgery failed. Lyman Bostock, the ebullient center fielder of the California Angels, was pronounced dead at 1:20 a.m., another victim of savage, senseless gun violence in the gritty, crime-ridden city. It was Sunday, September 24, 1978.

The slaying was a horrific end for one of the premier players of the era. Bostock could do it all—run the bases like Lou Brock, field like Willie Mays, and, above all, hit. He batted .323 and .336 in his first two full seasons with the Minnesota Twins. Orioles manager Earl Weaver predicted that he would likely win five or six batting titles in his career. The next year, under the sport's new free agency rules, he offered his services to other teams.

The Yankees and Mets wanted him badly, but he signed a five-year, $2.3 million contract with the Angels, making him one of the highest paid players in MLB. He had earned $20,000 in 1977 from Calvin Griffith, the notorious skinflint owner of the Twins. Bostock's future was so bright he had to wear shades.

He'd gone to Gary in the last days of the season to visit his uncle Thomas Turner after a day game with the White Sox at Comiskey Park in Chicago, 35 miles away. Joan Hawkins and Barbara Smith, the women in the Electra with Turner and Bostock, were sisters and longtime family friends of Turner. Smith was the estranged wife of the man driving the Ford. He'd caught a glimpse of them together on Turner's front porch shortly before the shooting and apparently assumed they were having some kind of affair. They weren't. Bostock had known her less than an hour. His presence in the back seat of the Electra was pure happenstance. He was in the wrong place at the wrong time.

The gruesome event left many Angels wondering if their team might carry a curse. Bostock was the fourth player to die in the 1970s. Infielder Chico Ruiz was killed in a one-car wreck near Anaheim in 1971. Relief pitcher Bruce Heinbechner perished in a head-on collision in Palm Springs during spring training in 1973. And in 1976 shortstop Mike Miley died in a one-car accident in Louisiana.

Nearly as sad as Bostock's sudden end was the circus that ensued with his killer. Leonard Smith, a man with seven previous arrests but no convictions, was picked up by police at his home the morning after the shooting. The 31-year-old unemployed steelworker entered a plea of not guilty by reason of temporary insanity. He claimed that his wife's many infidelities during their violent, dysfunctional marriage had transformed him at the moment he pulled the trigger of his shotgun into a person so off his rocker that he lacked the intention to take a human life. In nearly all states, including Indiana, intent to kill must be proven to obtain a murder conviction. Smith's claim enraged Bostock's family, friends and teammates.

The first trial ended with a hung jury. In his second trial, attorney Nick Thiros worked the insanity theme like a maestro and earned an acquittal for his client. Smith was remanded to the Indiana state mental hospital in Logansport, but he was released less than year later after doctors deemed him cured and sane. He never spent another day behind bars and died in 2010 of natural causes at age 63.

Lyman Wesley Bostock, Jr., is interred in Lot 342, Grave D, at Inglewood Park cemetery outside Los Angeles.

## Ron Settles: Jailhouse Shock
*College Football 1981*

Three years after the death of Lyman Bostock, a different brand of violence ended the life of another Black athlete from California.

Just before noon on June 2, 1981, Ron Settles was driving through the town of Signal Hill on his way to his summer job as a baseball coach at a junior high school. Settles was 21, a talented running back gearing up for his final season at nearby California State University, Long Beach, a young man with no criminal record and a promising future. He'd already received letters of interest from the Dallas Cowboys and Seattle Seahawks.

Signal Hill was a quirky piece of turf, a town of 6,000 embedded within Long Beach and dotted with oil rigs pumping black gold amidst swank condos and hardscrabble shacks. Imagine it as a little piece of Texas along the Pacific. Residents packed plenty of heat. Signal Hill issued more pistol carry permits per capita than any other jurisdiction in the state. And the place had never been noted for hospitality toward people of color. Between 1968 and 1980, 42 formal complaints of police misconduct were filed.

Officer Jerry Lee Brown pulled Settles over, ostensibly for speeding. Brown later maintained that Settle refused to show his driver's license, flashed a knife and had cocaine in his car. Brown called for backup and he and Officer Patrick A. Shortall cuffed Settles and transported him to the station house. There, they say he flew into a combative rage and had to be subdued with repeated heavy blows to the head and body. Two hours later he was found hanging in his cell, his broken neck wrapped in a noose fashioned from a mattress cover.

That was the official version of events The police immediately rendered their verdict—suicide.

Donnell and Helen Settles scoffed at that account. They said there was no reason whatsoever for their bright, focused, upright son to take his own life. They hired attorney Johnnie L. Cochran, later to gain renown in the O.J. Simpson trial, and filed a $62 million civil lawsuit against city and police officials. The suit claimed that Brown and police cadet Gerry Fleisher "severely beat, strangled and killed"[2] Settles.

What really happened during those two hours? Did Brown and Fleisher string Settles up in his cell themselves after they beat him to death to camouflage their own violent acts? Was the hanging story a total fabrication? Or did Settles succeed at the task, as the police claimed?

Nobody knows. No photographic evidence of the purported hanging, if it exists, has ever been made public. It seems that the cops were asking the world to take their word for it.

The parties proceeded to a coroner's inquest. All the public servants implicated had been advised to assert their Fifth Amendment rights and zip their lips. Which they did. Through nine days of testimony attorney Stephen Yagman insisted that a dejected, downhearted Settles hanged himself because he saw his NFL future evaporating in a cloud of ugly criminal charges. Yagman also took issue with the notion that the deceased was some kind of straight arrow Eagle Scout, pointing to an autopsy that found traces of PCP in his system. The chemical animal tranquilizer was widely used at the time as a recreational hallucinogen. That's a fancy medical term for a club or party drug.

By a 5–4 vote the inquest jury found that Settles died not by suicide but "at the hands of another other than by accident."[3] Was the arcane legal phrase a convoluted way of saying he was murdered? Not quite. It left open the possibility that the police officers had only acted negligently or recklessly in the hours leading up to Settles' death. The jury did not conclude that they intentionally killed him.

The case seemed headed to trial. Officer Brown said he was now eager to take the stand and clear his name. But that never happened. After the inquest, no criminal proceedings ever occurred in the case of Ron Reginald Settles.

The sudden end of the wrongful death lawsuit nineteen months after his death was a surprise. Donnell and Helen Settles accepted a sum of $760,000 as full and final payment. Given the heinous nature of the allegations, that amount seemed minimal to say the least.

Their decision came after Stephen Yagman produced a document, handed over to him by Donnell Settles that Yagman said established Ron's act as a "copycat suicide."[4] Who was he copying? Lee Shelton, a criminal and pimp who'd become a mythic figure in Black folklore after committing a murder on Christmas in St. Louis in 1895. Shelton was known by many names, most commonly Stagger Lee, the title of a 1959 hit song by Lloyd Price celebrating his legend.

Stagger Lee was thought to be imbued with supernatural powers. One example of those powers was that he'd hung himself in his jail cell for thirty minutes, cackled at the gaping guards, then cut himself down to tell the tale and go on with his life. In an essay he'd written for a high school English class, Ron Settles expressed admiration for Stagger Lee's deed. From that Yagman asserted that he was aware of the idea of jailhouse hanging, approved of it, and proceeded to commit the same act himself.

His conclusion was a real head scratcher. It just prompted more questions. Did Yagman actually believe that Settles hung himself thinking he was going to survive like Stagger Lee? Why did Donnell Settles hand over his son's essay to Yagman in the first place? And why did he and his wife agree to settle a $62 million lawsuit for $760,000?

The full story of the tragedy has never surfaced and never will. The one certainty that emerged from the events of June 2, 1981, is this—young, large, strong, muscular Black men like Ron Settles are frequently viewed as threatening. As they go about their daily lives they alarm and frighten people and attract the attention of law enforcement on a regular basis. That is as true today as it was 50 years ago. And it very likely will still be true 50 years down the road.

## Andrés Escobar: Brave to the End
*World Cup Soccer 1994*

Human lives can be snuffed out by many different kinds of people. In 1994, during the World Cup soccer tournament, the killer wasn't a radical terrorist or a jealous, demented husband or an unhinged cop. He was a fan, emboldened by other fans, all of them enraged by a player's big-time blunder on the pitch in a huge match. At least that's the prevailing theory.

As the tournament began in the United States, the 34 million people of Colombia were exuberant about the prospects of their national team. An array of brilliant players under the guidance of coach Francisco Maturana had forged a 28-game unbeaten streak in international play, including six matches in the World Cup qualifying round. One of those was a 5–0 thrashing of superpower Argentina on their home turf in Bueno Aires. Soccer icon Pelé believed they were the best team in South America. Expectations were feverishly high. Colombia had a legitimate chance to win the World Cup.

Rabid fans were shattered when their heroes became the first team in the field of 24 to be eliminated. They won only one of their first three round matches. The Colombian dream died hard on June 22 at the Rose Bowl in Pasadena, California. Playing the host United States team—a nation that had not won a World Cup game since 1950—Colombia stunningly, inexplicably lost.

The pivotal play was the accidental goal scored for the United States in the 35th minute by Colombian defender Andrés Escobar. Attempting to deflect a long, deep setup pass by American John Harkes, Escobar sent the ball bouncing off his own foot into the Colombian net. The final score—United States 2, Colombia 1.

Escobar was an unlikely goat. While flashier stars like Carlos Valderrama and Adolfo (The Train) Valencia grabbed the spotlight, the team captain was the rock of the Colombian defense. He was due to sign a long-term contract with superpower AC Milan in Italy. He also was preparing to marry girlfriend Pamela Cascardo, whose picture he carried with him to California in a Bible, along with one of his late mother.

After the defeat the nation's mood turned ugly. Some players delayed their journey home to let the anger subside. Escobar took the opposite path. He refused to wallow in despair and never watched a replay of the goal. He freely admitted his error and offered his apologies. He even composed an open letter to the nation for Bogotá's premier newspaper *El Tiempo*. "We have to go on," he wrote. "No matter how difficult it is we must stand back up. We'll see each other again because life doesn't end here."[5]

Life may not have ended for any of Colombia's crestfallen fans. But for Escobar it did. Early on the morning of July 2, 10 days after the match, he was accosted by three men and a woman outside the El Indio nightclub on the outskirts of Medellín.

"Thanks for the goal!" one of the men shouted, and then *"Higueputa!"* which means "son of a whore."[6] Escobar tried to calm the drunken men down and reason with them, but one pulled out a handgun and pumped six bullets into his chest. He was pronounced dead on arrival at a Medellín hospital.

Escobar was just one of many victims who paid the ultimate price in the death-drenched world of Colombian soccer. In the 1980s and 1990s, as thousands died during the country's cocaine wars and the government campaign against the drug cartel, a string of slayings plagued the game—the coach of the national youth team and seven others in 1986, the secretary of the Metropolitan Soccer League in 1988, referee Álvaro Ortega in 1989, the vice-president of the Millonairos club in 1992. The nation's murder rate was eight times higher than America's.

In 1993, 20 fans died during a celebration of Colombia's rout of Argentina. The national team routinely practiced under armed guard. Maturana, an assistant coach, and a player all received death threats faxed from their home country to their hotel in Los Angeles on the morning of the World Cup match against the United States.

No one could conclusively prove that cocaine traffickers were responsible for the carnage. But in a country where the passion for soccer mixes fluidly with the lust for money and drugs, there were many outward signs of the connection between cocaine and the game—favors sought and granted, friendships made and lost, politicians bought and sold.

Escobar shared a last name with the most powerful cocaine kingpin of all, the man believed to be lurking behind much of the violence. Pablo Escobar was killed by security forces just seven months before Andrés died. Soccer had been the consuming passion of Pablo's life. He frequently invited national team players to his fortress-like compound for makeshift games and extravagant meals. Andrés did not want to participate, but he felt he had no choice. After his death many people came to believe that if Pablo had been alive Andrés never would have died. Pablo would have used the full force of his power to prevent any harm to him and other national team members.

Two brothers, Santiago Henao Gallón and Pedro David Gallón, were arrested in connection with the slaying, along with Humberto Muñoz Castro, Santiago's chauffeur. Muñoz confessed to being the trigger man. The brothers were coffee growers and sports apparel merchandisers. They were also cocaine dealers. Rumors abounded that they killed Escobar because they and their friends had lost millions of dollars wagering on the match with the United States. For what it's worth, that theory was quickly squelched by law enforcement.

The Gallón brothers were released from custody after a few days and cleared of any wrongdoing. Castro was sentenced to 43 years in prison but was released after 11 years for "good behavior."[7] Make of that what you will.

After Escobar's funeral in Medellín's largest stadium, thousands of fans guided his casket through the streets to a cemetery 10 miles away. Many of his teammates, fearful for their own lives, stayed home.

"This country is a permanent madhouse,"[8] said Francisco Maturana, who resigned as head coach of the national team after the World Cup. Any sane observer of the Escobar tragedy and the cocaine wars of Colombia would find it hard to disagree with his statement.

## Dave Schultz: Pinned by a Madman
### *Wrestling 1996*

The thug who pumped six bullets into Andrés Escobar might well have been mad, insane, deranged. Or he could simply have been a dull normal brute obeying the command of his boss to shoot and kill a man who had just cost the boss and his cronies millions of dollars in lost gambling bets.

The man who shot and killed wrestler Dave Schultz 19 months later in 1996 was mad beyond a shadow of a doubt. John Eleuthère du Pont was a diagnosed paranoid schizophrenic. Mental illness is real, and he suffered from it. Du Pont also was an heir to a fortune courtesy of his ancestors, founders of the corporate behemoth that gave the world gunpowder, nylon, rayon and neoprene. The figure most often cited is $200 million, roughly $500 million in today's money. The largess allowed du Pont to march to the beat of a different drummer in life.

It was a strange, sinister beat. The list of menacing, bizarre behavior was lengthy. Dying his hair Ronald McDonald red. Brandishing assorted firearms at the many people who annoyed him. Declining to bathe or brush his teeth for months on end. Steering a brand-new Lincoln Continental into a pond. Dynamiting a den of baby foxes. Folding his wife up and stuffing her into a fireplace near the end of their very brief marriage.

When you tossed ample, steady consumption of alcohol and cocaine into the mix, you had one royal mess of a human being.

How in the world did Dave Schultz and John du Pont cross paths in life? Their common bond was wrestling. Schultz was an elite performer in the hugely demanding sport, one that requires physical strength, speed, technical skill, mental toughness and endurance.

He had dyslexia as a youth in Palo Alto, California, and Ashland, Oregon. Many studies link the learning disorder with ambidexterity and that appears to have been the case with Schultz. It helped him immensely on the mat because he had no weaker side that could be more easily attacked by opponents. He excelled at every level and won titles in high school, at the University of Oklahoma, the

Goodwill Games, the Pan-American Games and the Olympics. He earned gold in 1984 in the freestyle welterweight 163-pound class.

Du Pont thought of himself as athlete as well. He'd been a varsity freestyler on the University of Miami swimming team in 1962 and 1963. He also competed in the exotic pentathlon event—swimming, shooting, fencing, running and equestrian show jumping. Dogged enthusiasm was his strong suit. He lacked the skill set required to excel at the highest levels. And to many observers he seemed to both envy and resent those who did excel.

Schultz was handsome, affable and empathetic. Du Pont was none of those. Perched at the summit of his sport, Schultz could have been an aloof jerk, but he chose not to be. He wore his crown lightly and the wrestling world loved him for it. Du Pont had a difficult time getting along with people. His huge wealth and sheltered childhood stunted his emotional intelligence and turned him into an obsessive, obnoxious control freak. If he wanted respect, attention and friendship he had to buy them.

The huge differences in character and personality were trumped by the fact that Schultz craved a stable environment in which he could devote himself completely to wrestling. USA Wrestling did not pay their athletes a red penny. Yet they were expected to compete against men who lived on generous stipends provided by their governments, particularly the Soviets. In America it was every man for himself. Wrestling was an endeavor far removed from MLB, the NFL and the NBA, with their huge payrolls, strong unions, pervasive media presence and mountains of cash. Schultz's life with his wife Nancy and children Alexander and Danielle was nomadic. They lived wherever they needed to live. At one time they resided in his dad's attic in Palo Alto.

That's where du Pont entered the picture. He didn't spend all his time holed up and pacing the floors at his pad in Newtown Square, 13 miles west of downtown Philadelphia in tony Delaware County. The 44-room mansion was a replica of Montpelier, the Virginia home of James Monroe. He had a public, philanthropic side too. The giant flag that hung on the wall of his foyer was a gift from President George H.W. Bush. For many years he was a special, unpaid deputy with the Newtown Township police department. He founded the Delaware Museum of Natural History. He gifted a half million bucks to the International Swimming Hall of Fame in Fort Lauderdale and gave another half million each year to USA Wrestling. His pride and joy was the Foxcatcher Training Facility, a state-of-the-art complex he'd built for wrestlers on his 800-acre estate known as Foxcatcher Farm.

Schultz arrived there in 1990 with his family. He knew a bit about what he was getting into. His younger brother Mark, who won Olympic gold in 1984 as a middleweight, was tight with du Pont and had just left Foxcatcher after a stay of several years. There was an intense, often heated rivalry between the brothers, but they looked out for each other. Mark told Dave that he was departing on bad terms with du Pont and urged him to be aware of his vicious, vindictive side.

## 2. Spilled Blood

So like everyone else at Foxcatcher, Dave put up with the man. It was the price to be paid for being able to fully pursue the sport they loved. The predominant view was that du Pont was nuts, dangerous and violent, a powder keg poised to explode. But some people didn't see him that way. Eccentric without a doubt. Impulsive, rash and prone to lying, absolutely. At times downright scary. But was he actually capable of harming people? That seemed like a stretch.

Friends and loved ones urged Schultz to grab his wife and kids and be on his way. He stayed put. Despite the ongoing drama and emotional stress, he was in a good place. The family had a house of their own on the estate grounds. He was nominally a coach and received a salary of $70,000, but his real job was to train for the Olympics. He hadn't made the team in 1988 and 1992 and those failures haunted him. His goal was to end his career with a second gold in Atlanta, then leave Foxcatcher behind and return to his native Palo Alto to coach at Stanford.

When the nightmarish end came on Friday afternoon, January 26, it somehow wasn't all that shocking. It left many distraught people with the same thought—*we really should have seen this coming.*

In an undated photograph, wrestler Dave Schultz leaps playfully onto John du Pont at the Foxcatcher National Training Center in Newtown Square, Pennsylvania. Their volatile, complicated friendship ended in tragedy on January 26, 1996, when du Pont pulled into the driveway of Schultz's home at Foxcatcher and shot him to death. Despite his claims of insanity, du Pont was convicted of murder and died in prison in 2010 (AP Images / Bill Fitz-Patrick).

Schultz was lying on his back in the driveway of his house at Foxcatcher, installing a new radio in his Toyota Tercel. Du Pont pulled up at the wheel of a silver Lincoln Town Car and pointed a .44 caliber Magnum revolver at him through the open window.

"You got a problem with me?" he yelled.[9]

He fired three times at point blank range, hitting Schultz once in the arm and twice in the chest. As he fell face first into the snow Nancy rushed out of the house to cradle him. Du Pont pointed the Magnum at her but did not fire. The last thing Nancy heard was a deep, gurgling noise in her husband's chest, seconds before he died in her arms. He was 36 years old.

Du Pont's bodyguard, a man named Pat Goodale, was riding shotgun in the Lincoln. He did not intervene or attempt to stop du Pont. Why he didn't remains a mystery. Perhaps he thought that if he had, du Pont would have plugged him too. Terrified for his own life, he sat idly by and witnessed a cold-blooded murder.

Du Pont ditched Goodale, retreated to his mansion alone and holed up in the steel-encased library that was designed as a bomb shelter. He surrendered after a 48-hour standoff with SWAT teams.

At his trial a year later, the jury rendered a verdict of guilty of third-degree murder but mentally ill. Judge Patricia Jenkins explained that its decision meant that du Pont was both sick and bad. Yes, he was a medically diagnosed paranoid schizophrenic. But that wasn't enough to exonerate him. Despite his illness, he intended to kill Schultz and he was fully aware that what he was doing was wrong.

The verdict was a relief to the wrestling community. Many feared that du Pont's high-priced attorneys would find a way to keep him out of jail. After many rounds of legal wrangling over his mental state, he entered prison. The jury's decision was upheld on appeal twice. He died at age 72 in the State Correctional Institution at Laurel Highlands on December 9, 2010.

A motive for the crime was never firmly established. Several theories emerged. Du Pont was captivated by a new wrestler at Foxcatcher, Bulgarian Valentine Yoranov, who later received 80 percent of his estate. He was punishing Schultz for remaining friends with another wrestler du Pont had ordered off the estate at gunpoint some months earlier. He felt that Schultz was deserting him by accepting the coaching job at Stanford. And finally there was the notion that du Pont, the not-so-great athlete, had long seethed over Schultz's success and prowess.

People don't do things for just one reason. Causation is a far more complicated process. That's Psychology 101. In the end, it doesn't matter much why du Pont killed Dave Schultz. The result was the same. A beloved, accomplished human being was taken in the prime of his life by a sick and bad man.

## Greg Halman: Brothers for Life
### *Baseball 2011*

Greg and Jason Halman were as close as close can be. Born 18 months apart in the Netherlands, the brothers grew up with their parents and two sisters on the top floor of a row house in Haarlem, near the North Sea 11 miles west of Amsterdam.

If you saw one boy, you almost always saw the other. They seemed to be joined at the hip. When they got older and developed a taste for tattoos, they went to a parlor one day and got identical designs at the base of the neck. Above was a cross, and below it three words—*Brothers for Life.*

Their father Eddy Halman was a native of Aruba, a self-governing island territory of the Netherlands in the Caribbean off the coast of Venezuela. Their mother Hanny Suidegeest was a white native of Holland. The family passion was sports. Big sister Naomi played basketball at UC Irvine in California and then in the top-ranked Italian pro league. Hanny and her younger daughter were softball players.

Eddy was a baseball man. That's what brought him to Holland from his birthplace. The game debuted in the country in 1911 when a teacher from England who'd picked it up in America introduced it to his students. The first pro league formed in 1922 and the Dutch have dominated baseball in Europe ever since. They've won 24 of the 36 national team tournaments held since 1954, with considerable help from citizens like Eddy, transplanted from the talent-rich Caribbean region. He played for the national team in 1979.

As soon as they could walk, Eddy started his sons in with balls and bats and gloves. Older brother Greg was more talented. Tall, fleet of foot and very strong, the right-handed outfielder developed with astonishing speed and wowed fans with his towering home runs. When asked what he wanted to be when he grew up, his answer was always the same—a pro baseball player in America.

The accent was on America. Greg loved the place. That came from Eddy as well. He came close to a career in the big leagues himself, but it didn't work out. Posters of Barry Bonds, Chipper Jones and Ken Griffey, Jr., adorned the walls of Greg's bedroom. He learned English as a child and practiced it diligently to prepare for his future. When he was 12 his dad took him to the States and showed him Wrigley Field and Fenway Park. The boy was instantly smitten.

Eddy was a troubled, edgy dude. He believed that politics and racism had screwed him out of a deserved career in MLB and he brooded about it for the rest of his days, carrying a chip on his shoulder as big as a boxcar. His anger erupted frequently. When the boys were young, he would sneak up behind them in a field and fire fastballs into their backs to toughen them up and keep them on their toes. He was so violent with Hanny that she finally walked out on the marriage. He retaliated by roughing up her boyfriends and vandalizing her car. And in 2007, Eddy's half-brother was convicted of killing his wife.

In their younger days, Greg and Jason carried on in his wake. Jason brawled frequently and Greg broke a guy's jaw one night in a bar fight. Their racial heritage was a contributing factor. They were burdened by it. Jason said that when "whites looked at them they saw black and when blacks looked at them they saw white."[10] The only place they felt close to fitting in was on the baseball diamond.

When he was 16, Greg's life journey kicked into high gear. He joined Corendon Kinheim, a pro team in Haarlem, and played alongside grown men. The next year the Seattle Mariners signed him as a non-drafted free agent and he was off across the Atlantic, where he toiled in the team's farm system for six seasons, primarily in the Arizona League. In 2008 he was the Mariners minor league player of the year.

With his love of music and pop culture and fluent English spoken without an accent, he came across an all–American guy. His teammates were always amazed when they found out he was from Holland, a foreign country on a different continent 4,800 miles away.

His speed in center field and explosive power at the plate made him a solid prospect for promotion. Near the end of the 2010 season the Mariners called him up from the Tacoma Rainiers and he played in nine games. The next year he played in 35. On June 15, with Eddy and Jason in the stands, he hit his first home run in MLB in a 3–1 win over the Los Angeles Angels.

There would only be one more, just over a month later. Greg could handle fastballs and sliders, but like many hitters he had a devil of a time with curveballs. Once pitchers figured that out his strikeouts skyrocketed. He was sent back down to the Rainiers, where he finished the year.

At the end of the season he went home to Holland like he always did, sharing an apartment on Jan Sonje Street in Rotterdam with Jason. By that time Jason was unhinging. He'd spent all his life in Greg's large shadow, struggling to stay afloat in baseball while his brother flourished and became a celebrity. Greg had pleaded with the Mariners many times to give Jason a tryout and they finally did, if only to be nice guys. Jason wouldn't make the grade. Everybody knew it. He simply wasn't good enough.

He reached rock bottom after he was released from the Dutch national team in October. He crawled into a shell and holed up in the apartment, smoking piles of pot, staring at the tube, blasting music and posting streams of gibberish on his Instagram page.

Hanny arranged for a doctor to pay him a visit. The doctor talked to him one on one for 10 minutes before fleeing in fear. She told Hanny that the young man needed serious help from specialists that she couldn't provide. After the tragedy medical experts described his condition as undiagnosed bipolar disorder. But no one acted in time to save a life.

Early on the morning of November 21, Greg berated his brother about the loud music. The argument turned ugly. Jason flashed a butterfly knife, similar to a switchblade. He opened it with the flick of a wrist and slashed Greg on the left side of his neck. It was a short, shallow slit but it penetrated the skin in exactly the wrong place, piercing the carotid artery that carries blood to the head.

When paramedics arrived at 5:34 a.m. Greg was on the floor, bleeding heavily. He died shortly thereafter. Later that day, Hanny went to Jan Sonje Street to mop up the mess herself.

Halman's Mariners uniform arrived a few days later from Seattle via UPS. His sister dressed him in it before he was laid into his casket, sunglasses on his head. The Mariners arrived en masse for his funeral as thousands of Dutch fans mourned. Halman was buried in a grove in Westerveld Cemetery, along the sea in the village of Driehuis. His family picked the site because it reminded them of a baseball diamond.

Jason was confined to a medical facility and examined extensively. On August 30, 2012, he was released after prosecutors and defense attorneys agreed that he should be absolved of the killing because of mental health issues. They determined that he was in a state of "psychosis"[11] on the morning of November 21, triggered in part by heavy marijuana use. He had lost contact with reality, including the ability to distinguish between right and wrong. In American legal jargon he was judged to be not guilty by reason of insanity.

Many people were outraged. But the Halman family accepted the decision. They'd already lost one son and brother. Sending Jason to prison would be like losing another.

The situation calls to mind the case of John du Pont. He was a diagnosed paranoid schizophrenic, but judges and jurors never accepted his claim that his illness rendered him not guilty of his crime. Unlike Jason Halman, du Pont was sent to prison for the murder of Dave Schultz.

There also are echoes of the Lyman Bostock case, where killer Leonard Smith gained acquittal on the grounds of temporary insanity. He was released from a mental hospital after less than a year of confinement and remained a free man for the rest of his life.

Today Jason Halman is a free man as well. He returned to baseball in 2019, joining Greg's original team, Corendon Kinheim. It seems like a fitting finale to a story of brotherly love gone berserk.

## Celia Barquín Arozamena: Broad Daylight
*Golf 2018*

It was an odd sight for sure. A foursome of men walking up the ninth fairway came upon a golf bag in a pushcart, sitting unattended. Near it on the grass lay a baseball cap, a cell phone and a scattering of tees.

They knew the bag belonged to the focused young woman out on the course alone. She'd played through them earlier on the front nine but now she was nowhere to be seen. What in the world was going on?

At 10:30 a.m. Ames, Iowa, police arrived at the Coldwater Golf Links southeast of the Iowa State University campus. Jack Trice Stadium lay less than a mile to the west.

The pathway between the eighth green and ninth tee cut through a patch of forest. A lot of golfers thought it was kind of spooky back there in the thick woods in the middle of the mostly treeless course.

It was in a small pond surrounded by those woods that police found the woman's floating body. There were deep stab wounds in her chest, head, neck and left leg. Some of her clothing was missing. Blood was also found on the fairway. It looked as if the assailant had attacked her there and then forced her back into the trees.

Police K-9 units tracked the victim's scent to two tents pitched on the north side of Squaw Creek across from the golf course. They encountered a nervous man with a scratched-up face and a raw, nasty cut on his hand that he kept trying to hide. At that moment the cops figured they had their suspect, and they could see from his wounds that the young woman had fought boldly for her life. At the scene they recovered a knife and a pair of blood-stained shorts from his black backpack. The next day he was charged with first-degree murder. The judge set a cash-only $5 million bond.

The two 22-year-olds central to the tragedy could not have been more different. Their paths crossed on the morning of September 17, 2018, by pure chance. The encounter led to one of the most vicious acts of random violence ever seen in the sports world.

Celia Barquín Arozamena came to play golf at Iowa State in 2014 from Puente San Miguel in Spain, a village 270 miles due north of Madrid, where the Pyrenees Mountains meet the Bay of Biscay. She grew up with golf and won the Under-14 Spanish championship. Her idol was the late, great Spaniard Seve Ballesteros who died in 2011, and she played the game with the same passion. That morning in Ames she was riding the hottest streak of her career, winning the Big 12 title in the spring and then the European Ladies Amateur in July.

But her college years with the Cyclones were almost behind her. She was a semester away from earning a degree in civil engineering and she was at Coldwater Links that morning to get in a round before her afternoon classes. Her eyes were on the future. In 2017 she watched in Des Moines as the Americans defeated the European team in the Solheim Cup, the biennial competition for pro women golfers modeled after the Ryder Cup. That inspired her to make the effort to go pro herself. The next step was Phase II of the LPGA Q-School in October. She'd made it through the sectional qualifier and her goal was to finish in the top 20 in the final competition and earn a tour card, which would allow her to play in nearly every event without qualifying each week. None of her "Cyclonitas" teammates, whom she loved dearly, would be there with her for that adventure. She'd be going it alone.

Collin Daniel Richards was going it alone as well. But he was headed nowhere.

His horror story began at birth. His father was a vicious tyrant. His mother left him and married another man. Richards quit school after eighth grade and

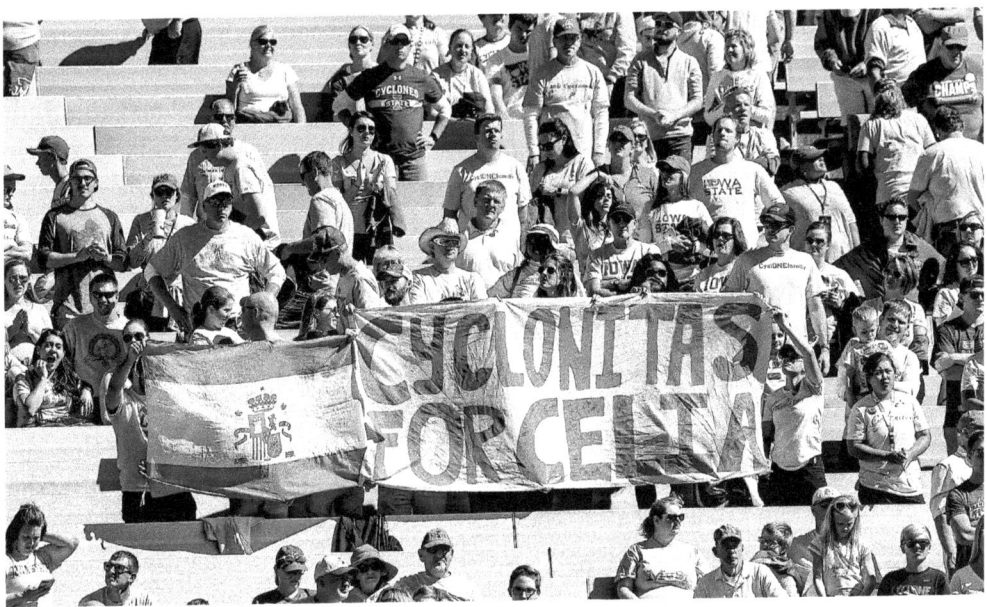

At Jack Trice Stadium during the Iowa State-Akron football game, fans unfurl a banner in memory of slain Cyclones golfer Celia Barquín Arozamena. The native of Spain was murdered on September 18, 2018, by a homeless ex-con and methamphetamine addict who attacked her on the Coldwater Golf Links near the Iowa State campus in Ames (AP Images / Charlie Neibergall).

lived a life of crime from that point on—three stints in reform facilities and convictions for domestic abuse, assault, theft, burglary and public intoxication.

He also had a vast appetite for home-cooked crystal methamphetamine—crank, ice, chalk, gak, cotton candy, white cross. In 2018, with society obsessing about the opioid epidemic, meth was largely overlooked. But the potent drug could inflict fearsome damage on the brains, mouths, teeth, lungs and stomachs of addicts, and the intense euphoric high it produced could quickly give way to paranoia, anger and violent rage. It happened to be in plentiful supply in Iowa because anhydrous ammonia, a key ingredient in the recipe, is a widely used farm fertilizer.

In the fall of 2017, Richards was booted out of his grandparents' house. He moved to the streets, landed in jail, and was released three months before the killing. After he was free, his meth use continued apace, and his rage intensified. In the days leading up to September 17 he made a horrific confession to a friend—he wanted to hunt down, rape and kill a woman.

At some point, with the help of someone, he might have turned his life around. But that never happened. Many blamed his family. If his mother and father and grandparents had not failed him, he might have changed his ways. Others found fault with "the system." If the schools had tried harder for him, he wouldn't have quit after eighth grade. If government provided more help for drug addicts, he could have gotten clean. If Iowa's prisons weren't overcrowded, he wouldn't have been released early and roaming Coldwater Links in broad daylight on September 17 tracking down a woman to rape and kill.

Those sentiments are understandable. But another thought comes to mind. Perhaps there are some human beings in this world who cannot be saved by their families or schools or social workers or drug rehab counselors or anyone else, and maybe Collin Richards is one of them.

A year after the slaying, he pleaded guilty to the crime. Iowa is not a capital punishment state, and he is now in prison serving a life sentence with no chance for parole. That is where he will die someday, largely forgotten.

On the other hand, Arozamena will live on in the hearts and minds of a multitude of people. After she died her mourners dressed up every corner of her world in yellow, her favorite color. But her legacy will endure far beyond that ritual of grief, and she'll be remembered more for the life she lived than for how she died. The same can be said of all of the other victims portrayed in this chapter.

That is at least a small measure of consolation.

## Mike Ryan: Covid Rage
*Hockey 2021*

The land of the free and the home of the brave was lurching into year two of the Covid pandemic. People were sick to almighty death of being cooped up and Herbie's on the Park in St. Paul was loud and alive as the Minnesota Wild notched a 5–2 win over the San Jose Sharks at nearby Xcel Energy Center. More fans made the scene after the game ended.

The NHL had kicked off its 2020–2021 season on January 13, three months later than usual, cutting the schedule from 82 to 56 games. Live attendance was limited. The vaccination campaign was up and running but mask and distancing protocols remained in effect in the Twin Cities metro area and throughout the country.

That didn't mean that the protocols were being followed. The divide in America that arose during the pandemic was on full display at Herbie's that Saturday night in April.

Bartenders and servers in the woody, upscale place wore masks. But only a small number of patrons did, a dozen or so out of the 50 people in the house. The rest were choosing to blow off the pleas of government and the medical establishment to cover their mouths and noses when they weren't eating or drinking. And they had no problem with getting right up into the faces of their cohorts.

Yes, the fans were cutting loose at Herbie's, founded by Wild owner Craig Leipold and named in honor of Herb Brooks, the fabled coach at the University of Minnesota who won three NCAA titles and led the U.S. team to Olympic gold in the 1980 Miracle on Ice at Lake Placid. They wanted to tune out the unholy mess the country was in and do what they did best—chow down, drink and watch hockey. It was a sign that the world might finally be heading down the path toward normalcy.

In the men's restroom some of the urinals were covered with cellophane to encourage distancing. Ryan Whisler, 43, didn't want to wait for an uncovered one to free up. Or maybe he decided to make a scene for the sheer hell of it. He stepped up to a covered urinal, punched a hole in the cellophane with his fist and took his pee, recording the moment on video for posterity with his cell phone.

A few feet away Mike Ryan, 48, looked on, totally disgusted. The head coach of the Bloomington Jefferson High School girls' hockey team was at Herbie's with two friends. Whisler was a total stranger to him. As repulsed as he was, Ryan stayed silent, left the restroom and went back to the bar.

We don't know exactly what went down between the two of them at that point, if anything. This much was verified by numerous eyewitnesses—as he and his friends were leaving, Ryan got into Whisler's face big time about his stunt in the loo, throwing a heap of abuse his way. Whisler responded in kind.

That seemed to be the end of it. But outside the bar, on a landing at the top of a flight of nine concrete steps, Whisler lunged at Ryan and grabbed his shirt. Ryan pulled away. Whisler ripped his mask off. As a third man stepped in to separate the pair, Whisler swung wide, landed a roundhouse punch in Ryan's face and shoved him backward, sending him flying through the air and down the stairs to the sidewalk. That's where police found him at 11:30 p.m., lying on his back and gasping for air in a pool of blood.

Whisler took off on foot, scampered back to retrieve an unknown object on the stairway, then hopped into a blue hatchback car with another man and fled the scene. At Regions Hospital, doctors discovered the worst. Ryan had a traumatic brain injury that he could not survive. He was placed on life support while his wife Julie and daughters Alyssa and Dana were notified. He died on Sunday afternoon, April 18, 2021.

After servers at Herbie's identified him through his credit card, Whisler turned himself into police on Sunday night. The next day, Ramsey County prosecutors charged him with second-degree unintentional murder.

They didn't think they could convince a jury that Whisler actually meant to kill Ryan. Maybe he did, maybe he didn't. His precise frame of mind was unknowable. But they could show that he acted recklessly and irresponsibly in a fit of rage. An ugly dispute in a bar on a Saturday night had turned violent in a heartbeat and ended in tragedy.

Sadly, it was just one of millions of Covid-induced confrontations throughout the country. And it was a sickening ending for a devout, Lutheran family man who loved hockey all his life. Ryan started playing as a youth in private leagues and for Bloomington Jefferson High School, then continued on at Gustavas Adolphus College. Four years later he began coaching boys' teams in Peewee and Bantam leagues and then at his alma mater.

When the girls' teams at Jefferson and Kennedy high schools merged in 2016, Ryan was named head coach. He strived to make his players not only winners on the ice but also in life. By day he was a salesman and manager for several top golf brands, including Calloway, at the time of his death.

There's a mourning ritual in the hockey community—when one of their own dies, people place hockey sticks by their front doors as a sign of remembrance and respect. Thousands of hockey sticks came out in the Twin Cities metro area on April 18 and the days following.

Michael G. Ryan is interred at Dawn Valley Memorial Park in Bloomington. Ryan Whisler pleaded guilty to manslaughter in May 2023 and faces up to seven years in prison.

# 3

## Dark Waters

### Ed Delahanty: Swept Away
*MLB 1903*

Niagara Falls is one of the most astonishing natural wonders on the face of the planet. It formed some 16,000 years ago when glaciers receded at the end of the Ice Age. Six million cubic feet of water pour over its crest every minute during periods of peak flow.

The three waterfalls that make up the system—Horseshoe (Canadian), American and Bridal Veil—won't be with us forever. Geologists predict that slow, steady erosion will wipe them away in 50,000 years. Whether any human beings will be around to witness their demise is anyone's guess.

The majestic, rushing waters have mesmerized onlookers for centuries. They've also spawned dark thoughts. Father Louis Hennepin, the missionary priest and explorer, put it this way 350 years ago: "the temptation to throw one's self down this incredible precipice is almost too great for resistance."[1]

Legend has it that Marilyn Monroe shared his perspective. She reportedly kept backing away from the churning depths while shooting the romantic melodrama *Niagara* in 1952. And Margot Kidder, who filmed portions of *Superman II* there with Christopher Reeve in 1979, confided to an extra on the set that the water kept luring her in time and time again.

Those anecdotes may be nothing more than revisionist history, brought on by the fact that both actresses died of drug overdoses deemed by coroners to be suicides. But since 1850, some 5,000 people have been found at the foot of the falls. Most of the incidents go unpublicized, and a large portion of them occurred before improved safety measures were put in place after World War II. But they still occur on the regular.

Some people plunge on purpose or fall by accident near the precipice. Others enter the water miles upstream. A few are daredevils, encased in wooden barrels or closed deck canoes, riding jet skis or clinging to giant inflatable balls. No matter how or why they go in, a fair number of them survive.

Baseball slugger Ed Delahanty was one who didn't make it out alive. On July 9, 1903, his mangled body, missing a leg, was discovered at the bottom of

Horseshoe Falls by the captain of *The Maid of the Mist*. Theories of exactly how he got there differ.

This much is known. Late on the night of July 2, he was on Michigan Central Railroad train number 6, traveling from Detroit to New York City. He was AWOL from the Washington Senators after playing his last game in Bennett Park in Detroit against the Tigers on June 25. On the train he got drunk as a skunk and became very belligerent. He brandished a straight razor at several passengers, smashed a glass case with an ax and tried to yank a woman out of her sleeping berth by her ankles.

Conductor John Cole assembled a posse and together they hustled Delahanty off the train, leaving him alone in the dark near the International Railway Bridge, a slender trestle structure connecting Fort Erie, Ontario, to Buffalo. A pedestrian walkway had been removed three years before, but he ventured across anyway. At that moment the bridge was drawn to allow a boat to pass beneath it. He soon dropped into the turbulent depths of the Niagara River, 20 miles south of the falls. His body turned up nine days later.

Did he jump? Did he slip and fall by accident, perhaps while running to elude a guard who was chasing him? Or was he pushed over by a thief who had just robbed him?

Delahanty's family cried foul play from the beginning, but there was no concrete evidence to support their claim. There also was no way to determine precisely when he died. Was he dead before he hit the water? Did the trauma of the plunge do him in? Or did he survive that and perish somewhere else on his journey downstream to the falls?

By any account, it was a jarring end to a spectacular career. Known as Big Ed to the public and Del to his teammates, he was a flamboyant, bold leftfielder and the oldest of five brothers from an Irish Catholic family in Cleveland to play in MLB. He was also a major league party animal. His constant carousing and prodigious use of alcohol impaired his performance on the field. Despite those handicaps, his numbers were remarkable. ESPN and the *Baseball Almanac* list his lifetime batting average of .346 as the fourth highest of all time. He hit .400 or higher three times in a 16-year career and remains the only player ever with both a four-home run game and a four-double game.

But by 1903 he was 35 years old and over the hill and he knew it. He'd bolted to the Senators in the new American League after 11 seasons with the Phillies when they offered him a $4,000 annual salary. He was making three grand a year with the Phillies. He'd jumped from one team to another in the middle of a season before. It was a common practice of the era, especially among talented players who thought they were being shortchanged by owners.

Perhaps Big Ed was growing despondent over the looming end of his career. It's a common state of mind in the sports world. NHL goalie Terry Sawchuk, MLB pitcher Don Wilson and NFL defensive tackle Jeff Alm found themselves in the same situation. They had little idea of what to do in the next chapter of their lives and it scared them. All three ended up dead before their time.

Despite all the unanswered questions, one sure takeaway from the freakish mishap is that water can kill. It's the substance that allows civilization to function and flourish, but it can also be lethal. And it doesn't have to be an overpowering force like the Niagara River or Niagara Falls. As you will read in his chapter, it can be a pond in rural Louisiana, a scenic waterfall in Hawaii, or one or another of the 30,000 lakes that dot the state of Florida. Water can indeed be dark.

## Joe Delaney: Great with a Capital G
### *NFL 1983*

The place went by a number of names—lake, water hole, drainage ditch, construction pit, pond. Whatever it was, it had swelled in size and depth from recent heavy rains and now covered roughly two football fields, with a maximum depth of 10 to 15 feet.

You couldn't really call it small. There was also a steep drop-off 15 yards from shore due to substantial dirt removal for a building project. It was strictly off limits to visitors at an establishment called Critter's Creek at Chennault Park in Monroe, Louisiana.

Critter's Creek was one of hundreds of aquatic amusement areas that sprang up in America in the 1970s and 1980s. Most of them are gone now, driven out of business by the sky-high cost of liability insurance. It was a private enterprise next to the city-owned park in Ouachita Parish and there was nothing fancy about it— several fiberglass water slides, a few concession stands and a small games arcade. The pond down the way gave the plain venue a bit of ambiance.

On the Wednesday afternoon of June 29, 1983, a boisterous crowd descended on Critter's Creek, drawn in by searing summer heat, free admission courtesy of a local television station and the debut of a new slide. Among the revelers was Joe Alton Delaney, 24, about to start his third season as a running back with the Kansas City Chiefs. He'd excelled at football and track at Haughton High School, 80 miles west of Monroe, and at Division I-AA independent Northwestern Louisiana University in Natchitoches. A second-round draft pick in 1981, he earned a Pro Bowl berth and AFC Rookie of the Year honors after rushing for 1,121 yards.

The 5–10, 185-pound scatback's second season was marred by the NFL players strike, a nagging ankle injury and surgery to repair a detached retina in his eye. He was looking forward to reporting to training camp in a few weeks at William Jewett College northeast of Kansas City. His goal was to get his groove back and reignite his stalled career.

The crowds got larger, the lines to get on the slides got longer, and around 2 p.m. three tween boys got tired of the wait and decided to slick by the *No*

*Swimming* signs and head to the pond. They weren't swimmers. They just wanted to goof off and toss a ball around in what they *thought* was shallow water.

Where were their parents? One mother was on the scene, but beyond that accounts of the incident don't say.

Delaney was hanging out with friends on the grass nearby and yelled at the boys to be careful. But a few minutes later they drifted out past the drop-off point and went under. Tyson Dickson, 12, made it back to safety by himself and screamed for help.

Even though he could barely swim, Delaney leaped into the muddy churn. He and another Good Samaritan, Keith Jakes, 17, tried to save the other two boys but their efforts proved futile. There would be no heroic ending that afternoon at Critter's Creek.

Jakes managed to pull Lancer Bernard Perkins, 11, to the surface and haul him to shore. He was taken to St. Francis Medical Center where he later died. In the pandemonium, people first thought that Delaney and the third boy had also returned to shore. But precious minutes went by, and they could not be found. As hundreds gathered in silence, divers recovered Delaney and Harry Leon Holland, 11. They both died in an ambulance on the way to St. Francis.

Delaney was survived by his wife Carolyn and daughters Tamika, 11, Crystal, four, and JoAnna, four months. He is interred at Hawkins Cemetery in the town of Princeton in Bossier Parish. Two weeks after his death, Vice President George H.W. Bush, on behalf of President Ronald Reagan, visited Haughton to present Delaney's wife and mother with the Presidential Citizens Medal, which is awarded to Americans who perform exemplary deeds or services for their country or fellow citizens.

Delaney's future in the NFL was very bright. When you think about what might have been, you could weep. During Delaney's rookie year, Oilers defensive end Elvin Bethea told the press that he'd played against the best—O.J. Simpson, Gale Sayers, Walter Payton—and that Delaney ranked right up there with them. In Bethea's words, he was "great with a capital G."[2]

As great as he was on the field, Delaney was even greater off of it.

## Craig Arfons: Last Run on Lake Jackson
### *Speed Racing 1989*

Jon Craig Arfons was born in 1949 into a family of speed racing legends based in Akron, Ohio. His father Walt introduced the first jet-powered dragster in 1960 and in 1964 he built a car for Tim Green, who set a world land speed record of 413.2 mph at the Bonneville Salt Flats in Utah.

Three days later Walt's half-brother Art surpassed that mark in a car called the Green Monster. Art set two more land speed records in 1964 and 1965 in a duel with Craig Breedlove. He also earned the distinction of surviving the first tire blowout ever at 600 mph.

At age 11 Craig watched his father wipe out on a course in Erie, Pennsylvania, and decided on the spot not to pursue life in the fast lane. But at some point, he dropped his qualms about following in the family tradition and made his first speed run on land in 1976. His mother Gertrude and Walt did not want him to race at all, but if it was going to be they preferred to see him on land instead of water. "I never liked the water," said Walt. "It's treacherous. When you hit the water it's like a million fingers tearing at you. At least on land you slide."[3]

His fears were well-founded. Piloting boats at ultra-high speeds may not be the most dangerous endeavor in the sports world. But it's definitely on the short list. The water itself is the menace. Unlike land, it's an inconsistent, unpredictable surface. In an instant a watercraft can hydroplane or collide with a small swell that can send it into a violent flip or cartwheel. And with an engine riding just inches from a pilot's head, a malfunction can be fatal.

In 1966, three-time national champion Ron Musson was killed in a crash on the Potomac River in Washington, D.C. Two years later American Lee Taylor died when his boat disintegrated during a test run. Donald Campbell's wreck in 1967 remains the most memorable of many mishaps. The only man ever to set world speed records on land and water in the same year perished at Coniston Water in England's Lake District. His headless, pulverized body was not recovered from the floor of the lake until 2001.

Despite parental misgivings, Arfons forged ahead. Intense and laser-focused, he seemed to harbor an inner need to match and even eclipse the feats of his father and uncle. He hung a sign in his office that read "Life Begins at 200 Mph." In 1979, he set a quarter-mile dragster record of 324 mph from a standing start, and in 1980 he broke his neck during a drag race in Detroit when his car flipped at 300 mph.

Arfons had limited experience racing on the water. But in 1988 he decided the time was right to attempt to break the measured kilometer speed record of 317.6 mph. Australian Ken Warby set the mark in 1978 and four men had died trying to break it.

His white hydroplane—the Rain-X Record Challenger—looked up to the task. It was a sleek, 26-foot, 2,600-pound unit fitted with an engine from an F-5 fighter jet, capable of unleashing 5,000 pounds of thrust. With his chief mechanic Fred Sibley Arfons picked Lake Jackson as the site for their run in the summer of 1989. It was a small, shallow, 3,400-acre body of water near Sebring in south-central Florida.

After two attempts on Saturday, July 8, were cut short because of six- to 10-inch waves, the team regrouped for a run on Sunday morning in front of a crowd that included Arfons' parents, son, daughter and brother. Arfons was in good spirits as he climbed into the cockpit. Conditions seemed perfect. He and his crew were supremely confident of reaching their goal. Perhaps too confident.

At 7:07 a.m. the Rain-X Record Challenger powered smoothly off the north shore of the lake and surged southward, peaking at a speed somewhere between 370 and 390 mph. As he approached the kilometer where his speed would be measured for the first of two times, Arfons turned on the afterburner, an auxiliary device fitted to the exhaust system of the engine to increase thrust.

In the next 10 seconds something went utterly haywire. He shut down the engine and released a drag parachute. But it was too late. The boat veered right, lifted off the water and cartwheeled madly before smashing the surface and breaking in two. The forward portion remained afloat. The rest, including the cockpit, sank to the bottom of the lake.

A rescue boat sliced through the fiberglass shards littering the water. Two divers extracted Arfons from the cockpit in less than three minutes and returned him to shore. On the way in a man pumped violently on his chest in an effort to revive him. On the beach, paramedics surrounded a gurney and wheeled his broken body past his hysterical mother and through the screaming crowd to an ambulance.

When he arrived at Highlands Regional Medical Center, Arfons was breathing with the aid of a life support system. But the damage inflicted on his body was massive—broken ribs, a fractured spinal cord, a shattered pelvis and a brain hemorrhage. He was pronounced dead at 8:38 a.m.

After the accident, Ken Warby called it "predictable from day one,"[4] saying his friend and rival did not have enough experience handling high speed on the water. Others joined the chorus of criticism. Arfons should have coasted to a stop instead of deploying a parachute, which increased the chances of a breakdown. The run should have been made on a larger lake. The boat was too light. It should have been tested in a wind tunnel or at least several more times on the water. In the end, experts could not pinpoint a definitive cause of the crash.

A memorial service for Arfons was held on July 13 in Manatee Village Historical Park in his hometown of Bradenton, 75 miles west of Sebring. Two days later there was a sunrise service on the shores of Lake Jackson. Community leaders in Sebring established the Craig Arfons Memorial Fund for his two children, Chad, 18, and Susie, 14. Arfons is interred at East Liberty Cemetery in the town of Green near Akron.

Chief mechanic Fred Sibley led a mission to retrieve the Rain-X Record Challenger from the bottom of Lake Jackson. Christened the JC-1 (for Jon Craig) it came to rest inside a Hooters jet-powered funny car. And despite the hopes and dreams and plans of many pilots and their crews, Ken Warby's water speed record set in 1978 still stands.

## Tim Crews and Steve Olin: They Never Saw the Dock
### *MLB 1993*

On a moonless March night in 1993, three Cleveland Indian pitchers sat in a boat on a lake in the middle of Florida. It was 84 miles north of Lake Jackson, where Craig Arfons suffered his fatal smash-up four years earlier. The guys were out in the darkness for some evening entertainment in the shallow, weedy water.

Around 7:30 they spotted vehicle headlights blinking at them from the far shore of the lake, half a mile away. Two friends were messaging them from a truck. They were ready to join the party and wanted to be picked up.

The driver revved his 150 HP outboard engine and roared toward the headlights. He was on the right side of the boat. One rider sat on the left side, and another was either in the middle between them or alone in a chair up on a higher tier, closer to the bow. The sources differ.

None of the three ever saw the dock. Other than a plentiful supply of hunker bass it was the lake's most prominent feature, jutting 175 feet into the water from the northeast shore. Long but legal, and not at all unusual in a state with 30,000 lakes. The rules did not require lights or reflectors, and the dock had neither.

The collision was horrific. The sleek, black, open-air craft rammed the dock head-high at a 90-degree angle, smashing three support posts and three cross beams. Investigators never determined the boat's exact speed but believe it was moving near 40 mph—far too fast for conditions. There was a deep, booming thud, like the sound of a gun going off. Then the engine died, and the boat drifted listlessly until the two men waiting to be picked up arrived and waded into the bloody water to pull it to shore.

Riding in the middle of the boat was Steve Olin, 27, a relief pitcher. He led the Indians in saves in 1991 and 1992 and had 48 in his career in 60 opportunities. He took the brunt of the blow and died at the scene of blunt force trauma to the front of the head.

The driver was Tim Crews, 31, a long reliever acquired by the Indians in December after spending three years with the Los Angeles Dodgers. He was pronounced dead at 5:40 a.m. at Orlando Regional Medical Center on Tuesday, March 23, the morning after the accident. The cause of death was the same as Olin's.

On the left side was Bobby Ojeda, 35, a journeyman left-hander in his first year with the Indians, projected to be the team's number two starter in his 12th MLB season. He was slouching low in his seat at the moment of impact and that very likely saved his life. He suffered a severe scalp wound and lost four pints of blood but made a full recovery.

It was a tragic end to a spirited, life-affirming day. That Monday was the only day off from spring training for the club, and Tim and Laurie Crews hosted a family picnic and cookout at their new house in Lake County, three miles south of Clermont and 40 miles north of the Indians spring training site in Winter Haven. They wanted their guests to let their hair down and have some fun before the team broke camp and headed north to start the season. They also wanted to show off their new place. They'd moved in just six weeks before.

It was quite a spread—a sprawling, two-toned 6,000-square foot ranch house on 48 acres that was once an orange grove, with horse stables and big gorgeous oak trees and plenty of pasture. Best of all was the water. Little Lake Nellie was small at 35 acres and shallow, with an average depth of 10 to 12 feet. Just south of it was Lake Nellie, eight times larger. Almost everybody who lived on Little Lake Nellie had a boat and a dock and most of them fished.

The festivities started around 3 p.m. The hosts had been working all day to prepare a feast of ham, grilled chicken, corn, beer, wine, vegetables and potatoes. Ojeda and his wife Ellen brought their 19-month-old daughter Katherine. Steve and Patty Olin arrived with seven-month-old twins Kayle and Garrett and their sister Alexa, one day past her third birthday. The Olins had gotten lost on the crazy roads coming up from Winter Haven and almost turned around and gone home. But Steve had promised Alexa a birthday horse ride, so they continued on. The Crews children were Tricia, nine, Shawn, four, and Travis, two. Indians strength and conditioning coach Fernando Montes was also at the gathering.

After a pop-up rainstorm and a 5:30 dinner, the men decided they wanted to go out bass fishing. Or maybe they really just wanted to go gator hunting. That's a term Florida boys like Crews use to describe motoring out onto the water in a fast boat and getting a little crazy. Crews certainly liked to speed, not only in cars but also in boats. That was well known. Whatever the guys had in mind, they'd been talking about it all day.

Perry Brigmond, a close friend of Laurie and Steve who'd built their house, wanted to join in. But he hadn't arrived home yet from Orlando and there was some additional gear for the boat that had to be rounded up. Ojeda, Olin and Montes played the childhood game rock, paper, scissors to see who would have to remain on shore to fetch Brigmond at his house and tend to the gear. Montes lost. It probably saved his life.

Laurie Crews did not care for the men's excursion at all. She made that abundantly clear. It was too dark and too dangerous, case closed. And she likely grasped the fact that her husband had had too much to drink. Her objections were duly noted. Then the three pitchers climbed aboard the fiberglass Skeeter boat and went out on the water anyway.

Fifteen minutes later they crashed into the dock.

The shock was immense. In the blink of an eye there were two huge voids in the team roster and two widows and six fatherless children in the Indians family. The goodbyes were numerous. A service in Portland, Oregon, for Olin and another at St. Luke's United Methodist Church in Cleveland for Crews. A third for both at St. John's Cathedral in downtown Cleveland and a fourth at the Chain O' Lakes spring training complex in Winter Haven.

Former Indian Andre Thornton, who lost his wife and daughter in a 1977 car wreck and became an ordained minister, presided at Chain O' Lakes. Dodgers manager Tommy Lasorda delivered one of five eulogies.

Bobby Ojeda was a beacon of light in the blackness. At least *someone* had survived. There's a photograph of Ojeda sitting in front of Crews' casket wiping away tears, his head wrapped in a bandana to hide the bandages covering his massive head wound. It's heartbreaking.

In the days and weeks after the accident the issue of alcohol flared up, as it so often does. A cooler found on the boat contained six full cans of beer, a nearly full liter of vodka, an empty beer can and a bottle of grape Gatorade. The BAC readings for Olin and Ojeda were .02 and .006. Olin probably had a single can of beer or a glass of wine or solo shot of hard stuff during his four hours at the party. Ojeda had no more than a few sips.

But Crews had a reading of .14. To reach that level a 6–0, 195-pound man needs to consume about eight standard units of alcohol in a four-hour period. A unit is defined as a 12-ounce beer with 5 percent ABV, a five-ounce glass of wine with 12 percent ABV, or a one-and-a-half ounce shot of 80-proof liquor.

The focus on alcohol consumption did not sit well with many Indians fans. The notion that they should be grieving less for the victims because Crews was drunk was insulting to them. A few of them verbalized an inconvenient truth—some people handle alcohol far better than others, even in large amounts. To conclude that Crews was out of control at the helm of his boat solely on the basis of his BAC reading was pure conjecture. They also blamed media for fanning the flames of the controversy. You will read in Chapter 11 of similar reactions to the deaths of runner Steve Prefontaine in 1975 and NHL goalie Pelle Lindbergh in 1986. Both were legally impaired when they died behind the wheel in one-car accidents.

Steve Robert Olin's cremains are interred at Skyline Memorial Gardens in Portland, Oregon. Stanley Timothy Crews was buried at Woodland Memorial Park in Gotha, Florida, near Orlando.

## Shannon Smith: Paradise Lost
*College Football 1997*

The secluded spot was far off the beaten path, up five miles of unpaved roads from the highway, then up another one by foot on a red dirt trail surrounded by thick, tangled vegetation.

Anyone hardy enough to finish the journey near the eastern edge of the island of Kauai (kow-EYE-ee) in Hawaii was rewarded with a beautiful sight—a 20-foot waterfall cascading over a rocky cliff into a small pool of emerald green water surrounded by wild ferns and guava trees. The official name of it was Waipahee (why-PAW-hee). The locals called it Slippery Slide.

The place was on private land, legally off limits to visitors since 1979. For good reason. Nine people had died there since 1962, including three on one day in 1971. But that didn't stop adventurous souls from trekking past the *No Trespassing* signs and across the one-time sugar plantation to take in its beauty—and take their chances in the water.

It could be that many of those souls weren't even aware of the deaths. On March 29, 1997, as a party of 11 made their way to Slippery Slide, 26 years had passed since the triple fatality incident.

The leader of the group was Shannon Smith, 20, a placekicker on the University of Hawaii football team. He'd lived on Kauai since he was two, when his parents Norbert and Rosemary bought and remodeled an old macadamia plantation house and converted it into a bed and breakfast called Rosewood. Shannon had visited the site many times, and he wanted to show it off to Hawaii head coach Fred vonAppen, his wife Thea and their son Cody, six, and daughter Kristan, 17. Two of Smith's teammates, strong safety Chris Shinnick and quarterback Tim Carey, were in the party as well. Shannon had convinced them all to fly in from Honolulu, 119 miles to the southeast, to spend Easter weekend at Rosewood. He wanted to show them the wondrous sites of his home turf, known as the Garden Island.

It was striking—a Division I head coach accepting such a personal invitation from one of his players. But Shannon could be very persuasive. Sullen and obnoxious as a young teen, he evolved into a friendly, exuberant guy who talked vonAppen into putting him on the Rainbow Warrior squad as a walk-on.

After a year on the bench except for one kickoff, he had a shot at becoming the starting kicker for the upcoming 1997 season. He'd only played one year of football at Kapaa High School after many years of soccer. As the only white kid on the roster he dropped the jaws of his Hawaiian, Filipino and Japanese teammates with his kicking skills. They called him Thunderfoot.

Shannon was also a daredevil and sky diver and cliff jumper. He was always game for a physical challenge. The tougher, the better. He possessed both the bravura and the physical skills to do things that other people wouldn't dream of doing.

He saved his favorite spot on the Garden Island for last. The group set out for Slippery Slide on Saturday, their final day on Kauai before they headed home. Four friends of the Smith family joined them.

Heavy rain had been falling for days in the mountains. The stream leading to the waterfall was way deeper than usual. Ankle-high had become waist-high, and there was no emerald green to be seen. The water was a mucky, muddy brown.

The 12-by-25-foot pool at the bottom of the falls was rough and churning and as brown as the stream. It was also deep, 20 to 25 feet instead of the usual 10. The force of the water was so strong that it was swirling in a vortex, like an underwater tornado that could yank people under the surface in an instant. Family friend Mike Law did not like what he was seeing at all. He told Shannon he was staying out and pleaded with him to do the same. The water was simply too treacherous.

Undaunted, Shannon plunged headfirst down the slide on a trial run, sprang out of the pool and hustled back to the top of the cliff. There he sat Cody down on his lap, strapped his right arm across the boy's chest and pushed down the slide again.

They were sucked into the vortex as soon as they hit the pool. On his solo dive, Shannon had skimmed the water then peeled off quickly to the right, away from the danger. But with 60-pound Cody in his arms they rolled hard to the left, directly into the swirling water. Their heads popped to the surface. They screamed for help, then went under. Seconds later, Cody popped up again, pushed to the surface by Shannon. As Shannon held him up, Fred and Thea and Tim Carey dove in, formed a human chain as best they could and relayed the boy to shore.

Shannon flailed and thrashed, exhausted and on the brink of collapse. But he refused to leave the water until Fred and Thea and Tim were safely on shore. Like the captain of a ship, he would be the last man on the watch. He treaded water, struggled to breathe and then went under for the last time.

Rescue scuba divers arrived and submerged quickly, their safety ropes attached to the thick limbs of guava trees. Ninety minutes later Shannon's badly bloated body appeared face up on the surface. A large contusion on his head indicated that he had probably slammed it into a rock wall and been knocked unconscious as he struggled upward from the depths of the water.

He died three days before his 21st birthday. At the time of his death his mother was shopping for his birthday gift. He was survived by his parents, three brothers and two sisters. Another sister died in 1969 at age three. On April 6, services were held at St. Catherine's Church in Kapaa on Kauai. His body was cremated.

Nearly three decades have passed since the tragedy, and the question remains—why did Shannon ignore the clear risks of what he was about to do? Why did he spurn the pleas of Mike Law to stay on shore? At the end he was beyond doubt a hero, and for that he deserves all the adulation he has received. But the decision to enter the water in the first place was a serious error in judgment that put not only himself but several others in harm's way.

Perhaps it's best to view the story as an ode to the fearsome power of water. Or a cautionary tale about thrusting yourself into a situation that you *think* you can control.

Whether you're Ed Delahanty above the Niagara River or Joe Delaney in a pond in Louisiana or Shannon Smith at a waterfall in Hawaii, water can be dangerous, terrifying and lethal.

## Marquis Cooper and Corey Smith: Engulfed
### *NFL 2009*

Marquis Cooper was the one with the boat, and before the 26-year-old linebacker left Florida for an off-season winter camp with the Oakland Raiders in 2009 he wanted to get out on the Gulf of Mexico for one last day of fishing with his buddies. They'd head out from Clearwater Pass to a shipwreck site 60 miles west, drop the anchor, and head home with a load of amberjack and maybe if they got lucky some small sharks.

Defensive end Corey Smith was set to go with him. He was Cooper's weightlifting partner, a veteran tight end of eight NFL seasons out of Richmond, Virginia, and North Carolina State. Like Cooper he was a journeyman, with stints at Tampa Bay, San Francisco and Detroit. At age 29 he was a free agent looking to sign with a new team.

They invited Nick Schuyler, 24, to join them. He was their trainer at LA Fitness in Lutz, 15 miles north of Tampa, the dude who was guiding them through some insanely hardcore workouts. Nick brought his best friend Will Bleakley, 24, a teammate from football at the University of South Florida.

So it was a gang of four that left the Seminole Boat Ramp at 6:30 a.m. on Saturday, February 28. All of their gear, tack, beer, food and ice was packed in on Cooper's boat—a 10-passenger, 21-foot, 3,400-pound Everglades with a 200 HP Yamaha engine. Everglades was a premium brand, known in the industry for their foam-filled fiberglass hulls. The foam increased buoyancy to the point where their boats were nearly unsinkable.

The sky was overcast, and the waves were high from the get-go. But they didn't pay it much mind. They were too busy enjoying themselves. And Corey didn't drink, so if things got too rowdy on board he could step to the console and take the helm.

Around three o'clock heavy rain, cold and fierce winds arrived, and it got very ugly very fast. They decided to head back to shore. But the anchor was snagged on something hard 140 feet below the surface, probably a coral reef. In an effort to dislodge it, Cooper revved the powerful engine full throttle. The stern squatted down low, frigid water poured in and the boat listed hard to the port side and capsized, throwing them all overboard.

They tried to turn the boat upright. But there was no place to grip it and get enough leverage to lift. They scrambled onto the hull. Bleakley swam under the boat and grabbed three lifejackets, a seat cushion and three strike flares. They cut the anchor rope and tried to flip the boat again. But it wouldn't budge.

Holding onto each other as the waves got higher, they placed themselves on and around the hull. Their cell phones were dead. The flares were soaked and useless. They soon saw the lights of rescuers in the sky, but the rescuers didn't see them. After darkness arrived, they recited the Lord's Prayer together, talked about their regrets in life and moved around as best they could to keep the blood flowing.

But they could only do so much. Their cumulative weight sank the boat lower until the water was up to their chests. Exhaustion, fear, dehydration and hypothermia took their toll. Sometime during the night, as Saturday became Sunday, Cooper crossed the bar. Schuyler held him in his arms as long as he could and then surrendered his body to the water. Hours later, as dawn broke, a delirious Smith pushed away from the hull and cast his fate to the sea.

## 3. Dark Waters

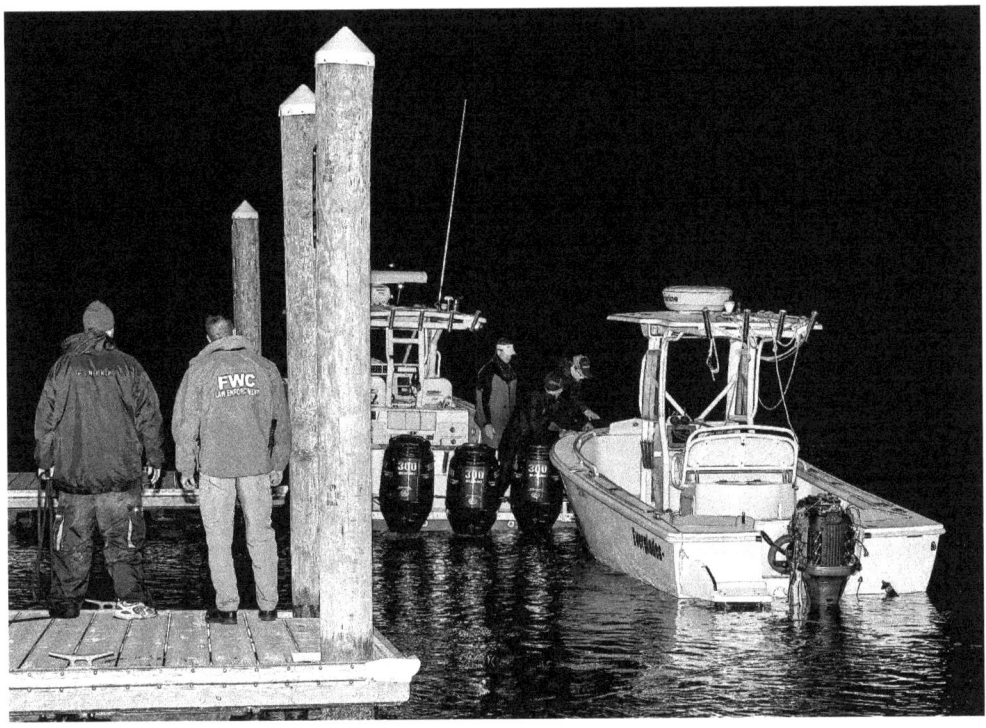

The boat belonging to Oakland Raiders linebacker Marquis Cooper arrives at the Bay Pines ramp in St. Petersburg, Florida, after being towed in from the Gulf of Mexico by the U.S. Coast Guard. Cooper, NFL tight end Corey Smith and Will Bleakley died at sea after the boat capsized in a storm on February 28, 2009. Nick Schuyler survived the ordeal and recounts it in his book *Not Without Hope*, written with *New York Times* reporter Jeré Longman (AP Images / Chris O'Meara).

Schuyler and Bleakley held on for the next 24 hours. Bleakley grew weak and disoriented and kept falling off the hull, and at dawn on Monday he drifted out into eternity. At 12:30 p.m. the Coast Guard cutter *Tornado* arrived on the scene. The Guard had been searching the gulf by helicopter, boat and plane from Cedar Key in the north to Fort Myers in the south. Schuyler was hoisted up to a chopper and flown to Tampa General Hospital after 43 hours in the water. Doctors said he would have been dead by nightfall.

Schuyler recounts the ordeal in his riveting book *Not Without Hope*, written with *New York Times* reporter Jeré Longman. The account above is Schuyler's version of what happened. Some people took issue with it, most notably Phoenix sportscaster Bruce Cooper, father of Marquis. He labeled it a bunch of self-serving bull and said the whole thing could not have gone down the way Schuyler claimed it did. His son was a strong swimmer and a fighter and never would have given up his life that easily.

Let's hope that the man's tirade calling out the sole survivor was no more than an anguished cry from a father in the throes of deep, overwhelming grief.

Regardless of what exactly transpired out on the gulf, the tragedy was an accident waiting to happen. Schuyler freely admits that in his book and lays out a long list of careless mistakes. No tracer or emergency beacon on board that would have helped the Coast Guard pinpoint their location. No detailed float plan filed with the dockmaster in Clearwater. Blowing off the forecast of stormy weather and small craft warnings that were posted the night before the outing. And yes, Schuyler confesses that he and Cooper and Bleakley consumed alcohol that day. But he insists it had nothing to do with the catastrophe that followed.

The worst mistake of all was lowering the anchor into the water off the stern because that can quickly destabilize a boat. It's a common mistake and it's not safe. Experts call it insanity, especially in turbulent seas. Despite that blunder, the men could have cut the rope as soon as the water got rough, sacrificed the anchor and headed back to shore without it. But they didn't do that.

The bodies of Cooper, Smith and Bleakley were never recovered. Their remains lie somewhere at the bottom of the Gulf of Mexico. What a tragic waste of young, vibrant lives.

Let's get out of the water now, dry off, and transition to the realm of flight. Come fly. But please—fasten your seat belt. These skies are decidedly unfriendly.

# 4

## Sound of Impact

### Knute Rockne: Dreadful News
*College Football 1931*

On the last morning of March in 1931, a red and silver airplane prepared for takeoff from Kansas City Municipal Airport. Flanked by two wooden wings, the "merchant liner" was bound for Los Angeles. There'd be stops in Wichita and two other as-yet undetermined cities to pick up mail. Those locations would be relayed from the ground to the pilot and co-pilot via a radio system that worked well. At least most of the time.

It was a miserable day for flying—cold, dark, wet, windy. The six passengers aboard the Fokker F-10 trimotor operated by Transcontinental and Western Air (TWA) would be roughing it. That was par for the course because they were more or less afterthoughts. The prime purpose of the flight was to move mail, not people.

Merchant liner was a term used by the press to conjure up a glamorous image of a flying boat, a kind of *Titanic* of the skies. It was a gross distortion of reality. The 10-seat cabin was frigid. There were no stewardesses or reclining seats or pillows, no food or drink unless you brought your own. Those perks would arrive in a few years, as would lavatories. For now you either held on until the next mail stop or did your business in a metal bucket or cardboard box behind a flimsy curtain at the rear of the cabin. And forget about trying to talk or sleep because it was loud as hell.

But traveling by air still had one huge advantage over the ground. Kansas City to Los Angeles via train took three full days, sometimes longer. On the road in an automobile it could take up to ten. NC-999—the Department of Commerce registration number for the plane—was scheduled to depart at 8:30 a.m. and arrive on the West Coast 23 hours later at 5:30 a.m. Pacific time.

That differential was an attractive, eyepopping temptation. On paper, it seemed alluring enough to draw travelers away from tracks and highways and into the skies.

But that wasn't happening. Flying was expensive. The passengers on NC-999 paid $130 each for their one-way tickets—$2,000 in today's money. Another hang-up was that flying scared the bejesus out of people. It was so new and different and strange. Western Air Express, America's first airline with a regular schedule, had been operating for just five years. In 1930, there were 417,000 commercial air passengers in the country. The pre–Covid pandemic figure from 2019—925.5 million.

Safety protocols were haphazard and the planes themselves were not of the highest quality. Despite those drawbacks, the number of accidents in the pioneer era of commercial aviation was actually fairly small. Just 12 were documented worldwide in the 1920s, with 84 fatalities. In 1930, 16 died when a Maddux Air Line Ford 5 crashed on the shore in Oceanside, California, on its way back to LA from the month-old Agua Caliente Racetrack in Tijuana.

Those lowish numbers didn't do much to soothe the fear. Long odds against catastrophe didn't mean squat if you happened to be one of the unfortunate souls losing out in the Grim Reaper's lottery. It was really quite simple. For millions of people the thought of being trapped inside a giant metal tube plunging through the sky toward Earth at 200 mph was utterly terrifying.

So in 1931 flying was largely for the bold and adventurous, the rich, and to an increasing degree the famous—Hollywood celebrities, civic and business leaders and stars from what would come to be known as the Golden Age of Sports.

Knute Kenneth Rockne was one of those stars. Like all teams in 1931, the Notre Dame footballers traveled by train. But when he was on his own their coach was an enthusiastic flyer. Rockne was frequently on the go, attending to a busy schedule. Time was always of the essence, and he was one of the six men boarding NC-999 that Tuesday morning in Kansas City.

It would be a stretch to call Rockne the *most famous* person in America at the onset of the Great Depression. That honor likely belonged to Charles Lindbergh, the Lone Eagle, or Rockne's friend Will Rogers, the Cowboy Philosopher, or Babe Ruth, the Colossus of Clout, or Henry Ford, the People's Tycoon. But Rockne definitely dwelled in the high rent district of Fame. The Fighting Irish were the New York Yankees of football—illustrious, hugely talented, intimidating. They'd posted five undefeated seasons in Rockne's 13-year tenure, including 1929 and 1930. Their list of vanquished opponents included a slew of prominent powers—Army, Princeton, Georgia Tech, Southern California, Stanford, Minnesota. His overall record was 105–12–5, a winning percentage of .881, still the highest in major college football history.

Rockne was not merely famous. Like Lindbergh he was revered, a living symbol of virtue and strength and honorable success, a Norwegian immigrant who'd risen to the highest levels of American life. A demigod, if you will. Was he really the magnificent human being that his public image suggested? Probably not. Even saints have their character flaws. Remarks were occasionally made about his sharp, acid tongue. But in the era in which he lived he was admired to a degree that isn't possible today. Fueled by bitterly divisive politics and toxic social media, modern America is too resentful, judgmental, cynical and negative for hero worship. Any person who approaches Rockne's stature these days is certain to be cut down to size in very short order.

He was taking a break from spring practice in South Bend for a quick trip out West. His agenda was full—consulting with Universal Pictures about an upcoming feature film, *The Spirit of Notre Dame*, speaking at the renowned Los Angeles Breakfast Club, revving up the sales staff of Studebaker with a pep talk, helping friend J.H. Happer, also on NC-999, open a new branch of the Wilson Western Sporting Goods Company. Rockne's business manager Christy Walsh planned on joining him on the flight but cancelled after his wife pleaded with him to take the train instead.

Flying, she said, was just too dangerous.

NC-999 departed 45 minutes late after waiting for mail connections. The horrid weather had not improved. At 10:31 the co-pilot radioed to Wichita that they were turning back to Kansas City.

Near the village of Bazaar in the Flint Hills cattle and corn country, workers in the fields heard a plane droning loudly overhead. The clouds were so thick they couldn't see it at first, but the engine didn't sound right. It was sputtering and groaning and whining.

At about 10:40 the Fokker burst out of the clouds trailing smoke and angling toward the ground as if the pilot was looking for a place to land. It pulled up again, and seconds later came an enormous bang. With its entire right wing snapped off, the plane lurched into a twisting nosedive and plunged 1,500 feet to the ground. Before it hit five bodies fell out. The severed wing floated like a butterfly in the stiff wind and landed a half mile away.

The engine conked out during the fall and after the booming sound of impact came silence. There was no explosion or fire, no flowing blood or seared flesh. Just the horrid stench of gasoline and eight badly mangled bodies, three in the cockpit and five scattered in the snowy wheat field, one with rosary beads wrapped around his fingers. After ambulances hauled the remains over 20 miles of muddy roads to the coroner's office in Cottonwood Springs, that man was identified as Knute Rockne. At the peak of a brilliant career, he was dead at age 43.

Through the wondrous, emerging medium of radio, news of the tragedy spread quickly. Rockne's mother and two of his sisters heard of his death on their home sets. The newspaper stories and newsreels for movie theaters would come later. Radio was immediate. For the first time in history, millions of Americans mourned a public figure almost instantaneously.

Will Rogers, who would die in a plane crash himself four years later, was among the thousands who offered condolences. King Haakon of Norway posthumously knighted Rockne. President Herbert Hoover, an avid fan of the game who served as student manager of the first Stanford teams in the 1890s under coach Walter Camp, was informed of the accident in the Oval Office. His face turned ashen. "What dreadful, dreadful news."[1]

The first plan was to hold Rockne's funeral in Notre Dame's new 54,000-seat stadium. But his wife Bonnie nixed that idea. She opted for an invitation-only service at the Basilica of the Sacred Heart on campus. On Saturday, April 4, the day before Easter, Rockne lay in state in a bronze casket at his home at 1417 East Wayne Avenue in South Bend until a 100-car motorcade proceeded to the church for the 3 p.m. funeral in front of 1,400 mourners.

CBS carried the service live on its 79 network radio affiliates across the country. There had been only one previous live nationwide broadcast—the parade in Washington in June 1927 to honor Charles Lindbergh three weeks after his solo transatlantic flight. The concept was so new that the press didn't quite know how to label it. One newspaper awkwardly described it as "a national hookup for a word picture of the services."[2] After the funeral, Rockne was laid to rest at Highland Cemetery in South Bend.

A Department of Commerce inspector and the Chase County coroner held an inquest in Cottonwood Springs the day after the crash. They quickly determined the cause to be structural damage due to the stress of ice. But the public remained captivated by the story and the incessant clamor for more details led government officials to launch a more thorough probe. Their efforts were hampered by hundreds of scavengers who flocked to the crash site and stripped the battered craft clean in search of souvenirs. All that remained were a few dozen chunks of mangled metal.

In the end, investigators could not definitely solve the mystery. But attention soon turned to the wooden wings as a likely culprit. The plywood wing panels were bonded to the ribs and spars with water-based resin glue. As rainwater and moisture accumulated over time the panels loosened and the glue eventually failed, causing the separation of the right wing.

The aftereffects of the crash reverberated for years. It almost sank TWA. All Fokker F-10s were immediately grounded and a new regimen of rigorous inspection was implemented. Those costs weighed heavily on the company's bottom line, but it managed to survive.

The crash did mark the end of the longstanding policy of the Department of Commerce that kept the official causes of plane accidents secret. It also hastened the demise of wooden wings. Airlines had long resisted vastly safer and more durable metal because of the sky-high price tag. But the new designs caused a dramatic increase in safety, which in turn prompted an astonishing boom in air travel. That led to the development of the 21-seat DC-3, the first plane to make airlines consistently profitable.

Another casualty was the Golden Age of Sports. The crash can be viewed as the symbolic end of the freewheeling, exuberant decade that featured many fabled superstars—Babe Ruth, Jim Thorpe, Bill Tilden, Red Grange, Man o' War, Johnny Weissmuller, Bobby Jones and Jack Dempsey.

Was the sports world really a greater, brighter, more exhilarating place a hundred years ago? Given the strong human tendency to romanticize the past, it's not likely. Be that as it may, the Golden Age was followed by the most severe economic downturn in American history, the rise of Nazism in Europe and the looming threat of another world war. Rockne's untimely death was a portent of more somber times to come.

## Thurman Munson: Out of His League
*MLB 1979*

The commuter jet was coming in way too low and slow, and neither engine was making any noise. Something was clearly wrong. To motorists cruising along the north boundary of Akron-Canton Regional Airport in Ohio the scene was something out of a Hollywood disaster flick, playing out live right in front of their astonished eyes at 3 p.m. on August 2, 1979.

Trailing heavy smoke, the plane mowed down 12 tall trees, smashed into a giant stump and bounced onto Greensburg Road, 870 feet short of the runway. As it spun wildly in circles a wing tore off and the back half of the fuselage ripped away and rolled into a ditch.

Up front, two burned and bleeding men staggered from the flaming wreckage and screamed to a gathering crowd that the pilot was still inside. The men had tried to yank him out of his seat but fuel leaking from the wing tank exploded and caught fire, forcing them to scramble away.

Firefighters arrived in three minutes, sprayed the battered hulk with foam to extinguish the flames and then approached it with axes, as if to break in. But they quickly backed off. The smoke was blinding, and the heat was beyond intense. They could feel it rising up from the pavement through their boots.

There was no hope for the man in the cockpit. He was still in his seat, consumed by an inferno. He was known to be an attentive pilot, but he wasn't wearing his shoulder harness that day and on impact with the tree stump his head slammed into the instrument panel, crushing his vertebrae and paralyzing him from the neck down.

As he sat there the flames surged time and time again and he was scorched to a charred black pulp, burned beyond recognition. The Summit County coroner said later that he might have remained conscious for three minutes after the crash, alive for as long as 10. Words can't describe the horrific last moments of his life. We can only hope that the end came quickly.

The dead man was Thurman Munson, 32, the catcher and team captain for the New York Yankees, the reigning World Series champions. The passengers were David Hall, 32, and Jerry D. Anderson, 31, two friends and fellow pilots from Munson's hometown of Canton. Hall was the man who taught Munson to fly.

The decimated craft was a $1.4 million, seven-seat Cessna Citation with the lettering N15NY, after Munson's jersey number. He'd only owned it for a month, but that's the way he was with planes. He'd bought and sold four in the 18 months he'd been flying. But those had all been props. The Citation was a jet.

It was a big step up, sort of like exchanging a Honda Civic for a Cadillac Escalade. Jets are made to fly faster, higher and longer than props, and pilots need to perform at an advanced level to guide them safely to their destinations. The Citation was a lot of plane, and it could be very harsh on pilots, particularly ones who hadn't clocked much time at the controls. Munson had 516 total hours in his log, but only 33 in his new ride. Most Citation owners hired professional pilots. Munson balked at that. He was determined to operate this flying machine on his own, just like he'd done with all the others.

He'd just flown home from Chicago after a night game with the White Sox, arriving at 3 a.m. Thursday. Something with the Citation didn't feel right. There was a malfunction warning light on the instrument panel, but it was more than that.

Thursday was an off day. He was flying to New York on Friday to begin a four-game series with the Orioles, and he wanted to check things out before he left. So after a lunch at Prestwick Country Club with his father-in-law Tony Dominick, Munson was in the air with Hall and Anderson practicing touch-and-go landings. Ascend to 2,800 feet, approach from the north, touch down, move along the runway for 10 to 15 seconds, then take off. Munson made five passes with no complications. He wanted one more before he packed it in.

On that sixth and final pass, disaster arrived in northeast Ohio.

Munson was in his 10th full MLB season, all with the Yankees, and his record of achievement was sterling—AL Rookie of the Year in 1970, AL MVP in 1976, World Series champion in 1977 and 1978, six All-Star games, five seasons as a .300 hitter. He also played through savage pain, handled pitchers like a wizard and absolutely hated to lose.

As accomplished as he was on the field, he was better known for the kind of person he was. His squat build, sloppy moustache, tangled hair and perpetual pout emitted a strong non-verbal message—don't mess. Few people did. You knew where you stood with Thurman, and for most that meant he didn't want anything to do with you. He just wasn't a mix-and-mingle-let's-tip-a-few-and-shoot-the-breeze kind of guy. His outlook on his profession was simple. Go full force, leave every ounce of your energy on the diamond, then go straight home to your family.

So no one was more surprised than Munson himself when owner George Steinbrenner and manager Billy Martin named him captain of the Yankees in 1976. The team hadn't had one since Lou Gehrig. Munson figured he was too abrasive for the role. He cussed at people and yelled at umpires and didn't get along well at all with reporters and fans. And he once laid hands on a college student in Minneapolis seeking an autograph.

Becoming captain didn't change him much. He brooded about being overshadowed by Johnny Bench and Carlton Fisk, the other two superstar catchers of the 1970s. He feuded frequently, most notably with Reggie Jackson and Steinbrenner. Jackson, who joined the team in 1977, royally dissed Munson by proclaiming himself "the straw that stirs the drink"[3] in the Yankee clubhouse. Steinbrenner incensed him by spurning his salary demands, and Munson retaliated by growing a beard in violation of the team's personal appearance code.

There was another side to the man, of course. There virtually always is. But the only place he could drop his guard and show his warmth and loyalty and compassion was at home with his wife Diana, their son Michael and daughters Tracy and Kelly. Getting back to them on a regular basis during the season was the main reason he'd taken to flying with such zest. To the end, Munson remained true blue to his hometown.

The outpouring of grief in Canton was the greatest since the assassination of their own William McKinley in 1901. At his funeral on August 6, the same reverend who married Thurman and Diana in 1968 delivered the eulogy. The organist featured many selections by Neil Diamond, Munson's favorite singer. Teammates Bobby Murcer and Lou Piniella spoke, and the entire Yankee team attended, including Jackson. Munson is interred at Sunset Hills Memorial Park in Canton.

The aftermath of the tragedy proved to be loud, long and ugly. It usually is when lawyers get involved. Diana Munson sued Cessna Aircraft, claiming that the company's sales reps unduly pressured her husband to buy an airplane they knew he could not fly safely. She also sued Flight Schools International for failing to provide Munson with adequate instruction. Cornhill, a British insurance company, denied the claims of the Munson estate, asserting that it had no responsibility to pay the million-dollar mortgage balance on the Citation because Munson was not flying with a certified jet instructor aboard on the day of the accident.

Some measure of clarity was achieved when the NTSB issued its investigative findings in April of 1980. Long story short, Munson screwed up. Badly. Three instructors had rated him above average as a pilot, but he committed "numerous errors"[4] on the final flight of his life. Making a very low approach to the runway and failing to correct for it. Falling below a safe air speed, which caused the plane to stall. Neglecting to lower the landing gear and wing flaps in a timely manner. Ignoring a written checklist that offered step-by-step guidance. Munson may well have been adept at flying prop planes, but the findings indicated that he was out of his league when it came to jets.

The $1.7 million payout that Diana finally received in 1984 was not an admission of wrongdoing by any party. It can be better described a move rooted in exhaustion, designed to put the endless haggling to rest. Which it did.

Thurman Munson was the first New York Yankee to get in over his head in the cockpit of an airplane. He wouldn't be the last. Twenty-seven years later, another Bronx Bomber found himself in the same situation.

## Davey Allison: Chopper Down
### *NASCAR 1993*

Thurman Munson died at the controls of a fancy flying machine that, for one deadly moment, he could not control. Davey Allison met the same fate.

The irony of Allison's demise is that he didn't die on the track like dozens of other auto racers who risk their lives day after day in one the world's deadliest sports. Instead he died in a helicopter, trying to land in the infield at Talladega Superspeedway in Alabama, 64 miles east of his residence in Hueytown outside Birmingham.

In the 1980s and 1990s it wasn't at all unusual for NASCAR drivers to get airborne. Most traveled to Winston Cup races, personal appearances and test sessions in private aircrafts owned by their teams and usually flown by hired pilots. Only a few drivers—Rusty Wallace, Ricky Rudd, Bill Elliott and Allison among them—flew their own planes. And just one, retired three-time Grand National Champion David Pearson, was known to fly a chopper.

Helicopters are different from airplanes. They can be a load. If a plane is mechanically stable and there are no strong winds, it can almost fly itself. Helicopters require more effort and diligence. Their ability to hover in the air often sparks instability. Pilots have to use their hands and feet almost constantly to stay in flight and maneuver the craft in and out of tight spaces. Allison had been flying for 10 years. But he had only logged 54 hours in helicopters and 45 of those had been in a Robinson R-22, which he'd replaced three weeks before his fatal crash with a more sophisticated Hughes 369 HS.

Allison's mother Judy didn't care for the Robinson or the Hughes one bit. She viewed them as extravagant, dangerous playthings that her son could do without. Despite her misgivings, Allison was proceeding whole hog. A friend described him as addicted to flying, especially in helicopters. On the day of his accident workers were installing a landing pad on his spread in Hueytown.

Purchasing and piloting the Hughes seemed to be a symbol of sorts for Allison's coming of age in his chosen profession. Early on he was a headstrong hothead, unable to handle setbacks and defeats. But in recent years he'd gotten his temper under control and his career was on an upward track. He had 191 career starts and 19 wins in Winston Cup races, including five in 1992. One of those five was the Daytona 500.

On the morning of July 12, 1993, Allison was headed to Talladega to watch a practice run by David Bonnett, the son of Neil Bonnett. They were close friends of the Allison family and members of NASCAR's illustrious Alabama Gang, which also included Jimmy Means and in later years the Stricklin family. With Allison was another gang member, former driver Red Farmer, who was now the crew chief for Allison's team on the Busch Grand National Tour, the level of stock car racing just below the Winston Cup. Farmer was taking his first ride ever in a chopper. It would be memorable.

## 4. Sound of Impact

Just after nine o'clock Allison attempted to land his 2,500-pound craft in a small, fenced-in parking lot in the infield. It came within a foot of the ground, then wobbled violently and lurched 25 feet into the air before spinning and crashing onto the pavement on its left side, where Allison was sitting. He was stuck in his seat belt and trapped in his seat, unconscious. Farmer busted a glass window open and crawled out.

At Carraway Methodist Medical Center in Birmingham doctors performed surgery to relieve pressure on Allison's brain. He never regained consciousness and died at 7:15 a.m. on July 13. He was 32. Farmer broke four ribs, his nose and his collarbone but healed fully after a long recovery.

Allison was survived by his parents Bobby and Judy, his wife Elizabeth (Liz) and their children Krista Marie, three, and Robert Grey, two. He was buried at Highland Memorial Gardens in Bessemer near Hueytown.

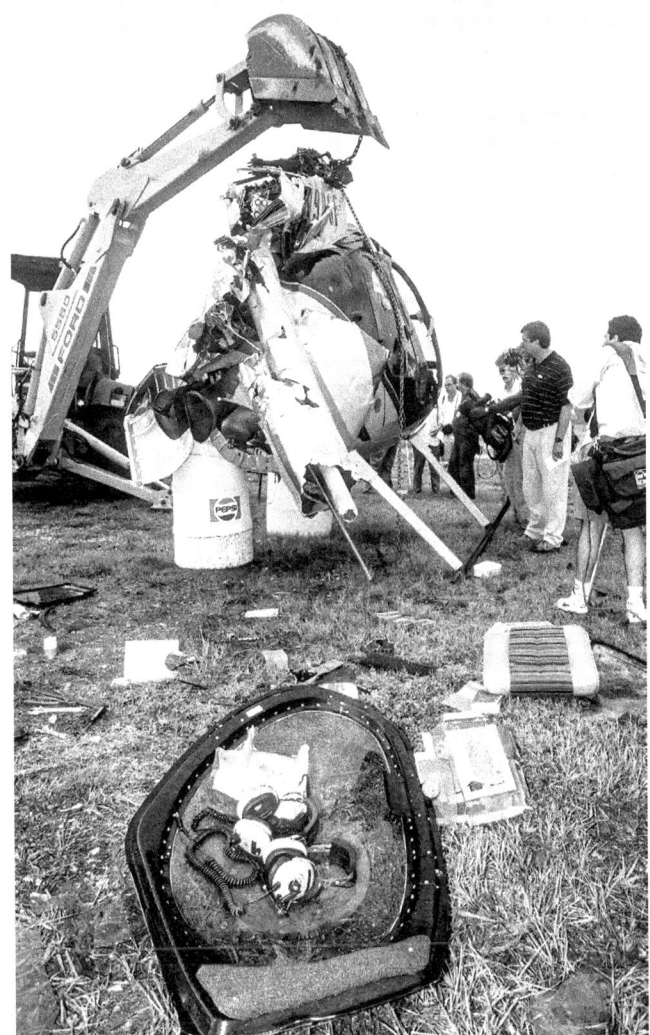

NTSB officials examine the mangled wreckage of Davey Allison's helicopter in the infield of Talladega Superspeedway in Alabama. The 1992 Daytona 500 champion was a veteran pilot but had only logged seven hours at the helm of his new Hughes 369FS chopper when he crashed attempting to land on the morning of July 12, 1993. Passenger Red Farmer survived (AP Images / Hal Yeager).

An NTSB investigation found no evidence of mechanical failure. Pilot error was determined to be the cause of the crash. Eyewitnesses said that Allison executed a downwind landing with the wind at his back, which is far more dangerous that landing into the wind. He also came in too quickly and too "shallow," meaning that he started his final descent to the infield too close to the ground.

It was the second air tragedy for NASCAR in less than four months. On April

1, reigning Winston Cup champion Alan Kulwicki died in a private plane with three others in a crash near Blountville, Tennessee.

Auto racing had seen its fair share of death in the air. In 1954, three-time Indy 500 champion Wilbur Shaw and a passenger died after falling into a cornfield in a snowstorm in Decatur, Indiana. In 1970, stock car pioneer and flying daredevil Curtis Turner died with golfer Clyde King after ramming a mountainside in western Pennsylvania. Five years later, Formula One and Indy 500 champion Graham Hill plunged onto a fog-shrouded golf course in London, killing himself and five others.

Then there were the numerous misfortunes of the Allison family. A year before his death, Davey hit a wall and flipped 11 times at Pocono International Raceway, breaking his arm and several ribs and fracturing his wrist. A month later, his brother Clifford died during a practice run at Michigan International Speedway in Brooklyn.

Before that, there was his uncle Donnie's smash-up at the World 600 in Charlotte that hastened his exit from competition. And in June 1988 at Pocono, Bobby suffered a horrific wreck, slipping to the brink of death before a paramedic climbed into his car and performed a tracheotomy that saved his life. He spent 108 days in the hospital and struggled for years to regain the basic human skills needed to function. As of 2024, both Donnie and Bobby were still alive.

Even for a family that long ago accepted the grave dangers of stock car racing, their suffering has been extreme.

## Rodney Culver: Nosedive
### *NFL 1996*

Rodney Dewayne Culver was a special kind of human being, cut from a different cloth.

His athletic achievements were distinguished enough. He was a three-sport standout in football, basketball and track at Saint Martin de Porres High School in Detroit. At Notre Dame the 5–9, 225-pound running back was a freshman letterman on the storied 1988 national championship team. He started for two years and was voted the sole captain by his teammates as a senior. In the NFL he played two seasons with the Colts, who acquired him in the fourth round of the 1992 draft, and two with the Chargers. He appeared in Super Bowl XXIX against the 49ers and scored 16 touchdowns in his four-year pro career.

But it was off the field where he truly stood out. He was a friend to all, a dedicated family man and a humble, devout Christian. He not only organized the Chargers' weekly chapel meetings, but he also took written notes as the chaplain spoke. Every autograph he signed included a verse of scripture.

Culver was also preparing himself for life after the gridiron. In college he said he had no intention of being one of those players "hung up on killing himself"[5] if he didn't make it to the NFL. After he did make it, he viewed his pro years as a prelude to what would come next—life as a father, husband and player in the business world, where he could put his finance degree from Notre Dame to good use.

He never got a chance at that life. He departed this world an eternity too soon at age 26. And for a human being of his caliber to die in the horrifying way he did seems utterly unfair, almost beyond comprehension. His death must have tested the faith of even the staunchest believers.

On the afternoon of July 11, 1996, Culver boarded ValuJet Flight 592 with his wife Karen, 25, at Miami International Airport. They were returning to Woodstock, Georgia, a suburb in Cherokee County north of Atlanta, where they lived with their daughters Briana, five, and Jada, 15 months.

Departure in the discount airline's 27-year-old DC-9 was delayed for an hour.

Ten minutes after takeoff, as the plane climbed to cruising altitude northwest of Miami over the Everglades, a nightmare erupted in a matter of seconds. There was a loud bang and then smoke and flames from the front cargo bay flooded the cabin. At 2:06 p.m. the pilot radioed the control tower that she was returning to the airport. Eight minutes later the plane disappeared from the radar screen. At a speed of 352 mph, it had nosedived like a bullet into a deep-water swamp with a bedrock base 20 miles northwest of the airport.

All 105 passengers and the crew of five perished instantly. Killed along with Culver and his wife was Robert Woodrus, Jr., an offensive lineman for the Miami Hurricanes who had just graduated. Pilot Candalyn Kubeck, 35, was the first female captain to be killed in a U.S. air crash.

Recovery efforts were a living hell. The site itself was virtually inaccessible. The DC-9 had disintegrated on impact with the bedrock below the swamp. Visibility in the water was zero. Divers donned rubber biohazard suits to protect themselves against burns from thousands of gallons of jet fuel. They struggled with sharp tangles of sawgrass, thick vegetation and muck deep enough to sink a man to his armpits. Mosquitoes, alligators and poisonous snakes swarmed to the site, attracted by mounds of decomposing body parts.

Only a smattering of fragmented human remains were recovered, along with pieces of luggage, toys, shoes, purses and other personal effects. The search for bodies was called off after 48 hours.

Culver was the second Charger to die tragically in 11 months. On June 15, 1995, starting linebacker David Griggs was killed in an auto accident in Davie, Florida, just 15 miles from the ValuJet crash site.

The 1988 Notre Dame national title team suffered yet another loss as well. In January 1989, only hours after returning to South Bend from a reception at the White House hosted by President Reagan, defensive back Bob Satterfield collapsed from a heart seizure and died. In 1993 defensive tackle Jeff Alm,

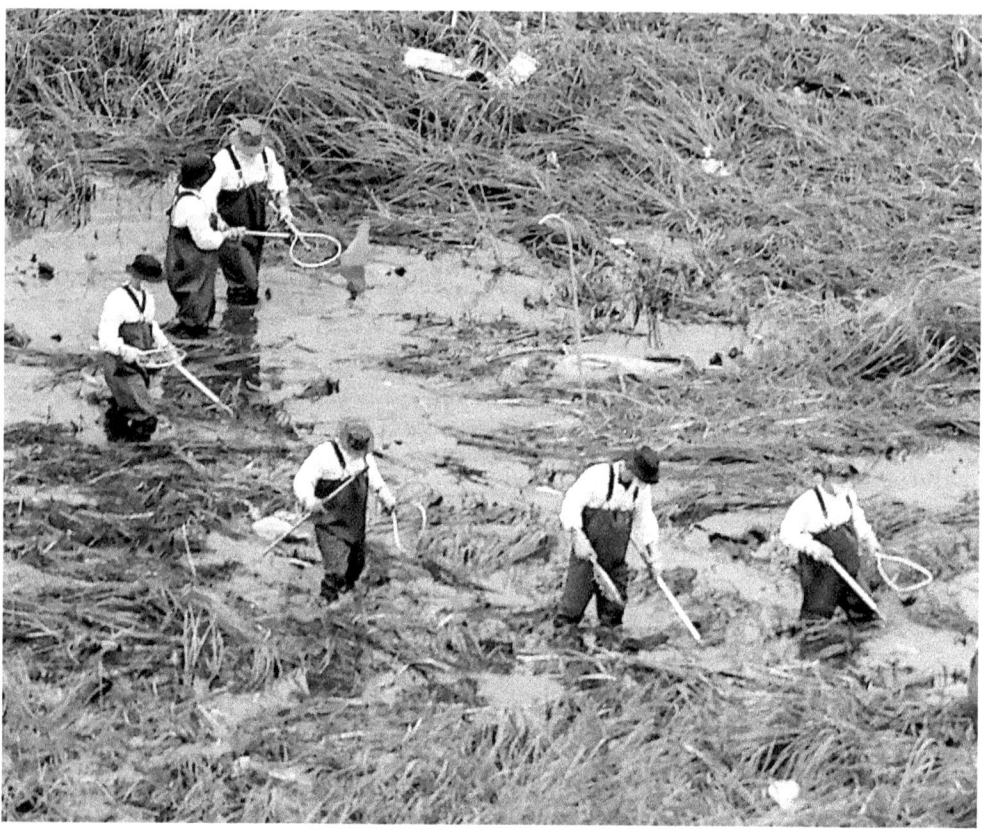

Dressed in hazard gear to protect them from heat, mosquitoes, snakes and gasoline burns, members of the Metro-Dade search unit hunt for remains of the victims of the ValuJet plane crash in the Everglades on July 11, 1996. Notre Dame and NFL running back Rodney Culver died in the DC-9, along with his wife Karen and 103 others. There were no survivors (AP Images / Candace Barbot).

despondent after killing his best friend in a car wreck, put a shotgun into his mouth on a Houston freeway. You will read an account of that hideous incident in Chapter 12. Then, a year after Culver's death, fullback Kenny Spears died of complications from a brain tumor. The heartbreak wouldn't stop. By the time the team assembled in 2018 for a 30-year reunion, eight members were gone.

Investigators later determined that Sabre Tech, the maintenance contractor for ValuJet, had improperly labeled and stored 140 oxygen canisters in the front cargo hold, which ignited the blaze. In 1997, Culver's family reached a $28 million settlement with both companies. It provided payments over the course of 40 years to Rodney and Karen's surviving daughters.

A memorial to the Culvers was erected in Woodland Park Cemetery South in Miami. On the third anniversary of the crash in 1999, another memorial consisting of 110 concrete pillars, one for each victim, opened along U.S. 41. The pillars point to the location of the crash site, 12 miles to the northeast in the Everglades.

## Payne Stewart: Flight of Doom
*Golf 1999*

On the morning of October 25, 1999, U.S. Air Force captain Chris Hamilton was practicing dogfights with another pilot over the Gulf of Mexico. It was a standard training exercise for flyers at Eglin Air Force Base in Fort Walton Beach, Florida, something they did two or three times a month.

Just before 10 a.m. he received an order to do something he had never done before—chase down a civilian Learjet flying north-northwest without radio contact across the heart of the Deep South, then try to figure out what in the world was going on. He hooked up with a tanker in midair to refuel and guided his F-16 fighter jet north toward Memphis.

Fifty minutes later he spotted the aircraft moving at 300 mph through the cloudless blue sky. There was no visible damage to it that he could see, and it was flying smoothly. Maybe *too* smoothly, as if there were no human hands on the controls.

He slowed down and eased within 20 yards of the Lear to take a closer look. He peered into the windows but saw nothing. They were all frosted over with a thin layer of whitish ice.

A feeling of horror gripped him. He described it later as something out of *The Twilight Zone*.

He knew exactly what the ice indicated. The plane's oxygen system had broken down, shutting off the ability to breathe. It was flying on autopilot and the people inside, however many there might be, were dead.

There were six. The best known was Payne Stewart. As he boarded the jet that morning in Orlando, Florida, he was on a roll in life. Best known for his tam o'shanter caps and loose "plus four" knickers, often in the colors of an NFL team, he had pulled out of a protracted eight-year slump in which he won only one golf tournament. He was now the reigning U.S. Open champion after winning at Pinehurst #2 in North Carolina in June. It was his second Open crown, third major and 11th PGA tour win. Then, in September, he'd been a member of the victorious American Ryder Cup team that defeated the Europeans at The County Club in Brookline, Massachusetts.

Stewart had at long last curbed the boorish, brash side of his personality. At age 42, he was focusing on his family—wife Tracey Richardson Stewart, daughter Chelsea, 13, and son Aaron, 10—and his rejuvenated faith in God. He started wearing a WWJD (What Would Jesus Do) bracelet, a gift from Aaron.

The twin-engine, high-altitude aircraft, partially owned by Stewart and operated by SunJet Aviation, was supposed to be headed to Dallas, where he'd be meeting with officials at his alma mater SMU to discuss the construction of a new course for the school's golf teams. After that the plan was to proceed to Houston for the TOUR Championship, one of the last events of 1999, with a field limited to the top 30 money winners for the year.

On board with him were his agents Van Ardan, 45, and Robert Fraley, 46, of Leader Enterprises and golf course designer Bruce Borland, 40, a rising star at Golden Bear International, the company headed by Jack Nicklaus. With pilot Michael Kling, 42, and first officer Stephanie Bellegarrigue, 27, the plane took off from Orlando at 9:19 a.m.

It never reached Dallas or Houston. Four hours later, after a 1,500-mile journey across eight states, the jet nosedived into a pasture on a cattle farm near the hamlet of Mina, North Dakota, 12 miles west of Aberdeen. It hit land at 100 times the force of gravity, leaving a burrow 42 feet wide and eight feet deep. Mercifully, all six on board had died long before impact.

The saga began shortly after takeoff. At 9:33 a.m., as the plane reached cruising altitude of 39,000 feet, air traffic control in Jacksonville lost contact with it. That jumpstarted a chain of events in which seven Air Force and Air National Guard jets from three bases went airborne to investigate and, if necessary, intercept the Lear. Hamilton got the closest, and he was the one who confirmed the horrific scenario. Despite rumors and media reports to the contrary, the military never considered shooting down the errant plane.

News of the situation quickly spread across the nation's airwaves. CNN and MSNBC picked up full live coverage. No one mentioned Stewart or any of the others by name at first because they didn't want a broadcast report to be the way the news reached the families of those on board. All they said was that a prominent golfer was one of the passengers.

But Tracey knew it was her husband's plane. She'd been trying repeatedly to reach him on his cell phone. All she got was his voicemail message, and she prepared herself and her children for the worst. She didn't know exactly when or where, but at some point, the plane was going to run out of fuel and crash.

At 12:13 p.m. Central Standard Time, state troopers in North Dakota watched through binoculars as it spiraled madly and plunged into the ground. A group of hunters were the first people to reach the crash site.

The cause of the tragedy was quickly apparent to aviation experts—depressurization in the cabin. Planes that fly above 12,000 feet are pressurized because at that level the oxygen in the air is too thin to sustain life. A cracked door or window or a faulty seal in the fuselage can trigger a catastrophe. Depressurization at 30,000 feet causes a drastic drop in cabin temperature and loss of consciousness in less than 30 seconds. After that the body shuts down and death due to hypoxia—oxygen deprivation—follows quickly.

As in all aircraft, oxygen masks were installed and available for use on the Lear. Why didn't the crew and passengers put them on? That was the biggest mystery. The likely answer is that depressurization occurred so quickly that they did not have enough time to react. A second possibility is that they did don the masks but blacked out anyway because of the severity of the situation.

And what caused the cabin pressure to drop in the first place? After a yearlong investigation, the NTSB found no definitive answer to that question. The total destruction of the craft and the lack of a black box on board stymied their efforts.

The flight of doom prompted a look back at an eerily similar incident in 1980, when a Cessna twin-turboprop jet carrying LSU football coach Bo Rein and pilot Lou Benscotter ran out of fuel and dropped into the Atlantic Ocean off the Virginia coast. Depressurization in the cabin was also the suspected cause of that crash.

At the request of the families that lost loved ones, a memorial was built at the crash site. It's a three-foot-wide gray slab imbedded in the ground. Inscribed on the stone are the names of the six victims, a Biblical passage from the Book of Psalms and the date of the accident. The one-acre site is cordoned off by a barbed wire fence to keep cattle away.

In 2000, the U.S. Open at Pebble Beach in California began with a golfing version of a 21-gun salute, with 21 golfers simultaneously driving balls into the Pacific Ocean in remembrance of Stewart.

The remains of William Payne Stewart are interred at Doctor Phillips Cemetery in Orlando. His epitaph reads "The Champion of Our Hearts."

## Cory Lidle: Manhattan Fireball
*MLB 2006*

Cory Lidle was crazy about flying airplanes. When the Yankee pitcher was up above the world, he left all the problems of his earthly existence down below on the ground.

One of those problems was that he'd been a replacement player during the 1994–1995 MLB player strike. He only pitched a single inning in a spring training game for the Brewers, but that was enough to make him a villain to many of his peers in the locker room. It wasn't easy being looked on as a scab, a me-first guy who climbed into bed with the bosses and hung his brothers on the field out to dry.

The air offered a refreshing escape from that chilly scene, if only for a moment. His wife Melanie put it this way—when Cory was in a plane he was in love. Like Thurman Munson and Davey Allison and millions of others, the righthander who'd played for seven teams in nine MLB seasons was hooked on the rush of being at the helm of an aircraft. Nothing else in life could compare.

Lidle (LIE-dul) was a newbie in the realm of flight. He started out renting planes here and there on a sporadic basis. After he signed with the Yankees in 2005, he laid down 187 grand to buy one of his own, a Cirrus SR20 single engine four-seater. It was the first time in his life that he felt he could afford it.

He earned his pilot's license in 2006 and by the end of the regular season that year he'd logged 100 hours of flying time, often with certified flight instructor Tyler Stanger, 26, in the co-pilot seat. Stanger was a close friend of a year or so, the first guy ever to take Cory up in a plane. He'd been training Lidle at his small flight school at Brackett Field, near Lidle's home in the San Gabriel Valley east of Los Angeles.

A hundred hours may sound like a lot of time. But it's not. Novice flyers generally need 300 hours under their belts before they've fully learned the ropes. Many aviation pros describe the period before that threshold is reached as one of extreme danger. They liken it to the years teenagers are behind the wheels of cars, trucks, and motorcycles. The chances of trouble arising are hugely magnified.

At 2:21 p.m. on October 6, Lidle took off from Teterboro Regional Airport in New Jersey. Stanger was with him. The NTSB never formally determined who was piloting, but after the accident it did affirm that Lidle was in the left seat of the cockpit. That's where the pilot virtually always sits.

The day was drizzly and cloudy with poor visibility. Conditions were not bad enough to require all pilots in the air to hold an instrument rating, meaning that they had the ability to fly the plane while staring through the cockpit window at nothing but gray fog, working only with the many instruments on the control panel. But the weather was still challenging, especially for a beginner.

The Yankees had just been rudely bounced from the AL playoffs by the Tigers. Lidle was on the mound for one and a third innings and gave up three earned runs. The 34-year-old would end his career with a won-loss record of 82–72 and an ERA of 4.57.

Now he and Stanger were prepping for a cross-country air journey back to SoCal in the Cirrus. Their wives and kids, who'd been visiting the Big Apple, were all flying home on the same commercial flight. Before their own departure, the two men took a quick sightseeing tour over Manhattan. They circled the Statue of Liberty, then flew north up the East River past the World Trade Center site, Brooklyn Bridge, Empire State Building and United Nations.

Twenty minutes into the flight, near Harlem, they approached a no-fly zone, reserved only for traffic in and out of LaGuardia Airport. The Cirrus stuttered into a sharp, 180-degree turn to redirect south. As it wobbled and spun out of control, a powerful east wind sent it careening into the Belaire Apartments, a 50-story building at 572 East 72nd Street, near the corner of York Avenue.

The first thought that sprang to many minds was terrorism. *Again.* September 11 was only five years in the past. Fighter jets scrambled above New York, Washington, Detroit, Los Angeles and Seattle.

At the crash site flaming chunks of metal rained down from the building to the streets below. The engine landed inside an apartment on the 30th floor. Shattered glass, water, fire and smoke saturated the structure, prompting evacuation. One hundred of the 132 units were damaged. Both bodies were found in the street, along with Lidle's passport. At that point the terrorist theory was dismissed. Sixteen people were injured—11 firefighters, five civilians, and a police officer. Miraculously, no one died on the ground or in the Belaire.

Melanie Lidle and Stephanie Stanger and their children were in the air themselves when the accident occurred. In a time with no on board Wi-Fi or iPhones, they were not aware of the tragedy until they landed in Los Angeles. Melanie's sister Brandy Peters met them at the gate to deliver the news.

The accident sparked a simple question. How in the world could an airplane be flying smack in the middle of America's biggest city, so close to so many skyscrapers of every height and variety stacked so closely together?

In fact, small planes like Lidle's flew up and down the East and Hudson rivers frequently, at altitudes ranging from 500 to 1,110 feet. Contact with air traffic controllers was not required, and pilots often operated under visual flight rules. That meant they looked out for other aircraft with their own eyes and did what they had to do to stay out of harm's way.

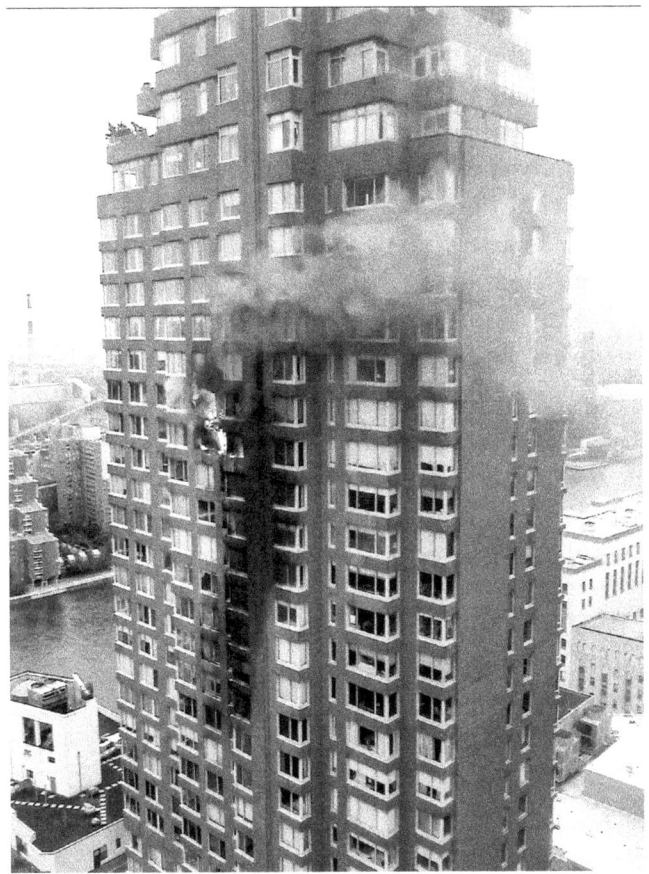

Flames billow from the interior of the Belaire Apartments on East 72nd Street in Manhattan. A single engine airplane piloted by Yankee pitcher Cory Lidle and flight instructor Tyler Stanger smashed into the 50-story building on October 6, 2006, while encountering stiff winds and thick clouds. Both bodies were found in the street. Sixteen people were injured on the ground and in the building (AP Images / Dax Gardner).

The crash also cast a harsh spotlight on the dangers of personal or general aviation. It's a world apart from the highly-regulated, safety-intensive commercial sector. In 2006, there were 1,573 crashes involving chartered and private planes in the United States, resulting in 706 deaths and 265 serious injuries. The comparable numbers on the commercial side—two crashes, 49 deaths, three serious injuries.

The number one cause of accidents in personal aviation is lack of pilot experience. That clearly seemed to be the case with the Cirrus. The NTSB described it as "inadequate planning, judgement and airmanship."[6] Caught off guard by the fast-approaching no-fly zone, disoriented in the thick clouds and unnerved by the force of the wind, the pilot executed the tight hairpin curve poorly and induced an engine stall, dropping the craft's altitude and pushing it into the north wall of the Belaire.

After an outdoor service at the Mausoleum of Christian Heritage, Lidle was buried at Forest Lawn Memorial Park in Covina Hills. An eight-foot statue of Lidle was erected at Cortez Park in his hometown of West Covina. Sadly, it was vandalized in 2014 by thieves scrapping for metal. They stole three bronze and copper plaques worth $7,000 and drilled into the base of the statue, sending it toppling to the ground.

It seemed like a fitting metaphor for a life cut cruelly short.

# 5

# Accidents Will Happen

## Terry Sawchuk: Senseless
*NHL 1970*

Once upon a time on Long Island, two hockey players were drinking together in a bar. They were roommates and teammates. Both were divorced from their wives. After several hours and who knows how many rounds, they started bickering about who had to clean up what and who owed how much on the bills in the rented house they were about to vacate.

It got so loud and ugly that the fill-in bartender asked the men to leave the premises. They took it outside to the parking lot and raged on. The bartender came out and told them to move along because he didn't *want* to call the cops, but he would if he had to.

The older guy in the argument was Terry Sawchuk, age 40. He started playing hockey on frozen ponds in his native Winnipeg, Manitoba, at age 10. He was so talented that he worked out for the Detroit Red Wings at 14 and quit high school to play in a minor pro league.

Sawchuk entered the NHL as a prodigy six years later in 1950. The accolades came early and often. The Calder Trophy for rookie of the year. Four Vezina trophies for best goaltender. Four Stanley Cup titles, three with the Red Wings and one with the Maple Leafs. His 103 all-time regular season shutouts still stands second to Martin Brodeur's 125. Sawchuk's ultra-low slung gorilla crouch in the nets was his trademark. Hunkering down was sheer hell on his knees but he endured it because staying low gave him a far better view of the puck and the players moving on the ice.

All of that was behind him on April 29, 1970, as he got into his roomie's face at E and J's Pub in Long Beach, 26 miles southeast of Madison Square Garden in Manhattan. His season with the Rangers had ended 13 days before. He'd spent nearly all of it on the bench as the backup to Eddie Giacomin, desperate for playing time that never came. He appeared in only eight games. The brilliant career that started with an enormous bang was ending with a whimper.

A boatload of careers in the sports world end the same way, but that wasn't any comfort to Sawchuk. He was edgy, anxious, moody—and angry. He'd always been like that but now it was magnified. So the bickering that started at E and J's dragged on in the backyard of the rental—a four-bedroom, white stucco house at 58 Bay Street in East Atlantic Beach, three miles west up the South Shore.

His roommate was Ron Stewart, a laid-back right wing and a veteran of 19 NHL seasons. He was one of the fastest skaters and cleanest players in the league, earning a mere 14 penalty minutes in the season just concluded. It was kind of funny that he and Sawchuk were living together again. They shared a house in Toronto when they were both with the Maple Leafs and it had gone well enough. That's why they were doing it one more time. But they weren't really friends.

The drunken tussle got rougher. By that time two people who hadn't been at the bar were on the scene—Stewart's girlfriend Rosemary Sasso, a nurse, age 38, and Benjamin Weiner, a close friend of Sawchuk. Stewart either fell or was pushed to the ground. Sawchuk pounced on him. He said later that fists flew, but no one else backed up his claim. Weiner leaped down to separate them, but they threw him off, stood up and carried on.

At some point they both stumbled backward and tripped over a barbecue pit, and it was then that Stewart's bent knee came into full hard contact with Sawchuk's gut and groin, inflicting the blunt force trauma on his gall bladder and liver that ended up killing him.

That's the official, reported version of what happened. The Nassau County district attorney called the incident "tragic, senseless, bizarre."[1] It was tough to argue with that. No one ever explained precisely how or why Stewart's knee ended up in Sawchuk's gut. In the hospital a week before his death, Sawchuk described it to a visitor as "a fluke, a complete fluke accident."[2]

The Nassau County grand jury agreed. The Rangers retained an attorney for Stewart the day after the incident, but he was never charged with any offense. After a hearing on June 8 that was short, sweet and to the point, the grand jury exonerated him, labeling the death accidental.

True enough to a point. But the word makes it sound as though the two men were just kind of horsing around and weren't really trying to hurt each other. Given the intensity and duration of their squabble, that seems like a stretch. There was also a piece of evidence that apparently was given short shrift—Rosemary Sasso's statement in a newspaper that Sawchuk had been spitting up blood for two weeks before the altercation. That could well have been a sign of a damaged liver or gall bladder, making the collision with Stewart's knee all the more damaging.

He lingered at death's door for 31 days. The public received no information about his condition until three weeks after the incident. That seems inconceivable today, but it was a different world back then. The media was far less pervasive and intrusive. Doctors removed his gall bladder and operated twice on his bleeding liver, the second time on May 30. He died the next day at New York Presbyterian Hospital in Manhattan.

It was the end of a troubled, painful life. Twenty-five seasons of hockey had taken a horrendous toll on his six-foot frame. His body weight in his prime was 195. In 1970 he weighed 20 pounds less. At age 12, he broke his right arm playing rugby. Fearing punishment from his parents for doing something he wasn't supposed to do, he hid the injury from them. Without treatment the arm didn't heal properly, and it remained four inches shorter that his left arm forever.

That mishap seemed to be a harbinger of all the hurt that followed. Severed hand tendons. Punctured lungs. Ruptured discs and a ruptured appendix. A shoulder injury that kept him from lifting his stick hand above his chest for the rest of his career. And 400 stitches in his face from uncountable run-ins with blades, sticks and flying pucks. In 1962, he started wearing a sinister-looking fiberglass mask, something out a slasher movie, with the eyes open and ventilation slits for the forehead, nose, mouth and cheeks.

His mind was as beat up as his body. His childhood was rough. Two of his brothers died before they were 18 and Terry started installing bakery ovens when he was 14 to help support the family. Hockey players are generally seen as a gregarious bunch. Sawchuk defied the stereotype. The quiet loner nicknamed Ukey because of his Ukrainian heritage avoided people as often as possible. If you approached him in a hotel lobby on the road, he might raise a hand in your direction. But he wasn't greeting you. He was shooing you away, lest you interrupt his work on his crossword puzzle.

He got even less friendly after the Red Wings traded him to the Bruins in 1955. It stung hard. He had loved the Red Wings since childhood and his extended family was settled in the Detroit metro area. His pride was grievously wounded. In 1957, halfway through his second season in Boston, he walked out on the team after suffering what he called a nervous breakdown. Many reporters dismissed that claim and called him a quitter, plain and simple, igniting a number of nasty feuds that lasted for the rest of his life.

In 1969, his wife Patricia finally divorced him, fed up with years of excessive drinking, infidelity and abuse. Then his dad got into a horrible car wreck. And now the 11-time all-star wasn't sure he'd find a place on any NHL roster come the fall. The only real ray of hope was the expansion draft on June 10, when the Buffalo Sabres and Vancouver Canucks would select 40 players between them. If he was one of them, he'd be joining his sixth NHL team.

Terrance Gordon Sawchuk died 10 days before that draft. A requiem Mass was held on June 5 in suburban Berkley, outside Detroit. His seven children wept quietly in their pews. Stewart attended, along with 10 other Rangers and Gordie Howe. Sawchuk was buried in Mount Hope Cemetery in Pontiac, sharing a plot with his mother. His father joined them there a year later.

With his volatile mood swings, anger and anxiety, Sawchuk was a textbook case of undiagnosed, untreated depression. His claim that he suffered a nervous breakdown in Boston in 1957 was essentially true. Antidepressant medications existed in rudimentary form in the 1950s and 1960s, but they were not prescribed to millions of people like they are today. Chuck Hughes was in a similar situation with statins, which might have impeded the heart disease that killed him at Tiger Stadium in 1971. If Sawchuk had been able to access antidepressants he might well have lived a longer and less traumatic life.

In 2021, another NHL goalie at the very beginning of his career would die just 15 miles southwest of Sawchuk's grave. You will read about his freakish demise at the end of this chapter.

## Don Wilson: Beyond Strange
*MLB 1975*

It's hard to find a sudden death in the sports world more curious and perplexing than Terry Sawchuk's. A contender in that regard would be one that occurred five years later in Houston, Texas.

Don Wilson was a tall, strong, right-handed pitcher with the Astros. At 29, he was on the backside of an impressive career, with a fastball and slider that could still be very effective. His lifetime ERA was 3.15, he threw no-hitters in 1967 and 1969, and his won-loss record of 104–92 was more impressive that it appears because he'd compiled it playing for a team that reached the .500 mark only twice in his eight full seasons.

If Wilson were playing today, he'd no doubt have a multi-year contract that paid him many millions of dollars, with a hefty pension awaiting at the end of his career. But in the era before the arrival of free agency in MLB, he earned a mere $40,000 per season. That's roughly $235,000 in 2024 money. A solid wage for sure, and enough to provide a good life for his wife Bernice and two children, Denise, nine, and Alexander, five.

But it was hardly a fortune, and at some point, his playing days would end and his salary would disappear. He wasn't as close to the end of the road as Sawchuk, but it was likely to happen sooner instead of later. He was growing concerned about how he could go about making a living for the rest of his life.

He'd discussed his predicament with several teammates, and it may have been weighing on his mind on the night of January 4, 1975. It was a Saturday. He and Bernice went out and returned to their house in Houston's Fondren Southwest neighborhood at 1 a.m. in a brown 1972 Thunderbird. The garage door was opened with an automatic hand opener. Bernice went inside and Don, heavily intoxicated, lay asleep in the reclined passenger seat. The radio was on, and the engine was running. It died some hours later when the gas tank emptied.

At 1 p.m. Sunday Bernice was awakened by the sound of her daughter crying. She calmed her down, then went downstairs to check the garage and saw her husband passed out exactly where he'd been 12 hours earlier. The doors of the

Thunderbird were locked and the windows were up. The keys were in the ignition and the garage door was down.

Traumatized, she ran inside and called a friend and then the Houston Fire Department at 1:24 p.m. to request an ambulance. Paramedics and cops arrived in five minutes, broke into the car and found Wilson dead, ankles crossed, hands in his lap, an open pack of cigarettes on the dashboard. He'd been overcome by carbon monoxide fumes flowing out of the T-Bird's tail pipe. The invisible, odorless poison seeped up into the bedroom above the garage and killed Alexander as well. Denise would soon fall into a coma in another bedroom. She spent several days at Texas Children's Hospital and recovered slowly but fully.

The police were baffled. Their questions were legion. Who drove the car home? Who opened and shut the garage door? Why had Wilson remained in the T-Bird all night? Why were the doors locked? Why hadn't Bernice suffered from the effects of carbon monoxide like her husband and children? Most critically, why was the left side of her face badly bruised and swollen?

Had she and Wilson gotten into a fight after they arrived home early Sunday, or maybe before? By all accounts he was not a violent man, and there was no record of domestic discord between the couple. But that didn't settle the matter. It wasn't what lawyers call determining. Were investigators dealing with a suicide, an accident—or a murder?

Bernice was the only person who could shed light on the situation, but she quickly retained the services of power lawyer Richard "Racehorse" Haynes and stopped talking, claiming she had amnesia and couldn't recall how she hurt her face. Much later when she started talking again, she said she'd slammed into a wall in a panic after finding her husband in his vehicle. Later on she called the injuries fallout from an infected salivary gland.

It may have been one or the other or a combination of both. Or something else entirely. Who knew? Only Bernice.

Several of Wilson's teammates vehemently disputed the theory that he had taken his own life. Given his zest for living and positive outlook, they called it downright impossible. That was useful information. But again, it wasn't determining.

As for murder, there wasn't a shred of evidence to support the idea. People who kill their spouses virtually never become hysterical afterward like Bernice did. On the other hand, if she did have murder on her mind, it would have been easy to accomplish that Sunday morning. No gun, knife, rope or sledgehammer was necessary. With the car engine running, the windows rolled up, and her husband passed out like a hibernating bear in the passenger seat, all she had to do was shut the garage door.

A month later, the coroner concluded that Wilson's death, along with Alexander's, was accidental. The finding didn't do much to clarify things. It all remained as clear as mud. In fact, mud was clearer. Five decades on, that description is still apt.

## Richard Wertheim: Lethal Ace
*Tennis 1983*

The tennis ball streaked across the net like a flaming rocket, landing in the service box and then spinning sharply toward the official sitting behind the baseline, crouched forward in a folding chair, hands on knees. He tried to dodge the ball, but it slammed into his crotch at 120 mph. He shrieked in pain, threw his arms in the air and fell backward in his chair. His head hit the hard acrylic surface with a sickening smack.

Unconscious and bleeding, he was placed on a stretcher and transported from the National Tennis Center in Queens to the Flushing Hospital Medical Center. The 61-year-old was an avid tennis player himself in his hometown of Lexington, Massachusetts. But he was far from healthy. He'd battled chronic cardiac issues since suffering a heart attack and stroke at age 40. The fact that he was on the court at all that day was a testament to his deep love of the game.

On September 15, 1983, five days after the accident, Richard Wertheim died without regaining consciousness. Traumatized by the brutal jolt to the head, his damaged heart had given out.

The server of the ace that killed was Stefan Edberg. The Swede was just 17 at the time, playing in the junior finals of the U.S. Open against Australian Simon Youl. Edberg was distraught about what happened. It was a ghastly thing to have to live with for the rest of your days, even if you did absolutely nothing wrong. He hadn't intended to hurt anybody, let alone kill them.

Edberg did go on to win his ill-fated match against Youl. That earned him the Junior Grand Slam for players 18 and younger—titles in the French, Australian, British and U.S. opens in the same year. He remains the only player to accomplish that feat. In his adult career he won 41 singles crowns, including two each at Forest Hills and Wimbledon. He also excelled in doubles play.

Wertheim, on the other hand, has become a quirky footnote in sports history. A year after his death, his family sued the United States Tennis Association (USTA), seeking $2.25 million in damages. The theory of their case was that a change in USTA procedures for linesmen contributed to his death. That change required them to sit, not stand, behind the baseline in the "ready position"—leaning forward in their chairs, with their hands on or above their knees when the ball was in play.

The purpose of the change was to make the linesmen look more involved in the match. Why that mattered to the powers that be as much as it apparently did is baffling. Under the old way of doing things, linesmen either stood behind the baseline or sat six to eight feet above it in elevated chairs. The family argued that if Wertheim had been sitting up high Edberg's ball wouldn't have come anywhere near him. And if he'd been standing, he might have been able to dodge it and avoid his fatal injury.

A trial court jury in New York agreed with the family to a point, finding the USTA 25 percent at fault under the state's proportional negligence statutes. The court awarded the estate $165,000 in damages.

In 1989, the Appellate Division of the New York Supreme Court overturned that verdict and nixed the award. The justices said it was a case of going too far. Sports officials assume the normal risks of the game when they sign up for duty. The new rule that required linesmen to sit on the court instead of stand or sit in an elevated chair came with the territory.

The change didn't constitute a breach of duty on the USTA's part, and it could not be construed as evidence of recklessness or gross negligence. It wasn't like a frustrated player intentionally slamming a ball into a linesman's head or chest or crotch in anger over a bad call. Nor was it a case of an official slipping and falling on a poorly maintained surface and getting hurt. In those situations, somebody did something wrong and damages would be warranted. But not here.

Simply put, Wertheim was the unfortunate victim of an accident that was nobody's fault.

The governing bodies of tennis did make a change after Wertheim's death. They shelved the sitting requirement. Officials stationed behind the baseline now stand during matches. The reversal can be seen as a tacit admission that they overreached. That was scant comfort to Wertheim's survivors. But no linesman has been killed by an errant shot or serve since.

## Owen Hart: Real as Can Be
*World Wrestling Federation 1999*

Owen James Hart was born in 1965 into a royal family in the kingdom of pro wrestling, the 12th and last child of Helen and Stu Hart, a trainer, wrestler, promoter and owner of the Stampede Wrestling Foundation. He grew up in Hart House, a 22-room Victorian mansion in the hills overlooking Calgary, Alberta. In the basement was a school and gym called Hart Dungeon, where he trained from an early age.

All eight of the Hart boys wrestled, but only two lasted in the sport—Owen and Bret, the number six son, eight years older, who would become Owen's best friend, tag team partner, rival and nemesis, both in real life and in the fictional world where they both performed.

At 18, Owen was ambivalent about following in his footsteps. It wasn't easy being a Hart. All eyes were on you, and there was pressure to uphold the family name. Bret was already established, looking down on his kid brother from a higher perch in the pecking order. That didn't help matters.

Neither did the fact that Owen's wife and high school sweetheart Martha didn't care much for pro wrestling. She disliked just about every aspect of it—the greed and arrogance of the owners, the ongoing physical dangers to wrestlers, crazed fans, financial insecurity, brutal touring schedules. Owen started in right after high school, anyway, wrestling incognito in college and then as Bronco Owen Hart in London before joining Stampede to apprentice with his father.

He yearned to do something different with his life. Because Helen was born in Pennsylvania, he was a citizen of both America and Canada. Perhaps that had something to do with his desire to become a U.S. customs agent. He also thought about working as a Calgary firefighter.

Those aspirations never materialized and in 1988 he signed with the World Wrestling Federation (WWF). In a business overflowing with scads of promoters, events and alliances, WWF stood alone at the top. Under the leadership of rock star CEO Vince McMahon it was entering its golden era, with Hulk Hogan as the marquee attraction.

Owen was now deep into a sport that is different from all other forms of athletic competition. There's an element to pro wrestling that you won't find anywhere else. It's scripted in advance. The outcome of virtually every match is determined before it starts. Wrestlers who generate press, vibe, chatter, sponsors and fans are the ones who usually win. Those who fall short in that regard usually lose. Performing in the ring is not as easy as many people think. The physical and mental aspects are challenging. But there is no pretense of any match being a true test of athletic skill.

To many observers that seems like a warped violation of a sacred covenant. Competition is spontaneous. Athletes give maximum effort every time they enter the arena. No one knows at the beginning of a match or game or race what the outcome is going to be.

Pro wrestling instead comes off as a cartoon, a fairy tale, a soap opera. It's a glitzy, garish spectacle that has little in common with *real* wrestling, the kind practiced by Dave Schultz and all the other competitors at John du Pont's Foxcatcher farm outside Philadelphia.

That's a fair enough description. Let's add in the theatrical element and call it performance art. The wrestlers are actors, throwing off an illusion of reality. Key to the enterprise is the concept of kayfabe (KAY-fawb)—carnival slang for protecting the secrets of the business. Play along with the ruse. Don't ever drop your pose. Never fall out of character in front of fans and the public, either inside or outside the ring.

There are heroes and good guys, fan favorites called faces. There are villains and nasty boys called heels. In both camps you will also find what the business calls "enhancement talent"—wrestlers set up to lose because in the eyes of promoters they lack star power.

Hart started out in WWF as a face. The bosses didn't want to promote him as Bret's little brother, so they created a character called the Blue Angel, a comic book figure with a mask and cape. The Blue Angel quickly became the Blue Blazer,

## 5. Accidents Will Happen

and as he morphed from face to heel and back again there was the Rocket, the King of Harts and the Black Hart. He wrestled in Japan and Europe and Mexico. He wrestled solo, in a tag team with his brother-in-law Davey Boy Smith the British Bulldog and with teams called the Hart Foundation and the Nation of Domination. He feuded with Bret more than once along the way, and the playacting was fueled by raw emotion. Owen deeply resented living in the shadow of his older brother.

By May 23, 1999, after 15 years in the business, he'd come nearly full circle, wrestling again as the Blue Blazer in a pay-per-view matchup with the Godfather before 18,000 fans in Kansas City, Missouri. This time around the role was more campy. At the open he was going to drop from the rafters of Kemper Arena via a harness and grapple line attached to a cable with a clamp. When he got five feet above the ring, the script called for him to activate a quick release mechanism, separate from the cable and fall flat on his face on the canvas like some cartoon goofball.

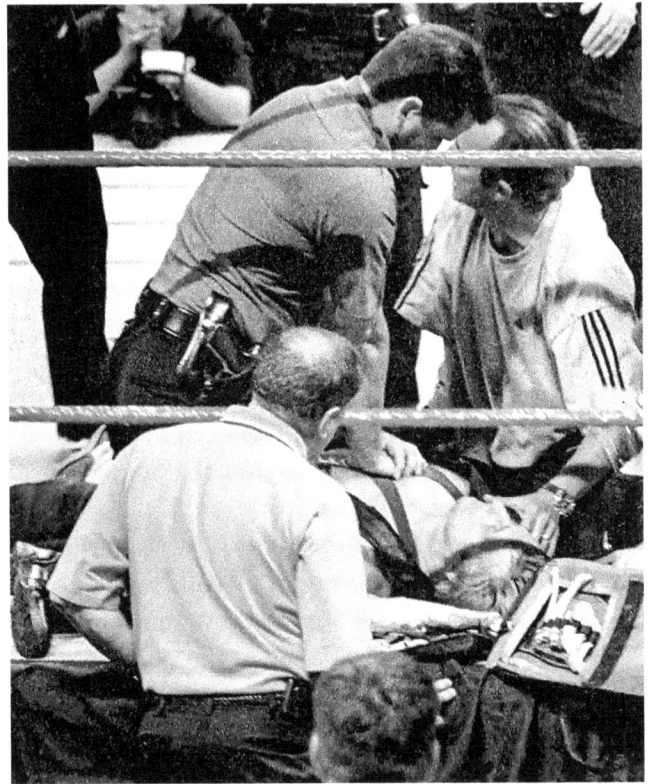

EMTs surround WWF wrestler Owen Hart on May 23, 1999, after his seven-story fall from the rafters at Kemper Arena in Kansas City, Missouri. His neck broke on impact, and he died several hours later at Truman Medical Center. Investigators blamed the accident on a faulty release mechanism that separated him from the cable that was guiding his descent into the ring (AP Images / Steve Meyers).

What happened instead wasn't fake or fictional or planned in advance. It wasn't a piece of performance of art. It was as real as real can be.

Seventy feet above the floor, just as he began to descend, the quick release activated out of nowhere, sending him hurtling downward at 50 mph. He crashed into the top rope, slammed his head on a turnbuckle and landed on his back in the middle of the ring. His neck broke on impact.

The TV audience did not see the fall or its aftermath, and the announcers reported the ongoing developments in shocked, hushed tones. After paramedics swarmed Hart and administered CPR, he was transported to Truman Medical

Center, where he was pronounced dead several hours later. The official cause of death was massive internal bleeding.

After a 15-minute delay, the show continued. The other matches on the card went on as scheduled. Vince McMahon's decision provoked a firestorm of criticism that smoldered as Hart was mourned by the wrestling world at an open casket service in Calgary and buried at Queen's Park Mausoleum, with his seven brothers serving as pallbearers.

Attention then shifted to the cause of the tragedy.

Who was in charge of setting up the stunt and what went wrong? How did Hart's harness separate from the cable? Was the release mechanism activated when it got tangled up in his cape? Did Hart himself pull it by mistake? Was the snap shackle strong enough to hold a 227-pound man in the first place? Why were there no back-up safety latches that would have stopped his free fall far short of the ring?

Then came a bombshell—WWF's number one rigger had flat-out refused to prepare the stunt, citing numerous safety concerns, forcing the bosses to bring in an inexperienced "hacker." At that point it became difficult to describe the incident as a simple accident. The investigation soon pointed to something different—a hurried, careless, haphazard job of preparation with substandard equipment and no oversight. A catastrophe waiting to happen.

Martha Hart was beyond livid. Her husband had been scraped off the floor of the ring "like a piece of garbage" and she swore vengeance in what she called a "David and Goliath" battle.[3] Seventeen months after the fall she reached a legal settlement with WWF for $18 million, $33.2 million in 2024 money. She also received compensation from Lewmar, Inc., the manufacturer of the harness system.

The standard wisdom is that money buys silence and time heals all wounds. In the case of Martha Hart that doesn't seem to be the case. Her anger at WWF and anguish over her loss continued for years. Her latest swipe came in 2018, when she refused to allow Owen to be inducted into the WWF Hall of Fame.

The title of her 2004 biography of Owen written with Eric Francis is *Broken Harts*. Nothing says it better than that.

## Matiss Kivlenieks: Fiasco
### *NHL 2021*

The party was hopping. Relaxation and revelry were the order of the evening, and Hawaiian dress was encouraged. There'd be a last shot, last beer, last cigar and a good night toast at some point, but at 10 o'clock, that was a while down the road.

The six dozen guests were having it large that night in the Village Oaks neighborhood of Novi, Oakland County, Michigan, 28 miles northwest of downtown Detroit. They were gathered at the lakeside home of Emmanuel "Manny" and Giana Legace. The main event was the backyard wedding of their daughter Sabrina and Nick Howell, followed by a reception.

It was also Sunday, July 4, 2021, with the nation mired in month 16 of the Covid pandemic. At that point the death toll in America stood at just over 600,000. But with no work on Monday for many, millions of shots in arms and the ugly memories of the 2020 shutdown starting to fade, the partygoers were more than eager to bust out.

Legace was an iron man of ice hockey. His career between the pipes spanned 23 years through 11 leagues with 20 teams, including six seasons with the Red Wings and shorter stints with the Blues, Kings and Hurricanes. In 2018 he joined the Columbus Blue Jackets as a goaltending coach.

Among the guests that day at his offseason home were two of his players—starting goalie Elvis Merzļikins, with his wife Aleksandra, and back-up Matīss Kivlenieks (kiv-LEN-eks). Both men were natives of Latvia, two of the half dozen or so who play in the NHL in any given year.

Their bond was strong, forged by the ongoing adventure of playing the game they loved 4,500 miles from home, a country of 1.9 million the size of West Virginia on the shores of the Baltic Sea. Elvis called "Kivi" his little brother. Kivi had crashed with Elvis and Aleksandra in Columbus during the Covid shutdown.

The soft-spoken 24-year-old with a radiant smile joined the Blue Jackets as an undrafted free agent in 2017. He spent most of his time with the Cleveland Monsters of the American Hockey League before making his NHL debut in 2020, a 2–1 victory over the Rangers in Madison Square Garden. He was prepping for his first full season in the NHL. Kivi spent a lot of his time in the summers at the Legace house in Novi, where he became a cherished member of the household. At the party he was really more of a host than a guest.

At 10:15 p.m. he was in a hot tub with several other people, on a wooden platform down a short flight of steps from the backyard and patio. Six feet below the tub, on a stone walkway along the lake, a family friend had assembled a huge arsenal of fireworks. Each unit of the product called Mars Retrograde included three rows with three mortar tubes each, all nine packed "cake-style" into a portable launching box. Each full box weighed 25 to 30 pounds. All of them were angled to shoot away from the party toward the lake.

We don't know how many units there were, but several had already been fired. Just as it was about to ignite, one of the remaining boxes shifted position so that it pointed not at the water but toward the hot tub and backyard. Exactly how or why is unknown. A witness later told police that he noticed the off-kilter tubes seconds before they ignited. It was, he said, "like having a gun pointed right at you." He screamed "Bail!" to alert the crowd and ran for cover.[4]

The first shot rocketed over the tub. Kivi and the others scrambled out and ran toward the house. As he ran, the second shot slammed into his chest at a very high rate of speed. The last seven shots then fired in quick succession. No one else was injured.

In a heartbeat, the joyous celebration descended into frightful, panicked chaos. EMS personnel arrived in less than five minutes after the first of three 911 calls. Kivi had been hit by a three-inch-diameter shell, the largest allowed for personal use in Michigan. Professionals generally use six- to 10-inch shells. He was transported to Ascension Providence Hospital in Novi. He very likely passed before arriving.

On July 15, a memorial service was held at Schoedinger Funeral Home in the Columbus suburb of Upper Arlington. Before an open white casket, family friends and invited guests mourned and celebrated the short life of Matīss Edmunds Kivlenieks, gone an eternity too soon.

At first it was thought that he'd been fatally injured after striking his head on the concrete surrounding the hot tub. But an autopsy revealed that the exploding shell caused massive internal injuries to the chest and stomach that led to his death. There was no head trauma.

When he was hit, Kivlenieks was a mere 19 feet from the launch site, a shockingly short distance. Experts interviewed after the accident recommended keeping people a bare minimum of 50 yards away. If a large crowd is present, the distance should be increased to 100 yards. They also believed that the launch boxes were probably not braced to prevent them from shifting angles or tipping over.

At some point after July 4, the man in charge of the fireworks display spoke by phone to Novi police. He had managed displays at the Legace home before. After the misfires he attempted to alter the angle of the launching box by hand but failed. There was no indication that he was under the influence of alcohol or other drugs that Sunday. His identity has never been disclosed to the public. Whether he was the person who actually ignited the ill-fated mortar tubes is unknown.

After investigating, the Oakland County district attorney filed no criminal charges, calling the incident a tragic accident. It was one of many that year involving fireworks. The U.S. Consumer Product Safety Commission reported 18 deaths in 2020, along with 15,600 emergency room visits. The numbers very probably spiked that year because the shutdown of commercial shows in the Covid pandemic led to far greater than normal use by individuals, many of them inexperienced.

Spiked or not, those numbers illustrate America's passionate, troublesome love affair with fireworks. They're loud. They can hurt people. They can start fires. And they frighten and annoy the living hell out of your neighbors. But in the eyes of millions, there seems to be an inalienable right to light the fuse and celebrate the big boom. Especially on the Fourth of July and New Year's Eve. If you're inclined to political correctness you can toss in Cinco de Mayo, Juneteenth and Chinese New Year as well.

The laws governing purchase and use are a bewildering maze of state, county and local regulations. Massachusetts is the only state that totally bans personal use. Roman candles, sparklers, poppers, snakes, helicopters and the like can be legally purchased in 46 states. In Oklahoma, Mississippi, and Arkansas the minimum age for purchase is 12. Most of the rules lean to the lenient side. Michigan, as an example, has no minimum setback distance to separate viewers from launch sites.

Prices are affordable, and despite the dangers involved, demand is high and getting higher. Manufacturers, retail sellers and commercial users see no cause for alarm. They say that the number of mishaps is minuscule. They insist that fireworks are safe and that virtually all accidents and deaths have two causes—misuse of the products and the undue influence of alcohol and other drugs. Fireworks don't kill people. Flawed, irresponsible, careless human beings kill people.

Let's put that another way. Fireworks pose no threat to anybody until the moment arrives when they do. The death of Matīss Kivlenieks starkly illustrates that point.

# 6

## Demons and Disease

### Flo Hyman: No Warning
*Volleyball 1986*

Growing up in the heart of SoCal a few miles east of LAX, Flo Hyman was toothpick thin and tall. *Very* tall.

She was six-foot flat in elementary school, where her nickname was Jolly Green Giant. She hated people staring at her all the time and making hurtful, lame comments. It stung hard. But she took the advice of her father George, a railroad janitor, and her mother Warrene, a café owner. They urged her to embrace her tallness as a blessing and turn it into a positive force in her life.

That she did. "Florie" grew up to be just about the greatest female volleyball player the world has ever seen.

The game was first played in 1895 at a YMCA in Holyoke, Massachusetts, just 10 miles from Springfield, where four years earlier James Naismith marked off a court and hung peach baskets from balconies at each end. It was called mintonette then, a riff on badminton, and designed as an indoor sport less demanding than basketball that could be played by teams of any size.

After World War II volleyball went mainstream, becoming a staple in high schools and colleges. Strangely, it was a fixture in many nudist colonies too, where co-ed teams were all the rage. Olympic play for men and women began in 1964, and in the 1970s it had a stretch in the spotlight when Wilt Chamberlain took up the game and became its face to the world. He'd loved it all his life, and after he retired from the NBA in 1973, he joined the Seattle Smashers in the short-lived co-ed International Volleyball Association. He also coached two barnstorming teams—the Big Dippers for men and the Little Dippers for women.

Hyman began playing at age 12. She'd started out with basketball and track because they were considered the "Black" sports. But after several excursions with her older sister Suzanne to the beaches along the Pacific Ocean she switched. At first it was simply about having fun in two-on-two matches. Then she got serious, and she began competing professionally at 16 while still a student at Morningside High School in Inglewood.

She became the first female scholarship athlete at the University of Houston in 1974. By then she'd grown to her full height of 6–5 and acquired the speed, strength and agility needed to excel in a demanding game that's a far cry from the laid-back version played at backyard barbecues in suburbia. She hit the floor hard and often, chasing down shots. Her ferocious spike was delivered at 100 mph in the manner of a power forward's slam dunk. Her wicked spin serve was likened to a pitcher's screwball.

In 1978 she left Houston and moved to Colorado to join the U.S. women's team. It was a unit in disarray. They'd tanked royally at the Olympics in 1964 and 1968, losing 11 of 12 matches, and they didn't qualify for the Munich or Montreal games. After she arrived, they didn't even have a coach until Arie Selinger took the helm three months later. With he and Hyman leading the way, the team morphed from a mediocre nonentity into a high performer on the world stage.

The turnaround was swift. In 1978 they finished fifth in the world championships and two years later they were considered a prime contender for a gold medal until the U.S. boycott of the Moscow games squelched that dream. With Hyman as captain, they won silver in Los Angeles, falling to China in the final match. Just turned 30, Hyman was the oldest—and best—player on the team.

After the Olympics she moved to Japan and joined Daiei, Inc., a pro team sponsored by the giant supermarket chain. She fell in love with the country. The feeling was mutual. The fans roared "Hyman! Hyman! Hyman!" whenever she entered an arena. She hung out with American baseball players and their wives and launched a modeling and acting career. Her first screen credit was a special appearance as Spike in the action thriller *The Order of the Black Eagle*. She planned to return home after the 1986 season to continue acting in Hollywood.

She never got the chance. On Friday night, January 24, Daiei played a match against Hitachi, Ltd., in Matsue, a city of 200,000 on the Sea of Japan, 380 miles west of Tokyo. After a routine substitution in the third game, she sat down on the middle of the bench and then slid to the floor unconscious.

At first her coaches and teammates thought it was a fainting spell. She'd had several through the years. But as she was wheeled off the court on a stretcher in front of 4,500 stunned fans, the feeling arose that it might be something more serious.

It was. She was pronounced dead at Matsue Red Cross Hospital at 9:36 p.m., gone at age 31.

All signs pointed to a heart attack. But an autopsy performed in Culver City, California, on January 30 at the request of Hyman's family revealed something shocking. Her heart was in superb condition except for one small flaw—a dime-sized spot in her aorta, the main stem of the organ that pumps blood to all parts of the body except the lungs. In a moment of extreme exertion, the weakened, enlarged aorta burst open and smothered her heart in blood.

The rare genetic malady is called Marfan syndrome, after Antonine Marfan, the French pediatrician who first noted it in 1896. It erodes and loosens the connective tissues of the body, making it vulnerable to the kind of traumatic physical shocks that Hyman experienced frequently as a world-class athlete. After her death many doctors were surprised that the end hadn't come sooner.

It's thought to afflict 50,000 Americans of all races and sexes at any one time, most of whom, like Hyman, don't even realize they have it. The mordant quip runs like this—the first person to make a diagnosis of Marfan syndrome is usually the coroner.

For reasons unknown, the afflicted nearly always exhibit several notable physical traits. Like Hyman, there are often tall and near-sighted, with long arms and large hands. They can also have curved spines; long, narrow faces; deep-set eyes and oddly shaped chest bones.

The National Marfan Association lists several prominent people on its website who had the disease, including British poet Dame Edith Sitwell; Russian composer Sergei Rachmaninoff; and playwright Jonathan Larsen, the author of the hit musical *Rent* who died in 1996 at age 35. It claimed the life of University of Maryland basketball player Chris Patton in a pick-up game in 1976. There is also unconfirmed speculation linking Marfan to Abraham Lincoln, Charles de Gaulle and Olympic swimmer Michael Phelps.

If the damaged aorta is discovered, it can often be surgically repaired. That's what happened with Hyman's brother Michael, who was examined after she died and found to have the disease. He then had open-heart surgery that almost certainly saved his life.

Sadly, that was not the case with his sister. Death blindsided her at the peak of her prowess in the cruelest possible way. Flora Jean Hyman is interred in a mausoleum crypt at Inglewood Park Cemetery, a few miles from her childhood home.

## Len Bias: Shock to the Systems
*Basketball 1986*

The celebration got rolling just after midnight on Juneteenth, six guys hanging out and eating fresh crabs in their dorm suite in Washington Hall on the University of Maryland campus in College Park. They were all members of the Terrapin basketball team, living together as they attended summer school.

The man of the hour was Len Bias, 22, just back from a quick, crazy trip up the East Coast. On the 17th he was in the Felt Forum at Madison Square Garden in Manhattan, where the Boston Celtics chose him as the number two pick in the 1986 NBA draft. The next day he was in Beantown with his dad, meeting with Celtics president Red Auerbach and then with Reebok execs to hear details about the endorsement deal the shoe and sportswear company was offering him.

Leonard Kevin Bias was going to be quite rich quite soon.

It wasn't like he didn't deserve it. The explosive forward was a colossal force on the court. He was Maryland's all-time leading scorer and a two-time ACC player of the year. His leaping ability was astonishing, his jumper was a work of art, and he could create a play any time he wanted. He was durable too. He didn't miss a game in four seasons. Bob Knight said he only saw one player in his coaching career he regarded as the equal of Bias—Michael Jordan.

It took him a while to develop. He was cut from his junior high team and at Maryland he was inconsistent and volatile as a freshman. But he worked hard and matured. His temper still sometimes flared when opponents tried to rough him up. You couldn't really blame them. It was the only real chance they had of slowing him down.

Around 2 a.m. Bias left Washington Hall alone in his newly leased steel gray Datsun 300 Z-X sports car. Where he went remains unclear. Someone saw him at a nearby gathering sipping pop. Somebody else saw him at another party chatting with some ladies. And an informant later told police he had spotted Bias and another man in the vicinity of New York and Montana avenues in northeast Washington, a neighborhood rife with drug dealing.

Bias returned to his quarters around 3 a.m. Or was it 4 or 5? Accounts differ, but one thing was certain. Phase two of the celebration featured cocaine. Who introduced the white powder into the setting has never been determined. Was it one of Bias' suitemates? His longtime friend Brian Tribble? Bias himself? A combination of all of the above? Someone else entirely?

However it got there, it was in plentiful supply, just as it was all across the country. Until the 1960s most Americans didn't even know what cocaine was. But by 1986, in the heart of the Me Decade, snow was everywhere. It had emerged from dank basements and trashy alleys and stinky toilet stalls to find a warm welcome in many segments of society, especially the adventurous young and the carefree rich seeking the latest, greatest, most mind-blowing buzz that ever was.

Sometime after 6 a.m. Bias started to have trouble breathing, lay down on a bed and went into convulsions. After suitemate Terry Long attempted CPR someone called 911 at 6:32 a.m. Paramedics arrived four minutes later. At 6:54 a.m. an ambulance with Bias inside left for Leland Memorial Hospital in Riverdale, a mile and a half away.

Doctors planted a pacemaker in his heart, to no avail. Bias never breathed on his own again and never woke up. With a swelling crowd of friends, fans and family gathered outside the hospital he was pronounced dead at 8:50 a.m. Following a viewing of his open coffin at Pilgrim African Methodist Episcopal Church on Capitol Hill and a memorial service at Cole Field House on campus, Bias was laid to rest at Lincoln Memorial Cemetery in Prince George's County, Maryland.

The tragedy triggered three aftershocks. One hit family and friends from his hometown of Landover and Northwestern High School in Hyattsville. When Maryland's chief medical examiner announced on June 24 that Bias had died of a heart attack induced by cocaine intoxication, they could hardly believe it. This was not the Len Bias they knew.

They stuck to their guns even after police found 12 grams of coke inside a baggie hidden under the dashboard of his Datsun. They insisted he wasn't a user, even though they admitted he likely had friends and acquaintances who were.

Bias took several drug tests at Maryland and passed them all. His test during a pre-draft physical with the Celtics on May 27 also came back clean. But even a small amount of cocaine can be lethal, especially for people with low tolerance. The fact that the coke Bias ingested on the morning of June 19 was found to be exceptionally potent lent some credence to the notion that, appearances to the contrary, he was inexperienced with the drug.

A second aftershock shook the Maryland athletic department. Just hours after Bias's death, coach Lefty Driesell met with Terry Long and David Gregg, another suitemate, in the basement of his home. They prayed together. Details of what else happened are hazy. Gregg might have confessed to scooping up all the powder on hand, giving it to Tribble in a plastic cup and asking him to dispose of it. Driesell might have asked Long and Gregg to clean up the premises, stay cool and be very careful about what they said to police. Then it came to light that Bias was 21 credits short of the number he needed to graduate. At some point he had stopped going to class and never gone back.

The situation was just plain foul. The stench of a cover-up was ripe. Looking on from a distance, the world saw a program out of control, with no rules, no oversight and no consequences for bad behavior.

Under pressure from Chancellor John B. Slaughter, athletic director Dick Dull resigned on October 7. Driesell followed suit on October 29, taking a position as assistant athletic director. It was a sad ending for the coach after 17 seasons with the Terps that included eight NCAA berths and an NIT title. Some observers called Driesell a scapegoat who took the fall for other people's sins.

Things proceeded downhill from there. Long, Gregg and Tribble were all charged with possession of cocaine and obstruction of justice. The charges against Long and Gregg were later dropped in exchange for their testimony against Tribble, who was also charged with supplying Bias with the cocaine that killed him. A year after the incident, Tribble was tried and acquitted by a jury and walked away free. But the cops didn't abandon their mission to bring him to justice. In 1990, he was busted and convicted for selling coke and sentenced to a 10-year prison term.

The final aftershock ripped through the nation's political system. The tragedy played out just 10 miles northeast of the White House and Capitol Hill, and the power elite viewed it as a death in their own neighborhood. President Ronald Reagan and House Speaker Tip O'Neill, who was from Boston, were appalled, as were many of their colleagues.

They'd seen quite enough. Along with the cocaine-induced death of Cleveland Browns safety Don Rogers on June 27 in California, Bias's passing galvanized

## 6. Demons and Disease

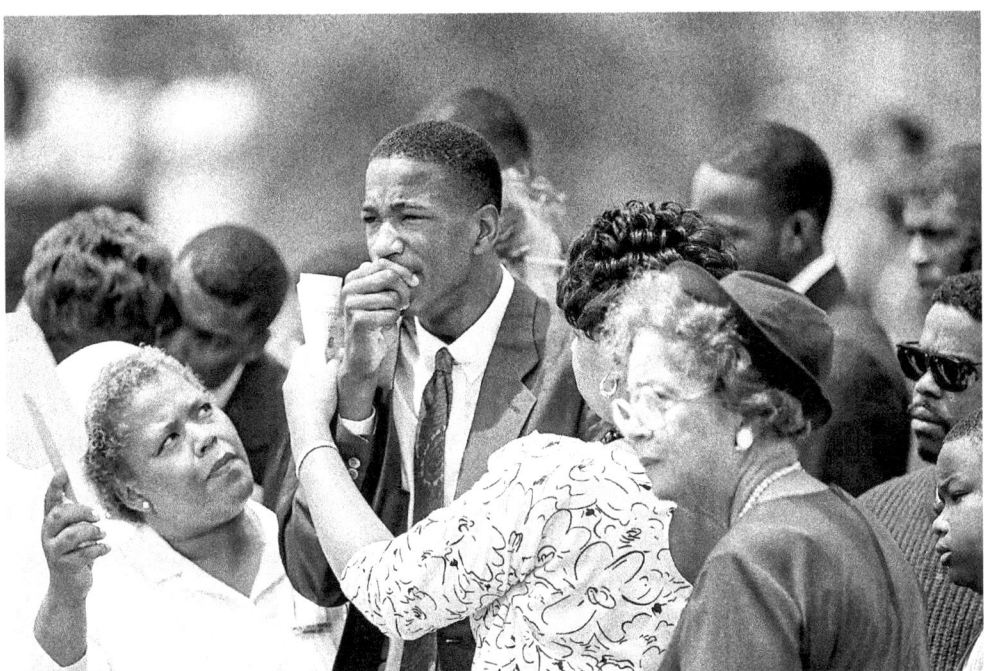

**James "Jay" Bias, Jr., is comforted by family and friends at a service for his older brother Len in College Park, Maryland, on June 23, 1986, four days after his cocaine-induced heart attack. Four years later Jay himself would pass tragically, the victim of a drive-by shooting in a shopping center parking lot. He died in the same emergency room as Len and is buried next to him in Lincoln Memorial Cemetery (AP Images / Bill Smith).**

them to strike a roundhouse blow in their War on Drugs. On October 27, Reagan signed the Anti-Drug Abuse Act of 1986. It became popularly known as the Len Bias Law.

The legislation ignited a firestorm of controversy. Critics accused O'Neill of using the bill to show voters that, contrary to their image, Democrats were indeed tough on crime. Then a nasty fight erupted over the law's grotesquely harsh treatment of "crack cocaine." Crack is a derivative of the drug that is combined with baking soda and cooked, creating hard, pebble-like crystals. The name comes from the crackling sound it makes when it's smoked. It first appeared in America in the late 1970s in Miami and made its way north and west from there.

Standard wisdom held that crack was far more dangerous than powdered cocaine, producing frightening, life-threatening highs on a regular basis and leading to the addiction of innocent "crack babies." Possession of a mere five grams of crack allowed offenders to be prosecuted under the new law in the federal system and mandated a minimum prison term of five years for those convicted. Possession of 500 grams of powder was required to trigger the same. There was no evidence whatsoever that Bias ever smoked crack but that didn't seem to matter.

The truth of the matter was that crack was no more addictive or dangerous than powder. That was a myth concocted by ignorant, white, overwrought law-

and-order zealots in search of a boogey monster. In the eyes of the critics, the real purpose of the distinction was to facilitate the round-up and lock-up of Blacks, who made up 80 percent of crack users in America.

They smoked crack not because of its potency but because it was cheaper. It didn't need to be refined and it was mixed with baking soda. Crack was discount coke for the serf class, not the fancy fine powder going up noses through rolled up C notes in Hollywood night clubs and prep school dorms and corporate hospitality suites.

If the Anti-Drug Abuse Act was indeed racist by design, the strategy worked. America's prison population doubled in the next decade. Most of the new convicts were nonviolent, young Black male offenders busted for possessing a few grams of crack. Although Congress dialed back the sentencing discrepancies during the Obama administration, they still exist today in the law. Efforts to remove them completely stalled in 2023.

Seven years after Bias died, the ugly cloud of cocaine would hover over another death in basketball. This time the deceased was not a Celtic-to-be. He was a Celtics captain.

## Reggie Lewis: Too Young, Too Soon
*Basketball 1993*

The first collapse came in April 1993, in the early minutes of a first-round playoff matchup between the Celtics and the Charlotte Hornets at Boston Garden.

As Celtics captain Reggie Lewis motored up the left side of the court, he stumbled and thudded to the floor. He sat there dazed and confused for a long moment, then got up and left the game. When he returned for six minutes in the third quarter, he felt dizzy and short of breath and his knees began to wobble. Coach Chris Ford brought him back to the bench. It would be the last basketball game of the 27-year-old's life.

The next morning he was examined by a team of 12 doctors at New England Baptist Hospital. They found scars on his heart that might or might not have been caused by cocaine. They asked him if he was a user. He said no. According to one of the doctors, who died in 1995, Lewis was then asked to take a drug test. He'd taken two in 1990 when the Celtics were seeking an insurance policy on his life. Both had come back clean. But this time he refused.

Three days later Lewis went to another hospital in Boston for a second opinion. He was told he had a treatable fainting disorder. He also sought guidance from a group of doctors in California. No consensus was reached on the cause or exact nature of his condition.

In July, Lewis started working out on his own, taking things very easy. On the 27th, he went to the Brandeis University gym with an unidentified friend to shoot baskets. He didn't break a sweat. At 5:07 p.m., after an hour on the floor, he collapsed again. Two police officers who happened upon the scene attempted to revive him with mouth-to-mouth resuscitation. He was taken to Waltham-Weston Hospital where he was pronounced dead at 7:30 p.m.

It was a devastating blow to the city of Boston, the team and its huge, fervent fan base. The soft-spoken forward-guard with a sly smile and fluid jumper was friendly, humble and generous with his time and money. He was also immensely talented. At Dunbar High School in Baltimore, he was the sixth man on two Poet teams that went 60–0 in his junior and senior years. He ended his career at Boston's Northeastern University as the school's all-time leading scorer. In his early years with the Celtics he played in the shadow of Larry Bird, Kevin McHale and Robert Parish, but by 1993 he was a star in his own right, averaging 20.8 points per game in his last two seasons.

He might best be remembered for a 1991 game against the Bulls in which he ate Michael Jordan's lunch. Lewis laughed off the superstar's silly trash talk, skied to block four of his jumpers and hounded him into a dismal 15 of 36 shooting night.

A crowd estimated at 20,000 filed by Lewis' casket at Matthews Arena on the Northeastern campus. Senator Edward Kennedy delivered one of the eulogies at his funeral service. Lewis was buried in an unmarked grave in Section 43 of Forest Hills Cemetery in Boston.

On November 19, almost four months after his collapse at Brandeis, a death certificate was finally filed. The official cause of death was adenovirus 2, a virus associated with the common cold and other, more serious ailments. It led to inflammation and scarring on Lewis' heart, eventually sparking cardiac arrest. But a cause of death pronounced by medical experts rarely tells the whole story. The finding struck many doctors as a gross oversimplification.

The Lewis family had a history of heart problems. Reggie's brother Jon was born with a hole in his heart and had corrective surgery when he was four years old. His mother suffered two heart attacks. Lewis himself was born with a heart murmur. The thought was that all of that clearly had *something* to do with his fate.

Then there was the ugly issue of cocaine. As in the case of Len Bias seven years before, it hovered over the story like a noxious cloud from the beginning. The substance can inflict serious damage on the heart, especially when used in large amounts on a regular basis. Donna Harris-Lewis fiercely denied the rampant rumors that her husband was a user. Many of his friends and teammates insisted that he, like Bias, had nothing to do with cocaine or any other drug. To back up their claims they pointed to the two negative tests in 1990.

But the cloud wouldn't lift. One of his college teammates indicated that he and Lewis snorted coke together many times. That statement was later recanted. And the former athletic director at Northeastern said that Lewis failed a drug test in his senior year. No hard proof or other eyewitness accounts of actual use ever surfaced.

An explosive *Wall Street Journal* story by Ron Suskind fanned the flames. It accused the Celtics front office, NBA brass and mainstream media of avoiding the issue, citing a see-no-evil, hear-no-evil mentality regarding drugs. The apparent strategy of choice was to sweep it all under the rug. No one's interest was served by keeping cocaine on the radar screen.

Some measure of clarity was achieved in 1995 when the Massachusetts public safety director announced that Lewis' autopsy showed no scientific evidence pointing to cocaine as the cause of death. That language neatly sidestepped the question of whether Lewis had traces of the drug in his system on the day he died. His death was attributed to hypertrophic cardiomyopathy, a congenital, structural defect that is one of the most common causes of death in young athletes.

Medical jargon can be tough to understand. In lay terms, Lewis had a bum ticker. The human heart is a highly complex piece of equipment and his was flawed. The muscles had thickened and hardened over time to the point where the organ had difficulty pumping blood. It could break down at any time. The fact that he was a professional athlete who stressed himself to extremes virtually daily made the situation all the more perilous.

There is no cure for the disease, and diagnosis is difficult because its most common symptoms—dizziness, shortness of breath, irregular heartbeat—are identical to many other less serious ailments. But early detection can be critical in controlling it. The best thing Lewis could have done for himself was quit basketball and switch to easygoing exercise habits for the rest of his life. He also could have adopted a leaner, fat-free diet and received a pacemaker or defibrillator to help control his heartbeat.

But Lewis was never diagnosed while he was alive, and he never quit basketball. So he moved closer to death every time he stepped onto the court. Suppose he had been a teacher or barber or dentist instead of a star on the world's most renowned basketball team. Might he still be alive today? All we can do is speculate. That goes for the issue of cocaine use as well.

One thing, however, is certain. Reggie Lewis left the world way too young and way too soon.

## Sergei Grinkov: Shattered Dream
*Pairs Figure Skating 1995*

On the morning of November 20, 1995, as Sergei Grinkov practiced in the rink at the International Skating Center in Lake Placid, New York, he was battling a bout of pain in his lower back, caused by the strain of repeatedly lifting and throwing his 90-pound wife and pairs partner Ekaterina Gordeeva.

The pain was sometimes mild, sometimes fierce. Grinkov tackled it head-on by lifting weights to build strength. He took no medications. To him it was simply an occupational hazard in the demanding discipline of world-class figure skating, even for a stalwart described by many as the strongest and healthiest athlete ever to perform in the sport.

As Grinkov hurled his wife through the air one more time, he felt dizzy and stopped skating. Ekaterina—known as Katya—thought her husband had hurt his back again. But a moment later he lay down on the ice and passed out.

Marina Zoueva, the pair's coach and choreographer, left the ice to stop the music. Paul Wylie, a friend of the couple and an Olympic skater, rubbed Katya's back to calm her nerves. Paramedics arrived and tried to revive Grinkov's heart, three times as he lay on the ice and twice more in the parking lot before taking him to Adirondack Medical Center. The staff there worked over him for an hour before Grinkov was pronounced dead at 12:28 p.m. He was 28. As Katya said her final goodbye she unlaced his skates, slipped them off his feet and carried them away.

It was the end of one of the most romantic stories ever in the sports world. Sergei and Katya met at the Central Red Army Club (CSKA) in Moscow when he was eight and she was four. Seven years later, as promising young skaters entering the authoritarian system of the old Soviet Union, they were placed together for the pairs competition against the wishes of the young man, who longed for a solo career.

For the next 14 years they were barely apart. They literally grew up in each other's arms. Considered an oddity at first because of the big difference in their heights, the 5–11 Sergei and the spindly 5–1 Katya evolved into a marvelous vision of grace and power.

"They never held anything back," said 1984 Olympic gold medalist Scott Hamilton. "They absolutely complemented each other mentally, physically, emotionally. They were a unit. Everything she needed, he had. Everything he needed, she had."[1]

Known as G & G in the skating world, they won nearly every competition they entered. In 1988, they captured the gold medal in the pairs competition at the Winter Olympics in Calgary. From 1986 to 1990, they earned four world crowns and then turned professional, joining the Tom Collins Tour of World Champions. By that time their partnership had blossomed into love, and they were married on April 20, 1991. Their daughter Daria was born on September 11 the next year. She shares her father's vivid blue eyes and crooked smile.

In the polarizing Cold War era, cynical observers might well have dismissed their marital union as a forced one, pressed on them against their will by the same authorities who ordered them to pair up in competition. But the Soviet Union was undergoing radical change. Four months after their wedding, Mikhail Gorbachev resigned as the leader of the Communist Party. By the end of the year the country no longer existed, with a plan in place to transform it into 15 separate nations. It soon became apparent that the G&G fairy tale matchup was for

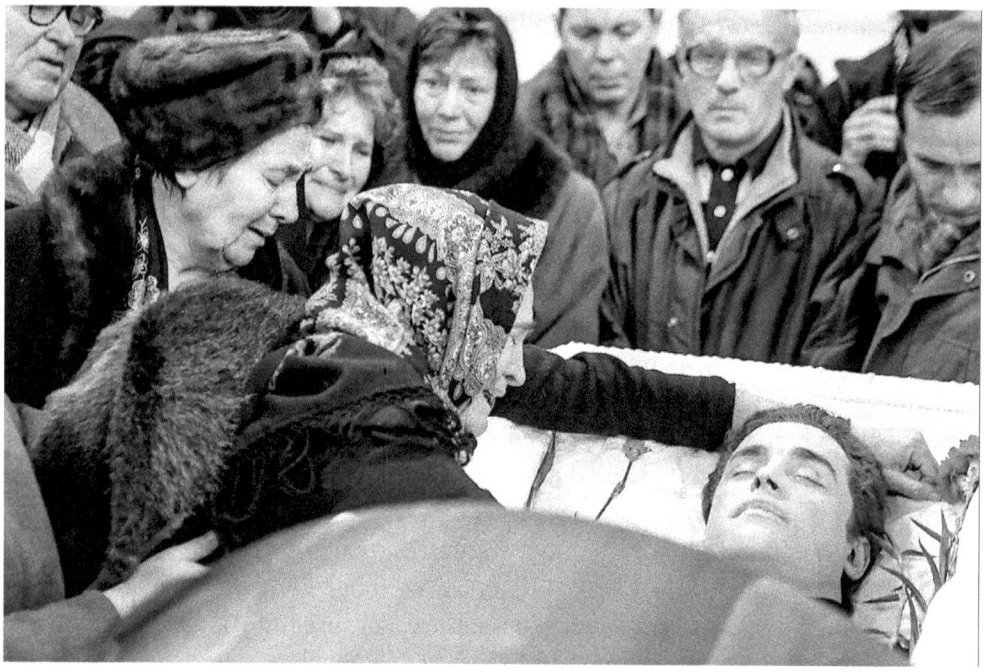

Anna Grinkov leans over the coffin of her son Sergei and bids him farewell at his funeral in Moscow on November 25, 1995. The service was held at the Central Red Army Club (CSKA), where Sergei met his future skating partner and wife Katya Gordeeva when he was eight years old and she was four (AP Images / Sergei Kivrin).

real. They became a kind of symbol and a beacon of hope in the new, freer Russian society that emerged in the 1990s under Boris Yeltsin.

In 1994, they took advantage of a one-time rules change that allowed professionals to compete in the Olympics and won their second gold medal in Lillehammer, Norway. After that the family moved to Simsbury, Connecticut, to train and live in the United States. They were in Lake Placid to prepare for a 55-city tour with the Discover Card Stars on Ice program.

Doctors attributed Grinkov's death to undetected coronary artery disease, very probably inherited from his father, who died in 1991 at age 56 after suffering his fourth heart attack. His condition was not cardiomyopathy, which causes irregular heartbeats, or Marfan syndrome, which swells the size of the heart's aorta and triggers aneurysms.

Instead, 24 hours before his collapse, Grinkov had a so-called silent heart attack, which produces only mild symptoms at the outset that are frequently ignored or dismissed as trivial. Medical research suggests that they account for roughly 25 percent of all heart attacks in America. The classic signs of cardiac breakdown—intense chest pain, profuse sweating, extreme dizziness and labored breathing—can arrive later, as they did with Grinkov, or not at all.

A private wake was held in Saranac Lake near Lake Placid the day after his death. Grinkov's body was then flown to Moscow for a funeral at the Central Red

Army Club, where his career began. On the cold, dreary afternoon of November 25, mourners gathered there for a candlelight service. He was buried in a simple wood coffin in Vagankovsky Cemetery.

On February 27, 1996, the cast of Stars on Ice skated in Grinkov's honor at the Hartford Civic Center. The participants included gold medalists Okansa Baiul, Viktor Petrenko, Brian Boitano and Scott Hamilton. Katya Gordeeva, a 24-year-old widow, performed alone on the ice for the first time in her life. To the somber strains of Mahler's Fifth Symphony, she gave a moving performance in memory of her husband.

## Andreas Munzer: Hunger Pains
*Bodybuilding 1997*

Fascination with the male body has deep roots in Western culture, going all the way back to ancient Greece, where it was exalted and celebrated, and nakedness was seen as a heroic state. Olympic athletes competed nude, and images of the male form could be seen everywhere in public and private spaces.

But events in which contestants displayed themselves in poses on stage to be relished by an audience and scored by judges did not arise until the 20th century. German bodybuilder Eugen Sandow and promoter Florenz Ziegfeld presented the first modern show at Royal Albert Hall in London in 1901. Sir Arthur Conan Doyle was one of the two judges. The first events in America were held in 1903 and 1904 in Madison Square Garden in New York City.

It wasn't like weightlifting. Contestants were not ranked on the basis of physical strength. How did they look? How glorious and breathtaking and deeply cut were the biceps, triceps and quadriceps? What about the abdomen, thighs, and calves and the rest of the corpus? That was what counted. You could call it the ultimate appearance sport, if you thought of it as a sport at all.

In the 1950s and 1960s, TV workout guru Jack LaLanne and movie idol Steve Reeves as Hercules gained renown for their physiques. The rise of Gold's Gym as a franchised operation brought bodybuilding to the masses in the 1970s, when women first began competing. The release of the docudrama film *Pumping Iron* in 1977 cemented its grip on millions of fans, many of whom were pumping iron themselves.

One of the hallmarks of the modern era is the utterly obsessive behavior of elite participants. All athletes who strive to excel can be counted on to go to extremes. That's the nature of the force inside them. But those who choose to excel in bodybuilding take things to a place beyond extreme. British journalist Jon Hotten calls it a sport without boundaries. That hits the nail on the head.

From an early age the obsessives dedicate themselves to building the perfect machine. Nothing is off limits. They vow to "stay hungry" and do whatever they need to do to gain an edge in competition. If that means turning themselves into liars, cheaters, criminals, drug addicts, violent social misfits and grotesque physical specimens, they live with it. In their view it's worth the price. A graphic exposé in the *Washington Post* in 2022 revealed that the "anything goes" culture has moved far beyond its roots and lurched into overdrive.

Andreas Munzer embraced the stay hungry ethos with tenacity. He was born and raised in the village of Pack in the rural region of Styria in southeast Austria, the son of dairy farmers. Andi was a quiet, serious kid who worked hard. He helped out on the farm, played soccer in the summer and skied in the winter.

When he was a teenager, he joined a gym and discovered his destiny. Arnold Schwarzenegger, 17 years older, was a native of Thal, just 35 miles away. As Andi began his career, the greatest bodybuilder ever had retired as a seven-time Mr. Olympia and the winner of a record 13 international titles. He'd moved on to Hollywood, where his roles as the Predator, the Terminator and Conan the Barbarian would earn him a fortune and pave the way for his election as governor of California in 2003.

The Austrian Oak was one of the most famous people in the world. Munzer idolized him. He hung a giant poster of Schwarzenegger in a glittery thong in his bedroom as a kind of inspirational guide. But there was more to his hero worship than that. Andi didn't just want to follow in his footsteps. He wanted to transform himself into the Second Coming of the man and become a sort of biological clone.

It was a tall order. At the end of the day, too tall.

At some point Munzer started juicing. That's a catchall term in bodybuilding for using performance-enhancing drugs. If you juiced you didn't talk about it much, but if you did talk, you were discreet because the practice was frowned upon by most people at the gym. Ingesting all manner of whatever into your system was viewed as unseemly, dangerous and demeaning. But if you were committed to getting your body totally dry and ripped—and Munzer was—you had to juice.

The hyper ambitious guys didn't view it as cheating. Their thinking ran like this—if everybody else going all out is doing it, and I just *know* they are, then I have to do it even if I don't want to. It's the only way I have to keep the playing field level and give myself a real shot at excelling in competition.

Anabolic steroids were the favored entrees on the juicing menu. Although nearly all forms of them were illegal unless prescribed by a medical doctor, they could be easily obtained on the black market and injected in liquid form by needle, swallowed as pills or powder, or applied to the skin as a gel or cream.

Steroids built bulk by increasing the amount of protein delivered to muscle cells. They also aided recovery after intense workouts and enabled users to begin their next sessions far sooner and in much better condition. When the cycle was repeated time after time, they could attain astonishing levels of strength and endurance.

In a sport with virtually no drug testing, steroids just laid the foundation. As Munzer's career blossomed and he began to compete in Europe and America, his training regimen included a staggering number of other substances. Painkillers to ease the suffering he faced on a daily basis. Insulin to improve metabolism. Five aspirin every morning to relieve pain and thin his blood. Ephedrine, a stimulant popular with baseball and hockey players, to increase workout intensity. Lasix, a diuretic frequently used on racehorses, to flush out water and reduce body fat and weight. The reduction in fat also helped develop the deep cuts that visually define muscles and impress judges at competitions.

His coup de grâce was growth hormones, in either human or synthetic form. They worked to build up not just muscles but bones, organs and soft tissue as well.

Juicing didn't guarantee great success. Far from it. Munzer learned that quickly. His native tongue was German and that was a plus because it was a long-held tenet in bodybuilding that Germanic and Black men stood at the top of the pecking order. But at 5–7, 230 pounds, he was lighter and shorter that nearly all of his rivals, and he never felt like the judges were giving him a fair shake. He was doing everything right, but his 58-inch chest and 21-inch upper arms just didn't measure up.

As he soldiered on through the 1990s, contestants with huge physiques of whatever shape and contour were coming into vogue with competitors, judges, fans, media and sponsors. Cynical onlookers labeled them "mass monsters." In 11 years Munzer won only one event, the 1989 World Games. His best finishes in Mr. Olympia, the sport's premier show, were ninth in 1993 and 1994. For someone dead set on finishing first every time he stepped on the stage, his career was one stinging disappointment after the next.

Being short and small wasn't his only handicap. He also may have been too decent of a human being to reach the summit in a sport brimming with nasty, raging, angry narcissists. Schwarzenegger hinted at that idea in an interview after Munzer's death. He considered Munzer a friend but said he may have lacked the "overall genetic makeup"[2] of a champion.

It's good that Munzer wasn't around at that point. He may have suspected the same thing about himself but hearing it from the man he admired more than anyone on the planet likely would have crushed him.

In March 1996, he entered his last competition, the Arnold Classic in Columbus. He finished sixth and won $5,000. He'd been in excruciating pain for months. Beneath his stunning exterior he was slowly bleeding to death. His stomach was swollen and hard. His blood was goopy and thick like Heinz ketchup and couldn't flow through his veins and arteries. His potassium levels were through the roof.

On March 12, he finally went to a hospital in Munich. He survived an operation intended to repair his stomach but remained in desperate shape. On the morning of March 14, he died of multiple organ failure at age 31.

An autopsy revealed traces of 20 drugs in his system. And the corpse itself was hideous. His testicles were shriveled up like rotten grapes. Half of his liver was a pulpy, shredded, plastic-like mess. The other half was full of tumors the size of ping pong balls. His heart was twice the size of an average man's. So were his kidneys.

There was also a shocking absence of body fat. It's frequently claimed that he died with absolutely none of it. Zero. That is hard to accept as true. No measurement was taken during the autopsy. The actual figure was probably somewhere between 0 and 3 percent. At that point the male body reaches a crisis state, spawning electrolyte imbalances and breakdown of the heart, lungs, kidney and liver.

In the end, the jarring visuals and numbers didn't matter much. Andi Munzer decided early on what he wanted to do with his time on Earth. He stayed hungry. He paid for that choice with his life.

## Korey Stringer: Water Is for Cowards
### NFL 2001

Like Andreas Munzer in the gym, Korey Stringer pushed himself beyond the limit on the football field—well beyond. He embraced the warrior code of his demanding, physical sport to the hilt. And like Munzer, the Minnesota Vikings offensive tackle paid the ultimate price for his devotion.

He was an enormous man at 6–4, 360, give or take 30 or so pounds depending on his calorie intake and the intensity and duration of his workouts. He loved meat and grease and carbs. A profile of him in *Esquire* magazine just months before his death featured a close-up photo of his enormous belly and a color spread of his favorite foods—French fries, chicken wings, barbecued ribs and chili cheese dogs.

He was also an extreme sweater. On a scorcher of a training camp day like the one that did him in, he could expel as much as three gallons of perspiration during the course of two 90-minute practices. His bulk made him highly vulnerable to heat illness. The larger the body is, the more heat it must expel to keep organs functioning. If the sweating machine ever conks out, mortal danger is sure to follow. Football gear, especially helmets and gloves, hold heat in and make the situation all the more dangerous.

Stringer was upbeat when he reported to camp in 2001 at Minnesota State University at Mankato, 90 miles south of Minneapolis. He weighed in at 335, his lowest number ever with the Vikings. In 1997 he played at 388. Being lighter made him feel agile, explosive, and energetic, and he was trying to hold on to that vibe in camp. Stringer was coming off an All-Pro season. But with 91 career starts in six years, he was feeling some serious wear and tear and he needed to maintain his edge. If that meant reducing his water intake to a bare minimum to keep his

## 6. Demons and Disease

weight down, he'd have at it. In the 2000 movie *Remember the Titans*, the warrior code's position on water was summed up well by tyrant coach Herman Ike Boone, portrayed by Denzel Washington: *Water is for cowards. Water makes you weak.* It doesn't get much more hardcore than that.

Stringer had his work cut out for him. The Vikings first day of practice on July 30 was brutally hot, with temperatures hovering in the 90s. The heat index was 110. The weather was so extreme that the state of Minnesota issued a livestock warning to farmers—keep all animals inside.

During morning practice Stringer vomited three times. He was taken to the medical trailer on a cart and missed afternoon practice. The next morning the *Minneapolis Star-Tribune* ran a wrenching photo of him from the day before, bent over at the waist, mouth agape, looking utterly wiped out.

The photo embarrassed and angered him. He showed up on July 31 determined to atone for his bad showing. The heat index was as high as the day before. He went through a full pads workout from 8:45 to 11:10, then lay down on the field and didn't get up. Five other players suffered heat distress as well.

Stringer spent 50 minutes in the medical trailer and passed out before being transported to Immanuel and St. Joseph's Mayo Health System Hospital. He was pronounced dead at 1:50 a.m. on the morning of August 1, 13 hours after arrival. He left behind his wife Kelcie, three-year-old son Kodie and at least one inconsolable teammate, wide receiver Randy Moss, who bawled his eyes out at a press conference later that day.

The official cause of death was multiple organ failure induced by exertional heat stroke. But that finding hardly settled the matter. Stringer had a long history of ingesting "dietary supplements," designed to boost energy and enhance on-field performance. He was particularly fond of a drink called Ripped Fuel. So were millions of other people. It was a hugely popular product, and if you were trying to drop weight, it was precious. His wife revealed that it was his habit to drink a bottle of it before every game during the season.

Did he drink one on the morning of his collapse? She didn't say.

You can fairly describe Ripped Fuel as a legal, liquid, chemical cousin of speed. It contains derivatives of ephedra, an over-the-counter herbal stimulant also known as Ma Huang, and it has a proven track record of raising blood pressure, skying the heart rate and, above all, triggering dehydration. It's the substance that played a key role in the death of Baltimore Orioles pitcher Steve Bechler in 2003. After Stringer's death the NFL banned the substance. Today it's off limits in virtually every major sport.

So the Vikings brass had their own take on the incident. It wasn't all about their guys dropping the ball in the medical trailer in camp. Stringer had been playing with fire for years, and his ongoing habit contributed in a big way to his death. They described it as the elephant in the room that Stringer's friends and family didn't want to talk about.

Kelci Stringer's attorney responded that the coroner's toxicology report came back "absolutely clean"[3] and that the front office was pathetically trying to smear the man's memory to divert attention from the irresponsible, careless behavior of their employees.

The Vikings replied that the report came back clean because the coroner never tested the body for the presence of ephedra or any other stimulants. They even broached the grotesque idea of exhuming Stringer's corpse and testing it to confirm their allegations.

It was all quite ugly. And this was *before* Kelci's grab bag of lawsuits alleging negligence were even filed. The rift put a distinct chill in the air at the Vikings ceremony to retire Stringer's number 77 at their Monday night game with the Giants on November 19.

After the Ripped Fuel hubbub subsided, the post-mortem review shifted to two questions. First, how common is it for a football player, even one who might be juiced up on some kind of speed, to exert himself on the field to the point of death? It doesn't happen *that* often, right?

As a matter of fact, it does. For the three decades or so that hard data has been compiled, two to three high school and college players have died each year due to heat illness. Most of the deaths occur in the Southeast on sunny days in the high heat and humidity months of August and September. Just six days before Stringer died, Florida Gators freshman lineman Eraste Autin perished following a punishing sprint session at a voluntary workout.

A heat emergency develops in stages. First comes profuse sweating, followed by painful muscle cramps. After that comes heat exhaustion, with dizziness, fatigue and a weak pulse. The final stage is heat stroke, where the body stops sweating entirely, robbing it of the only mechanism it has to expel heat. The heart pounds furiously, the skin turns red and dry, the mind goes fuzzy and body temperature soars. When Stringer arrived at the hospital his rectal temperature was 108.8 degrees. At that point life cannot be sustained.

The second post-mortem question was more specific. The NFL is not a rural high school in Georgia or a small college in Louisiana. How, then, in the presence of 100 or so coaches, staffers, medical personnel and players, could a 27-year-old man fry himself to death?

It happened because of the startling level of ignorance in the league concerning heat illness. The trainers in charge of treating Stringer in Mankato faced lawsuits from his wife and agent and a torrent of criticism for failing to recognize the seriousness of the situation. But they were never found to be legally at fault. In all fairness that makes a certain amount of sense because heat stroke was not on their—or the league's—radar.

The standard wisdom for decades was that air-conditioning, ice-cold towels and large amounts of drinking water were enough to cool down a seriously overheated player. In fact, immersion of the body in a cooling tub all the way up to the neck is what's needed. If that step is taken immediately after the rectal temperature reaches 104 degrees, deaths like Stringer's are entirely preventable. But the Vikings had no cooling tub on hand at Mankato. That's just the way it was in the NFL back then. If one had been available and utilized, Stringer would very likely be alive today.

The warrior code of football dies hard. There are still people in the sport today clinging to the ignorant outlook of coach Herman Boone. But there are far fewer of them. For that reason it can be said that Stringer did not die in vain. The powers that be in the NFL were chagrined and ashamed about what happened to him on that sweltering summer day. After Stringer's death the league adopted strict protocols for dealing with heat illness that include heat stress monitors, cooling tubs, urine tests to gauge dehydration and mandatory water intake. There have been no heat stroke fatalities in the NFL since.

Korey Damont Stringer is interred at Pineview Memorial Park in the city of Warren in Trumbull County, Ohio.

## Tyler Skaggs: Black Cloud
*MLB 2019*

Paramedics and police entered the upscale room at the Southlake Hilton just after 2 p.m. on July 1, 2019. An unconscious man lay sprawled face down on the bed, his cowboy boots dangling over the side. Repeated attempts at revival failed and he was pronounced dead at the scene.

The deceased was Tyler Skaggs, 27, a pitcher for the Los Angeles Angels. The Halos were in the Dallas-Fort Worth metro area for a four-game series with the Rangers. Skaggs was slated to start the Fourth of July game at Globe Life Park.

His wife of six months Carli always sent him a goodnight text when he was on the road. After he failed to respond on the night of June 30, authorities arrived at the Hilton the next afternoon and made the grim discovery.

Like Flo Hyman, Skaggs was a native of SoCal, born in Woodland Hills and raised in Santa Monica, where he grew up with the game. His father Darrell Skaggs and stepfather Dan Ramos both played, and his mother Debbie Hetman was the longtime softball coach at Santa Monica High School. He was a lanky, brainy, precocious kid who acquired many nicknames through the years—Ty, Pole, Skaggsy and Swaggy.

His seven-year MLB career was a struggle. First signed by the Angels in 2009, he rose through the Arizona Diamondbacks farm system, made his big-league debut with them in 2012 and returned to the Angels the next year. He underwent Tommy John surgery for a torn elbow ligament in 2014 and then battled frequent injuries as a key member of the Angels starting rotation. His lifetime record was 28–38 and his ERA was 4.41.

Those numbers are unremarkable, hardly the stuff of legend and lore. But Skaggs will be remembered for a long time. When the Tarrant County medical examiner released his report on August 30, it ripped through MLB like a Great Plains twister, leaving a trail of shock and grief in its wake.

The autopsy uncovered three substances in Skaggs' system—alcohol, oxycodone and fentanyl. He died of asphyxia after food particles and carbon dioxide flooded his lungs and supplanted the oxygen he needed to live. He suffocated on his own vomit and the death was ruled an accident.

The alcohol was not a factor. And Skaggs had been using oxycodone usually under the brand name Percocet on and off since 2013 to combat his physical ailments. It's an opioid-based analgesic and sedative taken by millions on a prescription basis to numb pain. But Skaggs didn't need to see a doctor. He could often score a more plentiful and potent supply on the black market.

He knew he was into Percocet way too deep and tried several times with family support to kick the habit, both by weaning off of it and going cold turkey. Like virtually everyone else who tries to quit opioids alone without professional intervention, he failed.

But it wasn't the oxy that killed him on the road trip to Texas. It was the fenty. The light blue pills he crushed and snorted up his nose on the last night of his life looked authentic, marked with the logo M/30 to signify 30 milligrams of oxycodone. But they were counterfeit, laced with tiny amounts of a drug 50 times more powerful than heroin and 100 times stronger than morphine.

Fentanyl is about the nastiest substance ever concocted by the human mind. Three milligrams can kill a 160-pound person. It's often mixed into street drugs to increase potency. The problem with that set-up is that buyers and retail sellers don't know it's there—until somebody dies. The situation begs a couple of truly disturbing questions. Are the drug dealers *trying* to kill their customers? If so, why?

In one sense the tragedy shouldn't have been surprising. There was no reason to assume that baseball players were somehow exempt from the scourge of opioid overdoses that has claimed more than half a million American lives since 1999 and shows few signs of abating.

It didn't help that Skaggs had unfettered, under the table access to what he craved. His go-to guy was Eric Kay, the Angels communications director and an opioid addict himself who was treated for an overdose just months before Skaggs died. They often snorted together, and Kay supplied several other Angels as well. One confessed to snorting in the dugout and in a bathroom stall in the clubhouse. It's a common dynamic in the drug world—codependent users bound together in an atmosphere of furtive conspiracy and edgy bonhomie. The one unusual feature is that Kay is now serving a 22-year sentence in federal prison after being convicted of selling Skaggs the drugs that killed him.

Ballplayers have long used legal and illegal substances to enhance per-

## 6. Demons and Disease

formance on the field and cope with long, exhausting seasons. The alarm sounded in 2019 because Skaggs was the first active MLB player confirmed to have died of a fentanyl overdose. With his death, the national pastime's rocky relationship with drugs entered a frightening new phase.

It started with alcohol. From the beginning booze was everywhere you looked in baseball, except on the field itself—at least most of the time. Drunkenness led to Ed Delahanty's fatal fall into the Niagara River way back in 1903. In 1960 Yankees manager Ralph Houk spoke for many when he called it all good. He said he'd take "nine whisky drinkers in his lineup over nine milkshake drinkers any day."[4] Alcohol's longtime companion was tobacco, be it smoked via cigarettes or cigars or chewed, chawed, dipped, rubbed or inhaled in smokeless form.

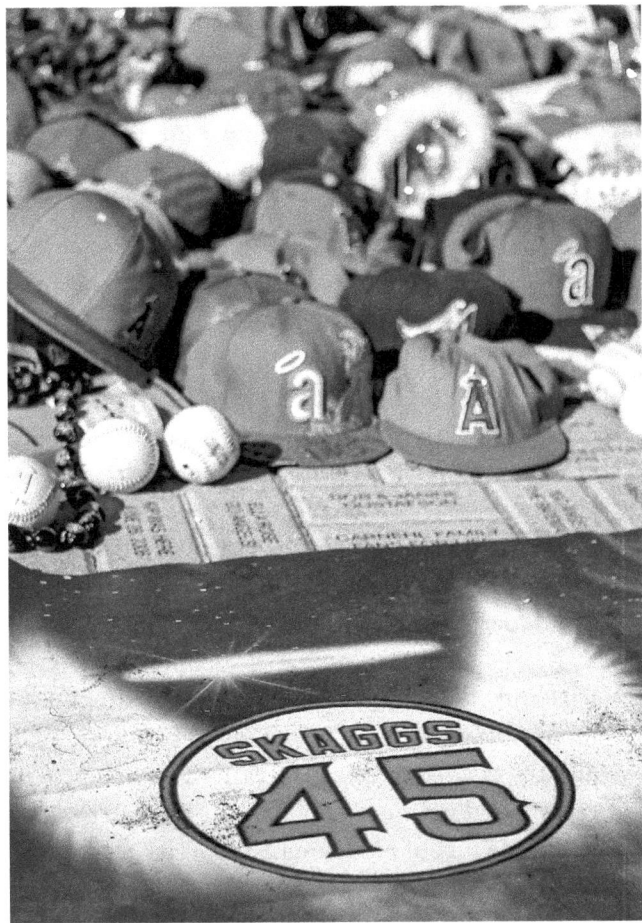

The death of pitcher Tyler Skaggs from a fentanyl overdose in July of 2019 shocked MLB to its core. This impromptu shrine to the veteran left-hander sprang up outside Angel Stadium of Anaheim before their game with the Orioles on July 26 (AP Images / Carrie Giordano [Jesenovec]).

The decades after World War II saw the explosive rise of speed. The most common form was the amphetamine Dexedrine. The powerful stimulant had been used in enormous quantities by American soldiers during the conflict, and it soon made its way from the battlefields to the playing fields, becoming a staple in every clubhouse. Beaning up with greenies wasn't considered a form of cheating. It was standard game day procedure. Speed was so common that a slang term arose to describe the bummer of having to take the field without the high it provided. That was called "playing naked."[5]

In the 1980s attention shifted to cocaine, the de rigueur drug of the day, and many stars were ensnared in snowstorms—Vida Blue, Steve Howe, Ferguson Jenkins, Dennis "Oil Can" Boyd, Dave Parker, Alan Wiggins, Keith Hernandez. After he retired, Tim Raines of the Expos confessed to snorting during games. He kept a vial of blow in the back pocket of his pants and always slid head-first on the basepaths to avoid breaking it.

Then came steroids, designed to transform the already large bodies of home run sluggers into Schwarzenegger-like hulks. Mark McGwire, Barry Bonds, Sammy Sosa and Jose Canseco showed that they could juice with the best of the bodybuilders.

Steroids and speed have been banned in MLB since 2006. Skaggs's death prompted a radical revamp of the sport's drug testing policy. Random testing for non-prescribed opioids and cocaine in spring training and the regular season began in 2020. Before that point testing had been allowed only with reasonable cause. Marijuana was removed from the list of forbidden substances. For the few violators, heavy fines and long suspensions were replaced with a treatment-based system.

So like Korey Stringer, Tyler Skaggs did not die in vain. Both of their deaths led to new protocols for handling dangerous, life-threatening situations. Those protocols may someday save human lives. Perhaps they already have.

Let's transition now to a second In the Arena chapter, with stops in Cincinnati and Aspen and four far-flung locales—an icy ski slope in Bavaria, a steep mountain pass in the Pyrenees in southern France, the frozen tundra of Alaska and the rugged, treeless terrain of Gansu province in China. Before we go, we'll relive a sad moment on a basketball court in the heart of SoCal, just miles from the home turf of Flo Hyman and Tyler Skaggs.

# 7

# In the Arena Redux

## Hank Gathers: Heart of a Lion
*Basketball 1990*

Hank Gathers grew up in North Philly in a crumbling brick row house in the Raymond Rosen housing projects, a once-vibrant complex of 500 homes built after World War II that had slowly gone to seed. As the 1970s arrived, the features of daily life included thugs, vagrants and druggies in the streets, garbage heaps and rat packs in the alleys, dirt lawns, gutted cars and gunfire.

When he was nine, Hank's parents split up and soon after he decided he needed to exit the depraved environment ASAP. Basketball was his path out. It was the path out for his mother Lucille and brothers Derrick and Charles as well. They were all counting on him to make it to the NBA and deliver them to a better place.

Many families with a baller in their nest share the same dream. It rarely comes true. But Hank was special. He excelled at Dobbins Technical High School and with teammate Bo Kimble earned a scholarship to USC in Los Angeles, about as far away from Raymond Rosen as you could get. Which suited Hank just fine.

After a year at USC they found themselves at odds with new coach George Raveling and transferred to Loyola Marymount, a Jesuit Catholic school in west Los Angeles with 6,200 students. Loyola had an underwhelming record of achievement in basketball, although it did produce two players who went on to win NCAA titles as coaches—Phil Woolpert with San Francisco and Pete Newell with California. They were teammates at Loyola in 1939 and 1940.

Things changed quickly when Gathers and Kimble arrived. They became the dynamic duo who spearheaded coach Paul Westhead's run-and-gun offense. Three pointers reigned down in torrents, most of them launched 10 seconds or fewer into a possession. At 6–7, 210, Hank dominated the paint, and on his best nights number 44 was virtually unstoppable. He cleaned the glass at will and his electrifying dunks brought the fans at Gersten Pavilion roaring to their feet.

In the 1987–88 season he led the Lions in scoring and rebounding as they went 28–4, the best record in school history. They won 25 straight before falling to North Carolina in the second round of March Madness. The next year he led all of Division I, averaging 32.7 points and 13.7 rebounds. After spending decades in the long shadows of UCLA and USC, the off-the-radar school from the West Coast Conference was having a moment in the spotlight.

On December 9, 1989, 24 days into his senior season, Gathers fainted at the free throw line during a home game against UC Santa Barbara. Doctors discovered a severe case of arrhythmia—irregularities in both the force and rhythm of the heart. They treated it with Ideral, a brand name for propranolol, one of the family of drugs called beta-blockers. They stem the effects of adrenaline on nerve cells, causing blood vessels to relax and dilate, which slows pulse and improves flow. Beta-blockers are also used to treat high blood pressure (hypertension) and angina (chest pain). He returned to action three weeks later after missing two games.

The episode rattled him greatly. Suddenly he felt like bruised fruit, damaged goods, a defective product. It didn't bode well for his NBA aspirations. He hated what the Ideral did to his body and mind. He felt sluggish, drowsy and disoriented. Before home games he would run sprints around the Marymount track to break a gushing sweat, flush the medicine out of his system and get to full strength before tipoff.

With the consent of his doctors he gradually scaled down his daily dose of 240 mg. His performance didn't suffer much. On February 3 he played brilliantly in a road game against LSU. Despite having five shots blocked by Shaquille O'Neal, Gathers refused to back down against a man who had five inches and 110 pounds on him. He racked up 48 points and 13 rebounds as the Lions took the Tigers to overtime before losing 148–141.

With the post season approaching, his doctors reduced his dosage one last time to 40 mg, on the condition that he submit to a treadmill test by the end of February. He never showed up.

Did anybody—coaches, doctors, family, friends, teammates—force the issue with him? We don't know. At this point in the story details get fuzzy. But one thing was for sure—Gathers was a player, and he was going to play. He loved the game too much to sit on the sidelines. And too many people he loved had too many hopes riding on him.

On Sunday, March 4, the Lions hosted the Portland Pilots in a West Coast Conference tournament semifinal. Before the 5 p.m. tip Gathers ran his sprints on the track. After a thunderous alley oop dunk early in the first half, he collapsed near midcourt, jumped up, then crashed to the floor again and went into convulsions, his leg twitching wildly. For reasons never determined a defibrillator kept on the sidelines was not immediately used. He was removed from the building on a stretcher and taken to Daniel Freeman Marina Hospital. Extensive, repeated efforts to revive him failed. He was pronounced dead at 6:55 p.m. Gathers was 23 years old.

The conference tournament was cancelled, and Loyola was awarded a berth in the Big Dance by virtue of their 13–1 regular season record. After a memorial Mass at Gersten Pavilion and a funeral in Philadelphia, the grief-stricken Loyola team continued their season. With millions of fans around the country pulling for them, they made a spectacular run, defeating defending champion Michigan in the Round of 32 before losing to eventual champ UNLV in the Elite Eight.

The tragedy was markedly similar to the one that would take the life of Reggie Lewis three years later. Gathers did not have a family history of heart problems like Lewis. Nor did the ugly cloud of cocaine hover over his death like it does with Lewis to this day. His autopsy found no traces of illicit drugs.

But both men died on a basketball court with defective hearts. Lewis had hypertrophic cardiomyopathy, a genetic disorder that causes an abnormal thickening of the left ventricle. Continual bouts of stressful exercise greatly increase the danger, and it's the most common cause of sudden death in high school and college athletes, claiming about half of the 15 to 20 who die each year. Gathers also had myocarditis, which inflames the tissues of the heart.

A second parallel to Lewis is that the situation soon descended into lawsuit hell. Hank was dead. Somebody somewhere dropped the ball big time, and Lucille Gathers was going to find out who it was and take as big a piece out of their hide as she could.

The gloves came off early. Lucille hired Beverly Hills lawyer Bruce Fogel and held a press conference to announce her intention to sue a mere three days after the funeral. That went over like a lead balloon. Then Marva Crump from the old neighborhood filed suit as well on behalf of her and Hank's son Aaron, who was born when Hank was 16. She claimed that he was the rightful recipient of any compensation that might be had. Marva and Lucille became bitter enemies as they angled for steep payouts from deep pockets.

The two women asserted that if the doctors had simply been upfront and honest about the severity of his condition, Gathers would have cleaned out his locker and walked away from basketball forever. That may or may not be true. It's also possible that the doctors weren't fully aware of the severity. Despite its modern focus on data, knowledge, precision and training, medicine remains an inexact science. In their minds they did everything they could under the circumstances to treat their patient. They hadn't breached any duty of care or committed any type of malpractice.

After all the clamor and finger-pointing subsided, out-of-court settlements were reached in both cases.

On February 29, 2020, a statue of Gathers was unveiled outside Gersten Pavilion. The event brought the focus back to a truth that seems to have been glossed over in the three decades since his death. In his unrelenting zeal to compete and excel in the arena, Hank Gathers was a warrior. He literally laid down his life for the chance to play.

Eric Wilson Gathers, Jr., is interred at Mount Lawn Cemetery in Darby Township, Pennsylvania.

## Ulrike Maier: No Chance
*Skiing 1994*

In January of 1994, as skier Ulrike Maier prepared for a World Cup event in the Bavarian resort of Garmisch-Partenkirchen, she was at a crossroads in her life.

"Ulli" was 26, in her 10th season on the World Cup circuit. She was one of the stars of the great Austrian team and a medal contender in the slalom races in the upcoming Olympics in Lillehammer, Norway. Maier also had a four-year-old daughter, Melanie, with partner Hubert Schweighofer, an Austrian police officer, and they were planning to marry in September.

A thought kept recurring. Perhaps it was time to retire. Her daughter was growing up, and she and Hubert were tired of leaving her in the care of her grandparents while they both traveled for work. She'd compete through the end of the season and attempt to make up for her so-so showing at the 1992 Olympics in Albertville, France. Then she'd return with Hubert and Melanie to her native village of Rauris, 100 miles south of Salzburg, and take over the skiing school run by her father.

Her career was already long and storied. She joined the Austrian World Cup squad at age 15 and made her racing debut at 17. Maier was three months pregnant when she won the super giant slalom (super G) title at the 1989 world championships. After her victory she said that she and her unborn child had skied "two as one."[1] Two years later she repeated as super G world champion. A week before the event in Bavaria she won for the fifth time in her World Cup career in a giant slalom in Maribor, Slovenia. At that point she stood fourth in the 1994 standings. She also remained the only mother on the tour.

An overnight storm on January 28 dumped a fresh layer of heavy snow on the fabled Kandahar course. The next day, as officials prepared for the downhill race, the start was delayed for an hour.

Of all the competitions on the Alpine tour, the downhill was Maier's weakest. She entered it only because she hoped to pick up a few extra points in the overall standings. She was far more skilled in the slalom, giant slalom and super G, which focus more on technical skiing. Weaving in and out of gates spread 10 or more meters apart, racers make their way down winding courses with a series of dips, turns and small jumps. Points are deducted for missed gates.

The downhill was different. The goal was to reach the finish line at the bottom as fast as possible in one run while staying within the borders of the course. Excessive speed was a constant concern. Between 1959 and 1993, five men died in downhill races. And as the years went on, the skiers kept getting faster. In 1994, the average top speed for male competitors often reached 80 mph. For women the number was 65 mph.

Many people thought the situation was spiraling out of control. The ominous presence of ice magnified the issue. Two hours before her fatal run, Maier expressed concern about it to race officials. Other skiers believed the run was too dangerous for the same reason. Officials responded by breaking up the icier stretches of the Kandahar course, but much of the ice remained in place.

A related issue was the use of a chemical called PTX3, designed to keep snow from melting in high temperatures. After Maier's accident American skier Picabo Street complained that the substance had "turned the course into a skating rink."[2]

As television viewers in Austria watched live, Maier was the 32nd skier down in a field of 67. Her run began smoothly, and she maneuvered well through the upper portion of the 1.7-mile course that contained the most ice.

Then, on a straight, seemingly safe stretch just 200 yards from the finish, disaster struck. Moving at 60 mph, she hit a patch of soft snow on the right side of the course and slammed into a pile of straw covered with hard-packed ice, which was serving as a mount for a timing post. Her helmet flew off and she somersaulted violently several times before sliding to a stop.

At first it was not clear how seriously she had been hurt. But after medics attempted to revive her without success at the scene, she was placed on a stretcher, winched up to a helicopter and flown 15 miles to a hospital in Murnau. Her neck was broken. The main artery in her chest was ripped open. Surgery was not possible, and she was pronounced dead three hours later. The chief doctor at the hospital delivered the horrible news to the world—"she had no chance."[3]

Hubert Schweighofer was outraged. He visited the accident site the next day and burst into tears. He blamed International Ski Federation (FIS) officials for promising to implement safety improvements and then doing nothing. He immediately threatened to file a lawsuit against them.

But after an investigation by the Munich prosecutor and German police found that all the standard safety measures had been in place, he backed off. The consensus thinking was that in downhill racing, risk is ever present. The accident that killed Maier could have occurred on any course in the world. Despite that, FIS in 1996 agreed to pay $496,000 in compensation to Melanie Maier. They characterized the payment as a moral, not a legal, obligation.

Before a crowd of 5,000, funeral services were held in Rauris on February 3. Eight members of the Austrian men's skiing team lowered Maier's wooden coffin into the ground in Ostfriedhof Cemetery.

## Fabio Casartelli: Deadly Descent
*Tour de France 1995*

Moving at a speed of 55 mph, the biker whisked through a series of tight bends as he descended a steep mountain pass in the Pyrenees in southern France, just miles from the border with Spain.

As he entered a left turn in the middle of the peloton, a huge spill erupted up ahead. Two bikers tumbled to the ground 10 yards in front of him. Trying to swerve around them, he lost his balance and careened onto the right side of the road, smashing his bare head into a block of concrete the size of a standard-issue gravestone. It was positioned there to keep cars from rolling down the ravine to the stream below.

Television cameras covering the race swooped in for close-ups as he lay curled up on the pavement, blood spurting from his nose, ears and mouth. Medics arrived in seconds, but there wasn't anything they could do. A bare human head meeting concrete at 55 mph is a mortal scenario. He died in a helicopter as he was being flown to a nearby hospital, 13 days shy of his 25th birthday.

The dead man was Fabio Casartelli, born and raised in the Lake Como region in Lombardy in northern Italy. His widow Annalisa laments the fact that he'll always be remembered for the way he died—on a mountain called Col de Portet d'Aspet on July 18, 1995, during Stage 15 of the Tour de France. She wished more people would remember him for the way he lived.

His amateur record was sterling, with five wins each in 1991 and 1992. The high point was a victory at the 1992 Olympics in Barcelona, where he finished the 194-kilometer (120-mile) road race with a time of 4:35:21. With his win he carried on in the grand tradition of Italian road race gold medalists—Attilio Pavesi (1932), Ercole Baldini (1956), Mario Zanin (1964) and Pierfranco Vianelli (1968).

He turned pro in 1993, joining the Ariostea team. In 1994 he moved to ZG-Mobil and the next year to Team Motorola, where his teammates included Lance Armstrong, the icon who would win seven Tour de France titles before being stripped of them all in a sordid doping scandal.

Casartelli's long-term goal was to race until he was 30 or so, then retire to a new life with Annalisa and their son Marco, born in April 1995. His timeline wasn't as firm as Ulrike Maier's, but he shared the skier's point of view. His sport was dangerous, with more than its fair share of pain and injury. Trying to ride forever was folly. Better to bow out sooner instead of later, with his mind and body at least somewhat intact.

Instead he became the third on-course fatality in the history of the world's greatest bike race, contested every year since 1903 except during the two world wars. In 1935 Spaniard Francisco Cepeda plunged down a ravine near Grenoble, and in 1967 British cyclist Tom Simpson died during a grueling ascent of Mont Ventoux, nicknamed the Killer Mountain, on the stage from Marseille to Carpentras. His death was attributed to heat exhaustion, spurred by the presence of amphetamines in his system. There also have been several other fatal mishaps involving officials, spectators and journalists, most notably in 1964 when nine died after a supply van smashed into a bridge in the Dordogne region in southwest France.

After Casartelli's death controversy arose over whether a helmet would have saved him. He usually rode without one, but on descents he often put on a hard shell. On that day he didn't. Why not? The punishing heat of the Pyrenees was the likeliest explanation. The short duration of the descent may also have been a factor. He might have thought that it wasn't worth the bother.

The tour's senior doctor said that because the point of impact with the concrete would not have been covered by a helmet, it would have done no good. The Team Motorola medical staff concurred, but the doctor who examined the body on behalf of the coroner strongly disagreed. In his view, the point of impact was clearly the crown of the head, and a helmet might well have reduced the chance of serious injury and possibly even kept him alive. But his opinion did not carry the legal significance of an autopsy, which was never performed, and the controversy lingered.

In spite of that, the tragedy did reignite the longstanding effort to make helmet use compulsory in the professional ranks. By 1995, they'd been around for 20 years or so, but they hadn't been embraced by riders. As in baseball and ice hockey, excess heat on the head was a major complaint, along with impaired vision and the sensation of feeling "hemmed in." There may well have been a touch of machismo involved too. Like many of their brethren in MLB and the NHL, a lot of bikers bought into the notion that helmets were unmanly.

At the time of Casartelli's death, helmets were compulsory for professionals in the U.S., Belgium and the Netherlands but optional in France and Italy. In 1991, when the International Cycling Union (UCI) tried to require them in the Tour de France, angry riders staged a wildcat strike and the union backed off. It wasn't until the death of Andrey Kivilev in the 2003 Paris to Nice race that UCI made them compulsory in all of its sanctioned events.

Near Casartelli's hometown in Lombardy there is a steep hill called Madonna del Ghisallo, named after the woman designated as the patron saint of cycling by Pope Pius XXII in 1949. At the top is a small chapel that also serves as a biking museum. Inside, among pennants, jerseys, photographs and memorabilia, is the crumpled bicycle that Casartelli was riding on the day he died.

## John McSherry: Last Call
### *MLB 1996*

John McSherry knew he had a weight problem. The commanding Bronx native known as Big John had struggled with it all his life. At age 26 in 1971, before beginning his rookie season as the youngest umpire in MLB, he was directed by the National League office to lose 50 pounds. He complied. But it was a temporary reduction. He gained it all back and then some, the struggle continued, and as the years rolled on, he suffered frequent bouts of dehydration and heat exhaustion.

In 1990 he took a leave of absence to enter a weight loss clinic at Duke

University. Two years later he was forced to leave Game 7 of the Braves-Pirates NLCS because of dizziness and shortness of breath. Former catcher and *Today* show regular Joe Garagiola mocked him with a cruel quip—"it looks like McSherry is getting *everybody's* meal money."[4]

As the 1996 season loomed, his "official" weight was 328 pounds. But that was a lowball figure. The real number hovered a shade south of 400. The huge discrepancy is a perplexing mystery and something to ponder. In any case, McSherry passed a physical in February and was medically cleared for duty.

April 1 was Opening Day at Riverfront Stadium in Cincinnati. This was back in the time when the Reds launched their campaign a day before everyone else in honor of their status as America's first professional team. It was always a festive occasion. Adding to the excitement was the managerial debut of former Reds third baseman Ray Knight. McSherry was not the kind to miss a day of work, especially one like this. But he told friends he was flying home to New York the very next morning to seek treatment for his irregular heartbeat.

The cold, blustery day that started with snow gave way to sunny skies in the afternoon, revving up the crowd of 53,000. McSherry seemed disoriented from the get-go. Montreal Expos coach Jim Tracy said later that he heard him slur his speech during the pre-game lineup exchange, perhaps indicating that his fatal seizure was already underway. After the playing of "O Canada" he put on his mask and went behind the plate, apparently forgetting that "The Star Spangled Banner" would also be played.

The first pitch of the game from Reds pitcher Pete Schourek was a perfect strike. He called it a ball. On the seventh pitch of the game to outfielder Rondell White he made no call at all. Then he wrenched his massive bulk upward, took several wobbly steps toward the backstop and slammed nose first onto the warning track.

Team trainers and paramedics encircled him immediately and four doctors bolted from the stands to assist. They turned McSherry over on his back; tore away his shirt, jacket and chest protector; then tilted his head back to try to create an airway. His thick neck made the task difficult. As they administered CPR and adrenaline shots in an effort to revive his heart, the lively crowd turned silent.

Accompanied by distraught colleague Tom Hallion, McSherry was wheeled from the field at 2:28 p.m. and taken by ambulance to University of Cincinnati Hospital. After he was pronounced dead there at 3:01 p.m., the flag in the center field stands at Riverfront was lowered to half-staff. Although several MLB umpires have died during their active careers, including Dick Stello, Lee Weyer and Nick Bremigan, McSherry was believed to be the first to suffer a fatal attack on the field. He was 51 years old.

Confusion set in at that point. There was no announcement of the death over the public address system. Officials from both teams decided to resume the game with the two remaining umpires from the crew, Jerry Crawford and Steve Rippley.

But they reversed their decision at the urging of Reds and Expos players, who believed that continuing to play would have been emotionally painful and inappropriate. The game was played in its entirety the next day, with the Reds winning 4–1.

As the cruel April Fool's Day scene unfolded, garrulous Reds owner Marge Schott lamented the "screwy decision"[5] to postpone the game and put her foot in her mouth in her suite at the top of the stadium. It was something she did often. This gaffe was not as appalling as her many slurs against Blacks, Jews, homosexuals and working mothers. But it was still glaringly off key.

"Snow this morning and now this," Schott grumbled. "I don't believe it. I feel terrible for him and his family but you don't do this to the fans. It's not fair to those who came here from so far away."[6]

The incident drew attention to other MLB umpires with weight issues. The public perception was that many of them were obese, and they were. Their appearance posed an image problem for the game and their lifestyle was at the root of it. Unlike players, there were no home stands for umpires. They traveled to a new city after every series during the six-month season, increasing temptations and opportunities to consume calorie-laden, unhealthy meals in hotels and restaurants.

Eric Gregg confessed in *Sports Illustrated* to a truly gluttonous level of daily consumption. Butter sandwiches from his room service tray, half a dozen beers to wind down after a game, a multi-course feast and a bottle of wine later on. He said that "every day was like New Year's Eve."[7] Two weeks after McSherry's death, he was granted a leave of absence to enter the Duke weight loss clinic. Gregg was forced to exit baseball in 1999 after he was deemed to be persistently over the strict new weight limit of 300 pounds.

His departure ushered in a new emphasis on physical fitness and weight control for umpires that continues today. You don't see any 400-pounders at ball parks anymore. Not even close. Today's umps are as trim and fit as the players, if not more so.

Services for McSherry were held on April 5 at St. Nicholas of Tolentine Church in the Bronx in New York City. Sixteen umpires, one from every National League crew, attended. Joining Yankees legends Babe Ruth and Billy Martin, Big John was buried at Gate of Heaven Cemetery in Hawthorne, New York.

## Caleb Moore: Fatal Obsession
*Snowmobile, X-Games 2013*

Caleb Moore hailed from north Texas, a part of America that rarely sees much snow. But the frame of mind that fueled his rise to stardom as a snowmobiler in the X Games was nurtured in the region's dry, brown, dusty hills.

He started out on trampolines and bicycles. Then he began racing four-wheel ATVs and left high school after his junior year so he could keep at it. Soon he got into motocross tricks. He described his first back flip on an ATV at 19 as the most exciting moment of his life. It provided the rush he craved, the monster high that kicked in each time he landed his quad in front of his fans on the Crusty Demons of Dirt Tour and elsewhere around the world.

When he was 23, he decided to switch from ATVs to snowmobiles. Never mind the fact that he'd never ridden one in his life. He was lured in by the rapid rise of extreme sports, including the X Games, a venture spawned by ESPN in 1995 that included ice climbing, snowboarding and snow mountain bike racing in its first winter competition. Snowmobiling was added in 1998.

He craved a piece of that action, and he practiced landing a sled in a $30,000 foam pit that his father built for him and his younger brother Colten in their back yard in the town of Krum. When he debuted at the Winter X Games, he was mocked as a Texas boy who had to huddle around a space heater because he couldn't handle the cold. He shut a lot of mouths by winning a bronze medal in freestyle snowmobile.

The machine itself—jet quick, nimble, and small and light at 450 pounds—was a big part of the appeal for riders and fans alike. Contestants had a minute and 15 seconds to perform a series of tricks on a variety of jumps. As in bull riding, figure skating and gymnastics, there were judges and rules and scoring systems to rank them.

But all of that somehow seemed to be beside the point. For Caleb and Colten and the rest of their danger-loving brothers in the trade, the gist of the thing was to pull off the trick. It didn't have to be perfect, and it wasn't about how the judges viewed it.

The fans felt the same way. And for many of them there was the added allure of maybe seeing someone crash onto the hard-packed snow and move closer to death's door right in front of their eyes. Or maybe even *through* the door. That outlook bothered many observers of the spectacle. But their beef didn't do much to stem its rising popularity.

The Winter X Games were held in Aspen in 2013. Before a crowd of 15,000 on Buttermilk Mountain on January 24, Moore attempted a jump called the Tsunami Indy Flip. It was a flamboyant stunt he'd pulled off uncountable times. But on this day that wasn't to be. Twirling in the air, his snowmobile under-rotated, and as Moore tried to land it, the ski tips snagged on the top of the approach ramp, pitching him forward over the handlebars and tumbling down the hill. The runaway machine then slammed into his upper body from behind. He blacked out and lay still on the snow face up, his arms and legs stretched out.

A few minutes later Moore came to and walked off the course to a medical tent clutching his father's arm. His brother—who would rupture his pelvis half an hour later doing the same trick—thought he looked OK. Caleb had already broken his ankle, pelvis, wrist, back and tailbone. He'd also suffered a dozen or so concussions. This appeared to be more of the same.

But at Aspen Valley Hospital doctors found bleeding in his chest. A blade on the snowmobile had pierced his heart. With his pulse soaring and his blood pressure diving, they ordered him airlifted to St. Mary's Hospital in Grand Junction, 125 miles west of Aspen.

Moore might have survived if Mother Nature had granted him quicker access to heart surgeons. Under normal conditions, the trip would have taken an hour by helicopter. But heavy snow, ice and high winds had grounded all choppers. That required a road trip by ambulance to the town of Rifle, 67 miles away, where a twin-engine turbo prop plane waited. By the time it finally took off with Moore aboard, six hours had elapsed since the accident.

Moore's heart stopped beating during transport, and he did not regain consciousness for the next seven days. He was pronounced dead at St. Mary's at 9:30 a.m. on January 31. The official cause of death was irreversible brain damage caused by lack of oxygen. His organs were donated. On February 7, Charles Caleb Moore, 25, was laid to rest in Wheeler County in the Texas panhandle.

He was the first competitor to die in the X Games, and a string of emotions ripped through the tight-knit community. Sadness, anguish, heartbreak, sympathy, anxiety, fear. Missing from the list was *surprise*. It was almost as if the tragedy was expected. And if it hadn't been Moore, it would have been someone else.

In the months following his death, critics of freestyle snowmobiling raised their voices. In their view it was pure daredevilry, gussied up to look like an athletic competition. The endeavor seemed designed to invite deadly disaster. The *Atlantic* implored the X Games to abolish it, saying the skills of the riders certainly could be put to better use in less risky arenas.

Snowmobiling wasn't the only event to draw scrutiny. Sarah Burke, 29, a Canadian freestyle skier who performed daring high-speed moves within the walls of a 22-foot half pipe, died in 2012 after wiping out during a training run in Park City, Utah. Then, 10 months after Moore's death, Nick Mevoli, 32, died in freediving's Vertical Blue Competition at Dean's Blue Hole in the Bahamas. In freediving, contestants set a target depth, stroke down through the water in an effort to reach it and then resurface, all in a single breath.

Mevoli's goal was to become "the deepest man on Earth," and he was gunning for a record depth of 236 feet. As his lungs shrank to the size of two baseballs, he turned back toward the surface after spending three minutes and 38 seconds underwater and reaching 223 feet. When he resurfaced, he passed out. He died several hours later at Vidd Sims Memorial Health Center on Long Island, 165 miles southeast of Nassau.

Moore, Burke and Mevoli put their lives on the line in an extreme way that went far beyond the dangers encountered in mainstream sports. To many people it all seemed like a decadent, senseless waste.

After a half-baked effort to remove freestyle snowmobiling from the X Games met with resistance from riders, the high-flying show went on. Organizers made a few changes in the rules, requiring riders to wear Kelvar chest protectors with foam padding and installing extra fencing along the course to protect spectators from wayward snowmobiles. Colten Moore won freestyle gold at the 2014 Winter X Games before a severe spinal injury ended his career three years later.

In 2021, organizers at long last nixed snowmobiling from the schedule of X Games events, citing budget constraints. It has not reappeared since. For better or worse, one act in the daredevil circus looks to be on its way to extinction.

## Oshi: Breaking Point
*Iditarod 2019*

The Iditarod Trail Sled Dog Race arose from the frigid, snowy climate and rugged terrain of Alaska, where dog teams have been ingrained in the cultures of Eskimo natives and white settlers for hundreds of years. Made up largely of Alaskan Malamutes and Siberian Huskies, the teams transported humans, food, mail and vital supplies to huge swaths of the vast land America acquired from Russia in 1867.

In 1925, the world was captivated by radio reports of dogsleds making the 647-mile journey from the village of Neena to Nome to deliver serum needed to quell a diphtheria outbreak. "The Serum Run" saved the lives of many children and transformed Balto, the lead dog on the final leg, into a canine celebrity second only to Rin Tin Tin. Today, a bronze statue of Balto stands atop a rock in Central Park in New York City.

With the advent of snowmobiles after World War II, sled dogs started to disappear from the landscape of the Last Frontier. To revive the heritage and commemorate the Serum Run, Dorothy G. Page and Joe Redington, Sr., put on a 50-mile race along the Iditarod Trail, named after a once-thriving gold mining center turned ghost town.

From those humble roots in 1967 the Iditarod grew into what is labeled the Last Great Race on Earth. The route runs 1,100 miles northwest from Anchorage to Nome, on the coast of the Bering Sea. Mushers and their dogs face every kind of challenge imaginable—subzero temperatures, gale force winds, chill factors close to minus 100, long hours of darkness, thick forests, barren tundra, and numerous species of gnarly wildlife.

In 1973, Dick Wilmarth, the first winner on the new route, covered the distance in 21 days. Today's elite mushers with larger teams and superior training and equipment can do it in close to eight.

The starting gun sounds in downtown Anchorage on the first Saturday in March. The southern route to Nome is run in odd years, the northern route in even years. Mushers start with teams of 12 to 16 dogs weighing 35 to 60 pounds each, pulling sleds with a total weight of 300 to 350 pounds. That number includes the sled itself, made of plastic and lightweight metals like aluminum and titanium, all gear and the musher. Wheel dogs, the largest and strongest, are harnessed right in front of the sled. Lead dogs, smart, light and fast, run in the front. Elite teams move at 10 mph, covering some 130 miles in a 16-hour day that includes mandatory rest stops.

Men and women compete on a completely equal basis. Does any other event in the sports world work that way? Libby Riddles was the first female champion in 1985. Susan Butcher won four out of five races from 1986 to 1990. Mushers from more than 20 countries have entered and Martin Buser of Switzerland has won four times.

In a typical year, 50 to 60 mushers start the race, most of them native Alaskans. The front-runners are full-time professionals, but the also-rans hold a variety of day jobs—lawyer, doctor, farmer, miner, fisherman, truck driver, teacher. Volunteers assume the bulk of the worker bee duties. The mood is merry and festive. The communal vibe is strong. For two glorious weeks the eyes and ears of the world are on them all as they bring off Alaska's signature event.

But there's a dark side to it all. There always has been. Death in the Iditarod is as constant as the North Star. No musher has ever died, but more than 150 sled dogs have perished in the history of the race. Those are just the documented deaths. Early records are sketchy. And how many more die at kennels in the off-season and during grueling training sessions? That's very difficult to determine. It's not the kind of information mushers are eager to share with the outside world.

Most dogs die of aspiration pneumonia, brought on by traumatic, intense physical stress. As they move, they ingest loads of germs and viral substances. The lungs become inflamed and infected and shut down. The digestive system unhinges and lurches into reverse and the dogs choke to death on their own vomit.

There are other causes as well. Some dogs freeze to death or expire from exhaustion. They collapse and never get up. Those deaths are often logged as *cause undetermined*. In 2013, Dorado suffocated in a snow drift in Unalakeet. In 2016, a dog was killed by a drunken snowmobiler who blacked out behind the wheel near Mulato. The next year a motorist struck and killed Groovey in Anchorage.

Hundreds of dogs who don't die break down from broken bones, pulverized paws and bleeding ulcers on the course. The winnowing of the teams only puts more stress on the dogs that continue. The numbers from the 2019 race are typical—726 started, 363 dropped out along the route, 362 finished and survived. And one died.

The casualty was Oshi, a five-year-old female on the Wildthingz team of rookie musher Richie Beattie. As he crossed the finish line in Nome at 10 p.m. on

March 14, eight dogs were harnessed in the front of the sled. Oshi was stashed in Beattie's thick fabric sled bag. It's really more of a roomy basket, large enough to hold gear, food and disabled dogs.

How did she end up there? Speaking to reporter Daniella Rivera from KTVA, Beattie pooh-poohed the question. "Yeah, yeah, she's just tired," he said.[8]

Vets who examined her at the last eight-hour rest stop in White River found nothing wrong, and she was moving well through the first part of the final 77-mile leg of the race. Then she started to falter. Her breathing was labored. Her gait was off. The peppy girl nicknamed Yo-Yo for her bounce suddenly had no bounce. Beattie unleashed her and relieved her of duty.

During the post-race check-up vets detected signs of pneumonia. She was taken to an animal hospital in Nome to receive oxygen and antibiotics. Her condition worsened and the next morning Beattie chartered a private plane to transport her to Anchorage. His wife accompanied her on the flight.

Oshi died of aspiration pneumonia on Saturday, March 16. Beattie claimed to be devastated. He said losing Oshi was no different from losing a member of his human family.

Under a new rule adopted in 2018, mushers who have a dog die during the Iditarod must withdraw from the race, unless the death was due to an "unpreventable hazard," such as being struck by a drunken snowmobile driver. Oshi's death did not meet that description and Beattie became the first musher penalized under the rule.

Because the death occurred after the finish he could not literally withdraw. But he forfeited his prize money, including a bonus for being the first rookie musher in the field to complete the race. At the same time, Beattie was not cited for any "deliberate misconduct," which would have drawn harsher punishment.

To the critics watching in disgust from the sidelines, it all seemed like so much nonsense. To them the Iditarod—and all the other dogsled races in Alaska and throughout the world—are exercises in deliberate misconduct by definition.

People for the Ethical Treatment of Animals (PETA) raised the most strident objections, just as they were doing 2,900 miles to the southeast near Los Angeles. It was a sad coincidence that at the time of Oshi's death thoroughbred horses were dying in record numbers at Santa Anita Park. On the very day the Iditarod began in Anchorage, a filly named Princess Lili B was euthanized after breaking both legs during a training run. Racing itself was in the middle of a three-week shutdown, prompted by the deaths of 21 horses in the first two months of the year.

In PETA's view, dogsled racing, like horse racing, cannot be "reformed" by fiddling with the rules. It cannot somehow be made "safe" for the animals who put their lives on the line solely for the benefit of human beings seeking fame, glory, riches and entertainment. That goes for horse racing as well, along with every other so-called sport that exploits animals.

All are examples of what they call speciesism, a world view that espouses the

## 7. In the Arena Redux

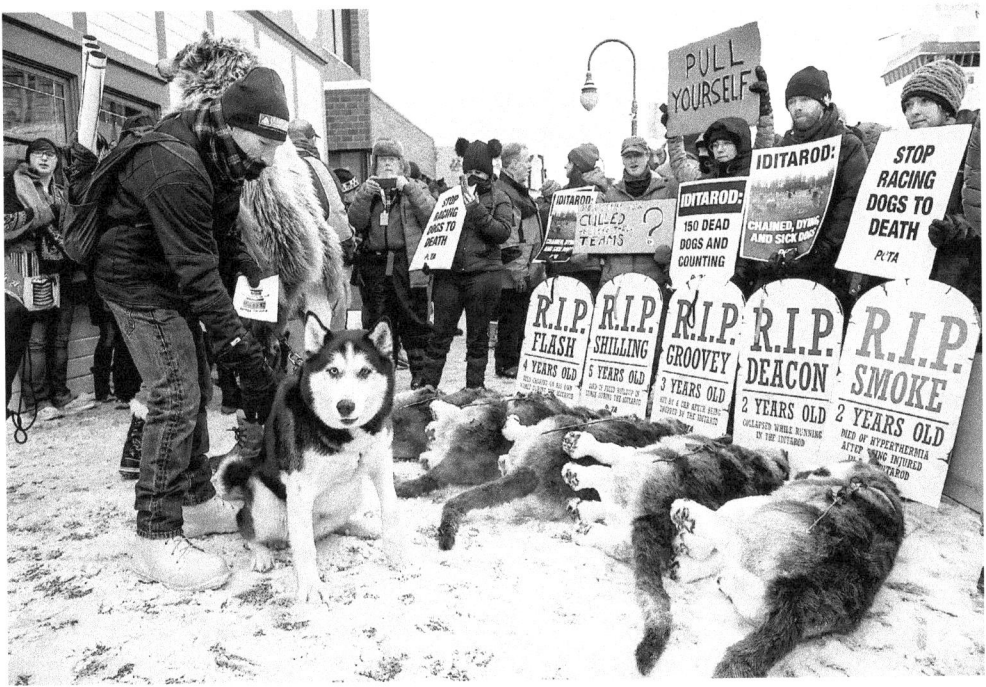

Anchorage resident Terry Fischer and his Alaskan Husky Litho cross paths with PETA protesters before the start of the 2018 Iditarod on March 3. The event is facing an ongoing storm of criticism over the brutal punishment it inflicts on sled dogs. More than 150 have died since the first race in 1967. Two thousand eighteen would see the death of Blondie, a five-year-old male in the team of Katherine Keith. He succumbed to aspiration pneumonia at the Koyuk checkpoint (AP Images/Michael Dinneen).

absolute supremacy of human beings over all other forms of creature life. *Let's get this straight once and for all. We didn't reach the top of the food chain for nothing. We are the lords and masters of the universe. Animals exist for our benefit. We can beat them, buy them, sell them, wear them, eat them, and kill them—whatever suits our fancy.*

To some extent PETA is getting what it wants. Bullfighting is now legal in only eight countries. Cockfighting and dogfighting are dwindling away to near extinction. So is greyhound racing. In the 1980s there were more than 50 greyhound tracks in 19 states across America. By 2023 only two remained, both in West Virginia. They operate with subsidies from casino revenue.

Will dogsled racing also face demise? The ongoing protests have prompted Exxon, Wells Fargo Bank, Jack Daniels and Alaska Airlines to drop their sponsorships of the Iditarod. A series of doping scandals, in which several dogs tested positive for opioids, has heightened the race's negative image. So have undercover exposés of pervasive brutality and abuses during training, including the outright killing of dogs deemed to be unfit for competition. The 2023 race included only 33 teams, a record low.

But total abolition seems like a longshot. Like horse racing, dogsled racing is entrenched, popular, and protected by government. At least in Alaska. So the best bet is that next year, on the first Saturday in March, the Iditarod will kick off one more time in downtown Anchorage. And like always, the deaths of any dogs that may occur will be viewed as acceptable losses.

## Yellow River Stone Forest: 21 Gone
*Ultramarathon 2021*

Roughly the size and shape of California, Gansu province lies in a remote region of north-central China, some 1,000 miles west of Beijing. Flat in the north and mountainous in the south, it has long been mired in poverty, with an economy centered on nothing much more than the mining of nickel, coal and copper. The province has been plagued throughout history by earthquakes, droughts and famines. In 1920, a series of landslides triggered by a single quake killed 180,000.

As the 21st century arrived, the economic outlook for most of Gansu's 25 million people was more of the same. One small ray of hope was China's physical fitness boom, spurred by a widespread desire among the population to lead healthier, more active lives.

Gyms and fitness centers were springing up everywhere, even in Gansu. Hiking had become a popular pastime and distance running was flourishing. In 2011 the nation saw 22 marathons. Eight years later there were 1,828. The number of ultralong trail running events skyrocketed from 16 in 2013 to 481 in 2019.

One of the most prominent was the 100-kilometer (62.14-mile) race through the Yellow River Stone Forest region in Jingtai County in Ginsu. The course wound on a sand and stone path through harsh, largely treeless terrain called karst, full of eroded limestone formations, sinkholes and barren, isolated hills. Parts of it were very steep. The ups and downs could exhaust even the most accomplished runners. The event had become a source of pride and a boon for stores, restaurants, hotels and tourist sites in the area. And for one weekend in the spring of 2021, the fifth edition of the race in Yellow River Stone Forest captured the attention of a large part of the world.

But it was hardly the kind of attention Gansu wanted. What played out at a place called Mijiashan Hill was a terrifying nightmare.

The first distress signals were received via WeChat at 12:17 p.m., three hours after the starting gun sounded on Saturday, May 22. Some 15 miles into the course, as they labored up a steep mountain pass 7,300 feet above sea level, runners in the lead pack were being assaulted by a fierce storm thundering in from Mongolia to the north. The chilly, overcast day had suddenly turned very nasty. The temperature nosedived, gooey snow pellets (graupel) and hail began to fall and wind speeds soared to 50 mph.

Most of the racers in the field of 172 were woefully underdressed, wearing only shorts and T-shirts or singlets. The few who were carrying emergency blankets saw them ripped to shreds by the wind. The runners were hung out to dry on the bleak landscape.

It would be more accurate to say they were hung out to *die.*

That stretch of the course was inaccessible by vehicle. Even though more than 1,000 responders eventually arrived on the scene with headlamps, flashlights and thermal imaging drones, the rescue effort was slow and ineffective. There was no coherent chain of command. Many responders got lost on the way to the danger zone. Helicopters were unavailable, and the urgency of the situation was not fully realized until 6 p.m.

By then it was too late. The slower runners managed to make their way back toward the start line and safety. But 18 males and three females from the lead pack were dead or dying. Some fell off the path into deep mountain crevices, but most perished from hypothermia. The condition can arise even in temperatures above freezing. It starts with shivering and brings on extreme fatigue, blurred vision, stiff limbs and mental confusion. Many victims foam at the mouth, and death can arrive within an hour.

Among the dead were two of the country's most renowned distance runners. Liang Jing, 31, nicknamed "Liang God" for his endurance, was a three-time winner of the Yellow River race. His stopwatch recovered at the scene displayed a zero pulse rate at 1:08 p.m. Huang Guanjun, 33, a deaf marathon champion in China's Paralympic Games, died running his first 100-kilometer event.

The most dramatic rescue was carried out by a shepherd named Zhu Keming. He was herding his sheep when the storm hit, and he managed to round up six soaked, shivering runners and guide them to his yaodong, or house cave. There, with pages he ripped from his books, he kept his small fire alive. As they all recovered, Zhu looked out the entrance of the yaodong and spotted three corpses lying on a nearby hillside.

Rescue efforts ceased at noon on Sunday. In its own way, the aftermath was as nightmarish as the calamity on the course. Media reports first indicated that there was no advance warning of the storm. That turned out not to be true. Forecasters had been calling for hail, falling temperatures and high winds on race day for nearly 72 hours.

Why did officials—and most of the runners, for that matter—ignore the predictions? What on Earth were people thinking? Maybe they weren't aware of the forecast. That makes absolutely zero sense, but it could still be true. A likelier explanation is that they knew about the potential danger but decided that, come hell or high water, the show would go on.

The utterly lax preparation for the race was also a mind-boggler. There were no staffers or first aid stations on the segment of the course where the runners were trapped. The two nearest checkpoints were located in mobile phone blind spots. Racers were merely encouraged, not required, to carry protective gear. The small race day crew was assembled just a week before the event. And the company in charge of the run had only one permanent employee—the owner.

Many commentators described the situation as business as usual in a country where lazy oversight and minimal regulation rule the day in every aspect of daily life, especially in the industrial sector. That laissez-faire philosophy is ironic in a nation with one of the most intrusive, authoritarian governments in the world, where an entire city the size of Chicago was shut down lock, stock and barrel in the early months of the Covid pandemic.

Could the deadly fiasco have occurred in the United States or any other advanced country? Never say never, of course. But that seems nearly inconceivable.

The staggering death toll and saturation media coverage compelled the Gansu provincial government to launch an immediate probe. Within a week, 27 local officials and race organizers were found to be negligent and faced punishment. On June 7, one of them, Jingtai County Communist Party Secretary Li Zuobi, committed suicide.

After the tragedy, the China Sports Administration indefinitely suspended all high-risk sporting events nationwide, including ultralong running races. That seemed like an empty gesture by nervous bureaucrats, designed to quell public outrage and save face. So did the pitifully small sum of $150,000 offered as compensation, to be shared by the surviving families of all 21 victims. What ultralong races will look like in China if and when they resume is anyone's guess.

Let's come back to America now and look at sudden death in horse racing. We'll visit Belmont Park, Yonkers Raceway, Kentucky bluegrass country, the bush tracks of the South and Santa Anita Park, where we'll learn more about the meltdown in 2019 that claimed the lives of 30 equine athletes.

# 8

## Win, Place or Die

### Frank Hayes: First Win, Only Win
*Steeplechase 1923*

Horse racing is a perilous enterprise. When a dozen or more animals weighing 1,100 pounds apiece circle a track in a tight pack at speeds of up to 40 mph, bad things can happen.

Racehorses are equine versions of teenagers, and like their human counterparts they can get bold and unruly. In a flash the powerful beasts can become very difficult to control. They can also crash and burn. Mishaps are inevitable, and sometimes people die. The Jockey Guild reports 144 deaths in North America since 1940. Thirteen professional jockeys have died worldwide since 2000. Nobody can predict when or where it might happen next. But death on the track is an ongoing feature of the Sport of Kings.

Most accidents follow a similar pattern. At some point in a race or workout a horse breaks a leg or a fetlock (ankle) or veers into the rail or trips on the heels of another horse or buckles and drops from sheer fatigue. Many times a breakdown in a race morphs into a spill that takes down up to half the field. The jockeys jump, fall or get thrown off their mounts and roll, run or curl up on the turf to protect themselves. They then get run over, stomped on and kicked by their own mounts or by an onrushing horse moving so fast that it can't be stopped or even slowed down much.

The death of Frank Hayes deviated from the norm. A lot of folks even call it one of a kind. He's the only jockey ever to win a race while dead. It doesn't get any more high concept than that. The fact that the death occurred at Belmont Park, one of the meccas of the sport, gives it an added dose of dash. The incident has become a treasured piece of horse racing lore.

Problem is, the story almost surely isn't true.

Hayes was an Irish immigrant and a stable hand and exercise rider who'd worked for trainer James K. Frayling for four years. Like many workers at the track, he was eager beyond words to get into a real race himself. He'd only been in one in his life. On June 4, 1923, he climbed on Sweet Kiss, an aged reddish-brown mare, one of five horses in a steeplechase, the second run on the Belmont program. The circular course was about two miles long. The purse was $1,000.

Sweet Kiss traded the lead gamely with betting favorite Gimme through 12 jumps, then won a sprint to the finish to prevail by a length and a half over the gelding. After Hayes crossed the finish line and slowed his horse to a walk, he slumped over her neck, as if to adjust a stirrup, then crashed onto the turf. As Sweet Kiss stepped around him into the grip of an exercise boy, a score of frantic onlookers surrounded Hayes. The track physician pronounced him dead on the spot. He was either 22 or 35 years old. The sources conflict.

Four days later he was buried in his racing silks at Holy Cross Cemetery in Brooklyn. His mount reportedly never raced again, but the incident earned her a lifelong nickname—Sweet Kiss of Death.

The question of the hour then presented itself—at what point did Hayes actually die? The *New York Times* reported on June 5 that he may have been first stricken by a seizure at the moment Sweet Kiss swerved into and nearly hit Gimme as they rounded the last turn on the course. But the *Times* concluded that he "undoubtedly died as he brought his mount to a walk *after* [emphasis added] passing the winning post."[1]

There's a different version of the event that has endured for a century. Wikipedia and *The Guinness Book of World Records* both assert that Hayes expired during the race and actually crossed the finish line as a dead man.

The claim seems spurious. If that were the case, how did Sweet Kiss slow to a walk after the race was over? And how could a corpse remain upright in the saddle through the last stages of the race? Hayes probably died when his head smashed onto the turf after he fell out of his saddle.

No concrete evidence of the mishap survives. There are no more living eyewitnesses. With that in mind, perhaps it's best to revise the record and put it this way—Frank Hayes is the only jockey to ever win a race and then die before weighing in. That's astonishing enough for him to keep his place in history.

There's another aspect of the story that is worth a look. The vital question for our time is not when Hayes died, but how and why. That's where the ritual of weighing in comes into play.

To be qualified to run a race, jockeys are required to weigh a specified amount. If they're above the number, they are disqualified. If they're below it, pieces of lead are packed into their saddle cloth to meet the mandated number. But trainers don't like the lead pieces. They think it's more efficient to carry all the weight in a human body because a body can move with the horse instead of just sitting there like, well, dead weight. So jockeys face intense pressure to hit the nail on the head when they step on the scale before the start. They weigh in with their saddles, helmets and other gear at that time and do the same after the finish to confirm that the horse did indeed carry the specified weight.

Hayes' assigned weight for his steeplechase at Belmont was 130 pounds. In the days before the race he weighed 142 pounds. A hundred years ago exercise riders were allowed to weigh more than jockeys. They still are. His difficult task was to drop 12 pounds in a very short period of time, thought to be about 48 hours.

All signs point to that reduction effort as the cause of death. There were opinions expressed that he may have had a weak heart to begin with and that his giddy excitement over winning proved to be too much for it to handle. True enough to a point, perhaps. But he also sweated profusely and recklessly in the summer heat, running for hours on end near the racetrack, all the while denying himself food and water. That is very likely what killed him. The root cause of his demise was extreme dehydration.

His ordeal was part of a tradition in horse racing that continues today. Jockeys have long engaged in many types of dangerous behavior to "make weight." They skip meals on the regular. They gobble laxatives to expel fecal waste and drink Lasix and other diuretics to leech water out of their thighs and bellies and butts. They induce vomiting, known in the trade as "flipping." They peddle stationary bikes in rubber suits and gloves and wool caps. They snort and swallow amphetamines and smoke cigarettes to suppress their appetites. Then they park themselves in the "hot box," a sauna heated to 140 degrees or so, for as long as needed to sweat out the necessary pounds.

When their efforts get too extreme, which is often, they endanger not only themselves but horses and other jockeys as well. They become so weak and disoriented that they lose their mental bearings on the track. They also degrade parts of their bodies, particularly shoulders and thighs, that must be in excellent shape to compete effectively.

Hayes is not the only jockey to die for the sake of a mount. More recently, Scott McKenzie, based at Penn National Race Course in Pennsylvania, starved himself to death in 2000. Five years later, Emanuel Jose Sanchez, a 22-year-old apprentice at Colonial Downs in Virginia, collapsed on a shower floor in the jockey room and died later in a hospital of dehydration. Randy Romero, who rode from 1975 through 1999 in his native Louisiana and Kentucky, ravaged his body so badly by reducing that he needed a kidney transplant and contracted hepatitis C. He died of stomach cancer in 2019.

In recent years, authorities in New York, California, Florida, and Kentucky have eased weight limits for jockeys, allowing them to carry up to six more pounds. There is also growing support for a requirement that they maintain a specified amount of body fat, such as 5 percent.

But wholesale change in the decentralized and often contentious business has proved difficult. The old way of doing things has its defenders. Most trainers and owners believe that letting jockeys carry even a few more pounds unduly stresses their animals. Many jockeys who weigh so little naturally that they don't need to engage in traumatic reducing are loath to give up their competitive advantage. And some people dismiss the reformers as a bunch of crybabies. You're either light enough to get to the starting gate or you're not. If you can't make weight, it's nobody's fault but your own. Go find another line of work.

So the frightful tale of Frank Hayes lives on. The beast that killed him—a compulsive, obsessive desire to drop body weight in exchange for a chance at thrills, riches, fame and glory—is alive and snarling in the racing world.

## Ruffian: She Reigns
*Match Race 1975*

The simple gravestone is embedded in the grass beneath the flagpole at Belmont Park on Long Island, the storied track that has brought glory to so many of the world's horses. Beneath it lies a horse who can surely be ranked among the very greatest and who may have been the greatest of all.

Ruffian was more than a star. She was a supernova who emitted a vast amount of brilliance and energy in her short life. In the end, the qualities that made her a legend were the same ones that led to her untimely death.

The filly was foaled at 10:10 p.m. on April 17, 1972, at Claiborne Farm in Paris, Kentucky, 20 miles northeast of Lexington in the heart of thoroughbred country. She ran for the first time less than 12 hours after birth, loping around the perimeter of the paddock with her mother. Twenty months later, owners Stuart Janney, Jr., and his wife Barbara sent her to the Marion du Pont Training Center in Camden, South Carolina.

There the gangly black horse with a white star on her forehead came under the tutelage of Frank Whiteley, Jr., who would train her for the rest of her career. At that point she had no name. People called her simply the filly; or Shenanigans, after her mother; or Sophie, as in sofa, a reference to her impressive, comfortable looking bulk.

Whiteley was a taciturn, driven man who had been in the business 40 years. He'd trained Tom Rolfe and Damascus in the 1960s and he knew he had a phenomenal pupil on his hands. After five months at Camden, Whiteley shipped her north to Belmont Park. On May 22, 1974, he entered her in a five-and-a-half-furlong race for fillies. On her entry form he wrote the name Ruffian, a takeoff on the Spanish word *rufián*, for bully or fighter. She won by a jaw-dropping 15 lengths in a time of 1:03, tying the track record.

She won four more races that summer. Crowds began lining up for her, chanting her name as if she were a rock star or an English princess, eager for a close-up glimpse of the horse that had the jaded racing press in a tizzy. In August, Whiteley discovered a hairline fracture in her right hind leg. He encased her foot in a pillow cast and confined her to her stall for eight weeks. It was not an injury that threatened her career, but he was taking no chances. Her two-year-old season was finished.

## 8. Win, Place or Die

As 1975 arrived, there was excited talk about a showdown in the Triple Crown races between Ruffian and Foolish Pleasure, the premier colt of the day. Whiteley would have none of it. He turned a deaf ear to the clamor. It would require too much effort too early in the season, especially after her layoff. What he and the Janneys had in mind was a run at the Triple Crown for fillies, a feat accomplished only four times.

Ruffian made it five. She won two early races, then the Acorn Stakes, the Mother Goose Stakes and finally the Coaching Club American Oaks, where she dispelled any doubts about her ability to win at long distances, finishing the mile and a half in a faster time that Avatar had posted in winning the Belmont two weeks earlier. She had started 10 races in two years and won them all by an average of eight lengths.

Trainer Lucien Lauren offered the ultimate compliment. "As God is my judge," he said, "she may be even better than Secretariat."[2] Lauren knew what he was saying. He'd trained Big Red himself.

The only thing Ruffian had not done was race against a colt. Foolish Pleasure stood at the ready. After his undefeated season as a two-year-old, he won the Kentucky Derby and missed the Triple Crown by no more than the length of his body, finishing second in the Preakness and Belmont.

Belmont Park and the New York State Racing Association proposed a match race between the two, to be broadcast by CBS television. The winner would receive $225,000, $15,000 more than Foolish Pleasure won at Churchill Downs in May. The loser would earn $125,000.

The status of Jacinto Vásquez was a sticking point. He was the varsity jockey for both horses, having ridden Ruffian in eight of 10 races and Foolish Pleasure in 10 of 14. Vásquez would have to pick one or the other. He chose Ruffian because of strong pressure from Whiteley and also because he thought she had a better chance to win. Aboard Foolish Pleasure would be Braulio Baeza, like Vásquez a native of Panama and a sterling professional.

The announcement of the Great Match Rate unleashed a flurry of anticipation and excitement. Head-to-head faceoffs between thoroughbreds were rare. There had been less than 10 significant ones in the 20th century. To experts they proved little about the true worth of the competitors, but to fans they offered great excitement. The strategy was always the same—start furiously and hold the lead. There had never been a come-from-behind winner.

This time there was the added allure of Boy Meets Girl. The standard view was that fillies lacked the size, speed and stamina to run well over the long haul against colts. But if there was ever a horse poised to challenge conventional wisdom it was Ruffian, and that turned the race into a symbolic event and a honky-tonk carnival, not unlike the Billie Jean King–Bobby Riggs tennis duel in the Astrodome in 1973. The racing association distributed 100,000 HIM and HER buttons. All true supporters of the blossoming women's liberation movement stood staunchly with the filly. On the other side were the traditional, the staid and stodgy, the unenlightened. As one man put it, "I'm for Foolish Pleasure because I'm a male chauvinist pig."[3]

It was all tremendous fun and a little bit silly. Ruffian was in fact a bigger horse than Foolish Pleasure. She weighed 1,125 pounds to his 1,061 and was nearly three inches taller and two and a half inches bigger around the girth. She also had the advantage of carrying only 121 pounds, the standard for fillies, against Foolish Pleasure's 126. As the hype reached its crescendo in the first days of July, she was the betting favorite of horseplayers and the overwhelming choice of trainers, who picked her to prevail in a *Daily Racing Form* poll by a three-to-one margin.

But there was one detail that worried Vásquez and the rest of Ruffian's human family. Their horse was larger than Foolish Pleasure in every measurement but one—shoe size. She wore a size five to his size six. And in the brutal pace of a match race, she would be pounding her bigger body on the hard, dry dirt with hooves that were significantly smaller than her opponent's. That might prove hazardous to the filly's health.

July 6 was a dark, humid Sunday, with lightning in the morning and a strong threat of rain in the afternoon. At Belmont, the Preservation Hall Jazz Band and the Duke Ellington Orchestra serenaded the crowd of 50,764, and as early evening arrived and the skies cleared, the place turned giddy and festive.

At 6 the contestants appeared on the track to wild applause. They circled the big oval and went into the starting gate nearly half a mile from the grandstand, HER on the inside, HIM on the outside.

It was all over in 40 seconds. At the bell, Ruffian slammed her shoulder against the side of the gate and came out almost perpendicular to Foolish Pleasure. Nose to nose they ran the first quarter in 22 and 1/5th, a pace even faster than predicted.

As they approached the half-mile pole, both jockeys heard a sharp crack, like the snapping of a thick tree branch. Ruffian leaned against the rail for a long moment and then pulled to the outside of the track as Foolish Pleasure surged away toward the buzz of the distant crowd and the finish line.

Vásquez hopped down and cradled the filly's right leg. He knew enough at that moment to fear for her life. She was in savage pain. When he heard the crack, he'd done everything in his physical power to stop her advance. But she was too strong for him. She powered on for another 50 yards, pulverizing her right foot and turning it into a pulpy mess of bone, ligament, tendon and muscle.

Sweating profusely, with her foot barely attached to her leg, Ruffian was loaded into a green horse ambulance by hydraulic lift and returned to her stall in Barn 34, where she was pumped full of drugs to combat the immediate dangers of shock, bleeding and infection.

Six doctors offered their unanimous advice to Whiteley and the

Janneys—operate immediately. That was dangerous because it would require anesthetizing the animal before she could cool down and stabilize. But waiting until morning was worse because it would delay the repair for 10 hours and increase the likelihood of even more damage and trauma.

Again Ruffian was loaded into the ambulance, this time for the short ride to the equine hospital of Dr. William O. Reed near the track. The procedure began at 8 p.m. Doctors cleaned the wound and tried in vain to piece together the shattered bones. A massive metal and plaster shoe-boot was placed on the leg. The only thing left to do was hope that Ruffian remained calm after she regained consciousness so the mechanism could do its work and begin the healing process.

When she awoke after midnight she spun wildly in circles. The men in the room tried to control her but she kicked violently and held them off. The operation had proved futile. Ruffian was no better off than she had been seconds after the horrible snapping sound on the backstretch. With her body dehydrated and withered by shock, she could not survive a second operation. Stuart Janney, who had taken his distraught wife home, issued his order by telephone—"please don't let her suffer anymore."[4]

At 2:20 a.m. on July 7, Doctor Reed administered a fatal dose of phenobarbital.

Joseph Durso of the *New York Times* lamented "the end of a gorgeous beast"[5] and asked—like everyone else—why? Vásquez blamed sheer, killing speed, fueled by the one-on-one intensity of the match race. In the end, some unalterable force within Ruffian herself compelled her to make the supreme effort that ended in tragedy.

The races went on at Belmont the next day. In the afternoon, a huge metal digging machine rolled onto the infield and started to turn up dirt near the flagpole. It dug a hole 12 feet deep and 12 feet square. Shortly after eight o'clock that night, as the sun was setting, a group of three dozen gathered at the gravesite. The Janneys had gone to Maine but the rest of Ruffian's family was there. Along the track rail, hundreds of onlookers pressed close, held at bay by Pinkerton guards, and in the grandstand, photographers set up their lights and threw an eerie glow across the landscape.

A moment later, the same ambulance that had taken Ruffian from the backstretch the day before pulled onto the infield, its headlights piercing the twilight. The back door was lowered to form an incline that led directly into the grave. Wrapped completely in white canvas, Ruffian was lowered gently to her resting place. There was no eulogy.

At Whiteley's request, his assistant Mike Bell climbed down into the grave and placed two blankets over the canvas. A single rose was dropped in, and the crowd dispersed. With that simple, silent ceremony, Ruffian assumed her place among the immortals of horse racing.

## Billy Haughton: Breaking Gait
*Harness Racing 1986*

Billy Haughton's career was unlike any other in the annals of harness racing. His record of achievement was extraordinary. With $40.2 million in total earnings, he led the U.S. in annual winnings 12 times, including eight straight years from 1952 to 1959. He might have earned twice that much if he hadn't given away so many drives behind high-performing horses to friends to help bolster their own careers.

Among his 4,910 victories were five Little Brown Jugs, America's premier race for pacers, and four Hambletonians, the leading event for trotters. He also won seven Messenger Stakes. The list of notable horses he drove includes Rum Customer, winner of the pacing Triple Crown in 1968, Green Speed, Handle with Care, LaVerne Hanover and Romulus Hanover.

Haughton was not only a driver but an owner and trainer as well. He trained all nine of his Little Brown Jug and Hambletonian winners. In 1986, he and his wife Dorothy Bischoff "Dottie" Haughton managed the largest racing stable in North America. They bred their love of horses into their offspring. Three of their five children got into the business, including son Peter, who'd already won 41 stakes races when he died in 1980 at age 25 in a car crash after a night of racing at the Meadowlands in New Jersey. Given the depth and breadth of his involvement, Haughton has been described as the greatest all-around horseman in the history of the sport.

It's a sport that differs in many respects from thoroughbred racing, its more prominent counterpart. The standardbred horses in harness racing are heavier and more muscular than thoroughbreds, with longer bodies and longer tails. Thoroughbreds are taller, slimmer and more athletic.

Harness racing is divided into two forms of competition, based on the gait of the horses. Trotters move with a diagonal gait—the left front and right rear legs lift off the ground together, followed by the right front and left rear legs. Pacers use a lateral gait in which the two legs on one side of the body lift at the same time.

About 80 percent of the harness races in America are for pacers. They're faster and more agile than trotters. But they're also more unpredictable and more likely to break gait. If that happens in a race, the horse has to slow down, often to a complete halt, refocus and resume the required leg movement to continue on. That's not a good scenario for its driver or for others approaching from the rear on the track.

Drivers sit behind the horses and guide them from thin, flimsy, two-wheeled, one-seat bikes called sulkies or spiders or race carts. They weigh about 25 pounds. The surface of the track can be composed of dust, dirt or clay, but it any case it's lighter and shallower than the surfaces for thoroughbreds, with much less cushion to buffer a horse or a driver crashing down after a spill.

The start is not stationary. Instead, the field falls in behind a motorized, moving starting gate that speeds ahead of the pack as the starting bell sounds. Standardbreds also race more often, usually three or four times a month. Thoroughbreds generally race once about once a month.

Despite all those differences, there is one great similarity between harness and thoroughbred racing—danger. Drivers and jockeys guide 1,000-pound animals wearing steel shoes around an oval at speeds of 35 mph or more. The packs can get very tight. Sometimes spills can't be avoided. And as in baseball and hockey, the competitors were very slow to embrace the practice of wearing helmets to protect themselves. There seemed to be a cavalier, fatalistic disregard for the risks involved. Lady Luck would keep you and your bare head up and running on the track as long as she deemed appropriate. When it was your time to go, it was your time.

Billy Haughton's time arrived on the night of July 5, 1986, at Yonkers Raceway in New York, 16 miles northeast of the Empire State Building. He was seated in a spider behind a colt named Sonny Key in the first elimination heat of the $600,000 Lawrence B. Sheppard Pace. Eliminations are run to pare the field down to a specified number of horses for the final race.

Haughton was wearing a helmet, and he had been for years. But it resembled the ones worn in baseball, and it didn't offer as much protection as the newer models, which had resilient fiberglass shells and a thicker Styrofoam liner inside. They were very similar to motorcycle helmets. Haughton had looked at a state-of-the art product just a few weeks before and was so impressed he ordered one for himself. But it hadn't arrived from the factory yet.

Switching out helmets was a big step. Like many other athletes—and human beings in general—he was used to doing things a certain way. Change was a challenge. Perhaps mortality had something to do with his decision. He was 62, and if you started counting with the horses he mounted as a boy on his family farm in Gloversville, New York, he'd been in the game for more than half a century.

He was no doubt feeling his age. He won the Hambletonian at 56 in 1980 with Burgomeister, but since then the marquee wins had proved elusive. The end of his career was in sight, and he wanted to make sure he reached it.

On the track that night at Yonkers, a two-year-old colt named Crimson broke pace and slowed to a near stop. The driver was thrown from his sulky but unhurt. Boxed in along the rail, Sonny Key slammed into Crimson at nearly full speed and went down. Haughton's sulky had no seat belt, and he catapulted out of it backward and landed on the track. His head snapped back and struck the surface so fiercely that his helmet split in two.

At Lawrence Hospital in Bronxville he underwent a CT scan. His skull was fractured. His brain injuries were beyond severe. After transfer to Westchester County Medical Center in Valhalla, he was in a coma for 10 days and never regained consciousness before dying on July 15. Haughton was the sixth harness racing driver to die in North America since 1979.

The world mourned the man sometimes called the Babe Ruth of his sport. There will never be another like him. His funeral was held at St. Paul the Apostle Church in Brookville on Long Island. Burial followed at the Cemetery of the Holy Rood in nearby Westbury.

## Mary Bacon: Riding Is Living
*Off Track 1991*

Mary Bacon was a tabloid fantasy done up in broad, bold pastels, a sassy, sexy 98-pound dynamo with an overpowering need for attention and the magnetism to attract it. Her craving for the spotlight was so strong that it obscured her huge talent and impressive if erratic career as one of the first female jockeys in America.

In 22 years, she rode in 3,526 races and won 286. But the numbers don't tell half the story. She ran full throttle, and her death at age 43 was the jarring finale of a life lived outside the limits.

Born in Chicago and raised in Toledo, Mary Steedman fell in love with horses very early on. Inspired by the movie *National Velvet*, she nurtured ponies in her neighbor's farm fields and began working at Raceway Park as a stable hand and outrider in high school.

After graduation she went to England and earned an instructor's degree at a riding academy. But her heart wasn't in teaching. She was hooked on the vibrant, intoxicating lifestyle of the track. Back home she found work as an exercise rider at the Detroit Race Course. There she met her first husband, Johnny "Pug" Bacon.

Her burning ambition was to be a jockey like him. Standing in her way was a big sign posted on the door into that profession—*No Females Need Apply*. You might spot a rogue woman riding now and then at one of the dingy bush tracks scattered around the hinterlands. But America's mainstream racing establishment required licensed jockeys, and the regulatory bodies in the 50 states only granted licenses to men.

Using the 1964 Civil Rights Act as her foundation, equestrian and show rider Kathy Kusner lawyered up and ended that injustice in 1969. She never raced herself, but the ruling she won paved the path for a wave of female jockeys. The stars included Diane Crump, the first woman to ride in the Kentucky Derby in 1970, Barbara Jo Rubin, the first to win a race at Aqueduct, and Robyn Smith, a close friend of Alfred Vanderbilt and later the wife of Fred Astaire.

Bacon was right there with them. Nineteen sixty-nine was a busy year for her. In March she gave birth to a daughter, Suzie, who she promptly handed over to her mother to raise. Three months later she won her first pari-mutuel race at the Finger Lakes track in New York. There would be 54 more wins that year in 396 races.

Along the way came an attempted kidnapping. A track employee in Wilkes-Barre, Pennsylvania, named Paul Corley Turner didn't care for her smartass attitude and the way she was always showing up the guys. In an effort to teach her some manners, he held her at knifepoint in the woods for several hours before she escaped. Two years later Corley reappeared in the bathroom of her motel room in Louisville. How he got there remains a mystery. She attacked him with a pair of scissors. He fired shots from a handgun and bolted. The FBI launched a manhunt, busted him, and sent him to prison for 12 years.

Bacon's career peaked in the early 1970s. She graced the cover of *Newsweek* and appeared in *Vogue*. Her charisma and looks snagged her endorsement deals with Revlon and Dutch Masters. In June 1973, she boldly took it all off for a spread in the *Playboy* feature "Women's Work." She continued to ride and finish in the money at tracks all over the country, breaking numerous bones and often sporting the flowered underpants she wore under her white jockey shorts to give the boys in the saddles behind her something to gape at. Roses and daisies were her designs of choice.

Things unraveled with lightning speed in April 1975. While riding at the Fair Grounds Course in New Orleans, she attended a Ku Klux Klan rally in nearby Walker. She was recognized, and she got up to say a few words to the crowd. The microphone was hot. The TV cameras were rolling.

"We're not just a bunch of illiterate Southern nigger killers," she said. "We are good, white Christian people working for a white America. When one of your wives or one of your sisters gets raped by a nigger maybe you'll get smart and join the Klan."[6]

Was the woman, on some subliminal level, *trying* to destroy the career she lived for? Might it be that she didn't think anyone would pay much attention to her remarks? Or did her lust for the spotlight push her beyond the bounds of propriety into a display of very bad behavior?

As a firestorm erupted, she tried to walk the comments back, insisting that some of her best friends were Black and that she loved the music of Barry White and Marvin Gaye. It just sounded lame. She had 323 mounts in 1974. In 1975 she had 143, and in 1976 a mere 38. Her endorsement deals were canceled.

She carried on, racing anywhere a trainer was willing to overlook her heavy baggage. Her quest for rides took her to Europe, South America and Japan. In 1979, at a small track in East St. Louis, Illinois, her mount flipped in the starting gate and landed on her. In 1981 she wed jockey Jeff Anderson and she stayed married to him until the end. The next year, she went down in an ugly spill at Golden Gate Fields in California. She suffered severe head injuries and lay in a coma for eight days before reviving. In the view of many, she never recovered from that trauma.

But she refused to walk away from the track. In her own mind, her career was not over. Nor would it ever be. On September 8, 1990, she won her last race at Bandera Downs, a quarter horse track in the Texas town of the same name 47 miles northwest of San Antonio.

By then, she'd been diagnosed with terminal cervical cancer. Even that didn't deter her. She was climbing the walls because she wanted to race. She wasn't so great with people, but she was still great with horses.

In June 1991, she left Jeff in Kansas City and headed back to Texas in her blue Oldsmobile Toronado, seeking one last chance at a mount. She never found it. In Fort Worth, she checked into a room at a Motel 6 and purchased a blue steel .22 caliber pistol at a pawn shop for $59.95. Just before noon on June 7, a maid opened the door and found her lying on the floor in a pool of blood. She died at John Smith Hospital at 1:45 the next morning. The cause of death was a self-inflicted gunshot wound to the head.

Sixteen days later, her remains were spread over the grave of Ruffian in the infield at Belmont Park. It's a fitting resting place for a woman who spent her life playing fearlessly in a man's game.

## Santa Anita Meltdown: How Many More Have to Die?
*Thoroughbreds 2019*

It was a four-year-old filly named Let's Light the Way who kicked the crisis into high gear. With four career starts, one win and $18,500 in prize money, she was hardly a superstar, just one of hundreds of thoroughbred horses racing throughout America on any given day.

Her last race had been a month before at Santa Anita Park in California. On the morning of March 5, 2019, she was working out there on a dirt track when she staggered and pulled up lame. The diagnosis after X-rays—a fractured sesamoid bone in her right front leg.

Her career was over. So was her one and only life.

A broken leg in a racehorse is a serious crisis. Their bodies are heavy, but their legs are slender and delicate, and each one contains 80 different bones. Most of the time they don't just break. They shatter. The healing process is slow and traumatic. Pinning and splinting don't work on horses like they do on humans. They rarely lie down, even when sleeping, and like Ruffian, when they revive after surgery burdened with a heavy cast, they often go berserk and further damage themselves.

It's not written in stone that a thoroughbred racehorse with a shattered leg must be "put down," as it's called in the business. But that's almost always what happens, and so it did with Let's Light the Way. She was euthanized a few hours after her breakdown.

The Stronach Group, the Canadian-based entity that owns Santa Anita, had seen enough. They felt the need to act. On December 30, after an injury in a race on a dirt track, Psychedelicat was the first horse to be put down during the 2018–2019 season. Ten more were put down in January and another eight in February. When the death toll for the season reached 21 with Let's Light the Way, Stronach shut down racing for three weeks. Before it resumed another horse died during a workout and then eight more perished in May and June.

The media zeroed in with a harsh, unrelenting glare. Satellite trucks and TV reporters arrived daily in the parking lots. So did PETA and other activists waving provocative signs. *Horses Want to Live. It's Not Sport, It's Violence. How Many More Have to Die?*

This was, after all, no out-of-the-way track in the South or Midwest. It was Santa Anita, the storied, picturesque venue 15 miles northeast of downtown LA, smack in the middle of a tony, affluent neighborhood at the foot of the San Gabriel Mountains. Opened in 1934, the park known as the Great Race Place attracted the glitterati of Hollywood as horse owners and fans from the beginning—Cary Grant, Clark Gable, Lana Turner, Bing Crosby, Spencer Tracy, Errol Flynn. Portions of Shirley Temple's 1949 movie *The Story of Seabiscuit* were filmed there. So were segments of the 1937 Marx Brothers classic *A Day at the Races*. The park is the site of many marquee events, including the Breeder's Cup world championships, the Santa Anita Derby and the Santa Anita Handicap.

What sparked the alarming string of fatalities? Determining a direct cause of death in each of the 30 horses was virtually impossible. But a close-up look indicated that a number of factors were involved. As the racing season began, they converged in a kind of perfect storm.

The metaphor is appropriate because the weather itself seemed to be at the heart of things. In the winter of 2018–2019, torrential rains punished SoCal on a record scale. The month of February alone saw 11.5 inches. The average amount is 3.1. Temperatures were also much cooler than normal.

The rain and cold inflicted heavy damage on the track surfaces at the park. In the first months of 2019 the mix of sand and dirt was lumpy, inconsistent and dangerous. Heavy sleds used to compress the excess moisture turned it all rock hard. After the spate of injuries and deaths, experts hired by Stronach analyzed the tracks and deemed them fit for racing. But the perception that they were a key part of the problem persisted.

A second factor was Stronach's relentless pressure on vets, trainers and owners to race their horses more frequently. More races meant more publicity, more spectators and more opportunities for bettors, all of which increased revenues. The pressure often came in the form of a take-it-or-leave-it proposition—pick up your pace or lose your stalls here. Get with the program or we'll replace you with someone who will.

Santa Anita's location played a pivotal role in Stronach's lust for cash. Real estate developers have coveted the 320-acre site for decades, with an eye toward leveling it all and building expensive luxury homes. In 2019 the land in the city of

Arcadia was estimated to be worth $500 million. Stronach chairwoman and president Brenda Stronach insisted that she didn't *want* to sell the property her company bought in 1998 for $126 million.

But the temptation was there, staring her in the face every day. Her way of beating it back was to maximize profits at the park to the greatest extent possible. It was a tough spot to be in, especially with her own father suing her for $400 million. Auto parts billionaire Frank Stronach, 86, was convinced his daughter was stealing the company from him as his health declined.

The third factor was the physical condition of the equine athletes. An investigation by the California Horse Racing Board put it his way—the main cause of the slew of deaths was "pre-existing pathologies"[7] in the horses. That's a fancy medical way of saying they were diseased or infirm or chronically fatigued or riddled with pain. Or any combination of the above.

It's not hard to see how they got that way. Their human overseers were forcing the strong but fragile animals to run too often and too fast on legs, ankles and hooves too small for the task at hand. Horses are not "born to run," at least not in races. That's a fantasy concocted by people who make their living at the track. They have to be taught how to compete against and beat other horses, which is a far cry from loping around a grass pasture a few hours every day.

The competitive culture is fueled by the pervasive presence of performance-enhancing drugs. Horses can take any drug that human athletes take, and they do. Some are legal, some aren't. There are amphetamines to improve speed and endurance, steroids to build muscle mass and increase strength, and painkillers to numb the hurt inflicted by the rigors of racing and training. There have even been some cases of blood doping, the switch out technique that brought down biker Lance Armstrong.

The most notorious drug is Lasix, a trademarked name for furosemide, given to horses in liquid form in the hours before a race. The purported purpose is to prevent bleeding in the lungs that arises from intense exertion. But the reality is that very few horses bleed severely enough to require medication. Lasix also functions as a diuretic, causing horses to expel epic amounts of urine. The most common number cited is 20 to 30 pounds. Dumping pee is a surefire way to drop weight in horses, just as it is with jockeys. It's also effective at flushing out traces of any illegal drugs that may be in the body.

But there's a downside to the drug too. It can trigger electrolyte imbalances and severe dehydration. Although it's banned in Europe, Asia and Australia, it has been a staple for decades at tracks in the U.S.

Despite all the attention it received, Santa Anita was hardly a special case. You could describe it as the whipping boy for the sins of the system. Racehorses with shattered legs are euthanized in numbers that can astonish people unfamiliar with the sport. The Jockey Club reported 441 thoroughbred deaths in 2019. That number could well be on the low side. Activist Patrick Battuello, founder

## 8. Win, Place or Die

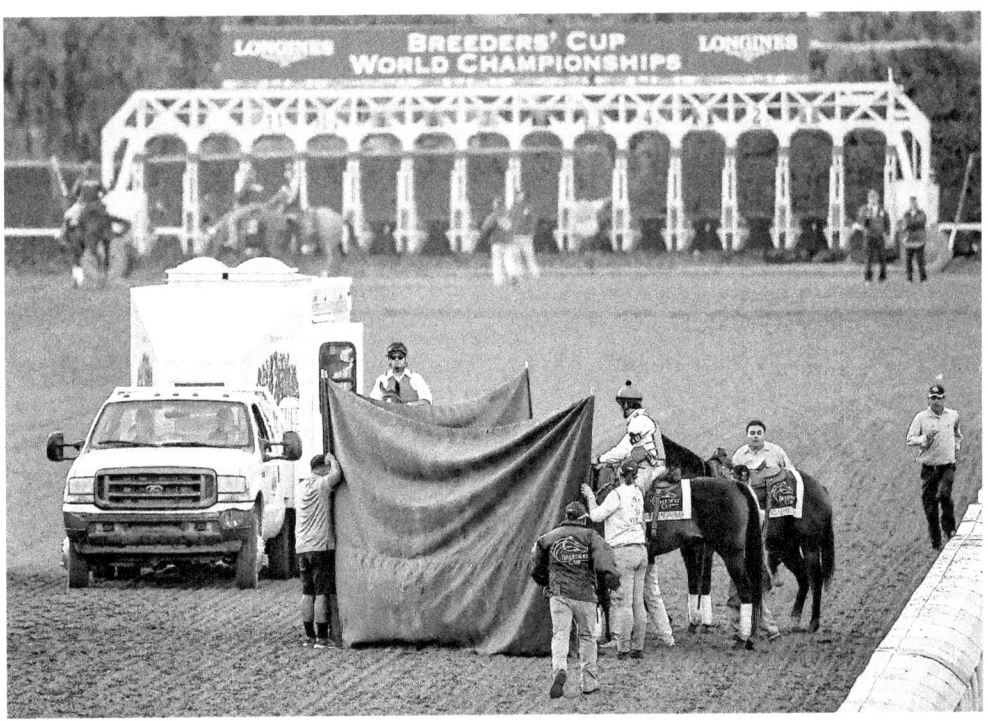

**Mongolian Groom is treated after his breakdown in the Breeder's Cup Classic at Santa Anita Park on November 2, 2019. The four-year-old gelding broke his left hind leg in the final stretch and was later euthanized. It was yet another death in the continuing string of equine fatalities that peaked with a three-week shutdown of racing at Santa Anita in March 2019 (AP Images / Mark J. Terrill).**

of Horseracing Wrongs, documented 1,100 deaths in 2019 and claims there have been more than 5,000 fatalities in America since 2014. In Battuello's view, all the fretting about track surfaces, corporate greed and performance-enhancing drugs is beside the point. It's a distraction from the real issue.

Like boxing, horse racing by its very nature is gruesome and barbaric. It cannot be effectively "reformed." Inflicting incessant grinding on the unformed skeletons of animals from the first days of their existence is wrong. So are shoving them into stalls to spend 23 hours of each day alone after their workouts, lashing them with hard leather whips, forcing them to wear blinders and jamming razor sharp metal bits into their mouths to bolster "communication" with jockeys.

And it's all done in the name of entertaining hordes of human beings in the grandstands or at off-track betting facilities, most of them waving little pieces of paper in the air, whooping like happy idiots and hoping for a windfall that will allow them to pay off their credit cards or buy a giant screen TV or take a trip to a sunny beach somewhere on the Gulf of Mexico.

The goal of Horseracing Wrongs is to abolish the pastime entirely. To them it's a relic of the past, existing today on life support. Racing was once the biggest spectator sport in America, but its popularity has been declining for years. Its monopoly on legal gambling is ancient history. From 2000 to 2020, the total amount of money wagered at all American tracks—called the handle—fell by 50 percent. Racetracks are increasingly dependent on government subsidies and tax breaks for survival. Adding to their woes is the meteoric rise of online gaming, which has created an almost infinite number of new outlets for people who want to wager.

The meltdown at Santa Anita led to a concerted crackdown across the country. Fatalities have declined sharply nationwide since the park's winter of discontent, and there were only five at Santa Anita in 2022. Jerry Hollendrofer, who trained four horses there in 2019, has been banished for all time from all Stronach tracks, including Gulfstream in Florida and Pimlico and Laurel in Maryland. Bob Baffert, the trainer of Triple Crown winners American Pharoah and Justify, was slapped with a 90-day suspension for doping violations, and 29 indictments were handed down nationwide. Race-day Lasix is now banned at all three Triple Crown races and at numerous tracks throughout the U.S.

The future of equine-based sports entertainment in America is not as clear as it used to be. Enacted by Congress in 2021, the Horseracing Integrity and Safety Act created a private agency overseen by the Federal Trade Commission to craft and enforce uniform anti-doping and medical control programs designed to replace the existing mishmash of state laws and regulations. But that move has been blocked by federal judges in Louisiana and West Virginia, who objected to placing enforcement powers in the hands of a non-governmental entity.

If federal oversight does indeed become an everyday reality, it may signal the dawn of a new era in the Sport of Kings, one in which many horses will be spared the fate of Let's Light the Way and thousands of others. Or it may simply mean business as usual. That seemed to be the case in 2023 when racing was suspended at Churchill Downs after seven horses died in the week leading up to the Kentucky Derby. Time will tell.

# 9

## Motorsport Mishaps

### Bill Vukovich: The Fearless One
*Indy 500 1955*

Bill Vukovich owned two gas stations and operated one in his hometown of Fresno, California, where he had lived since he was a small boy. He was also the most renowned auto racer in America. The fact that he was both at the same time illustrates how different the sports world was in the years after World War II. Such a double life for an athlete of his prominence is unthinkable today.

He lived an ordinary existence in many respects as a businessman, neighbor and churchgoer. He was a devoted husband to his wife Esther and a doting father to his children Bill Jr. and Marlene. But his mind was often elsewhere. His competitive fires blazed brightly, and he was focused on one thing—driving as fast as he needed to drive to win any race he entered.

At the same time, he had no interest in being a celebrity. That was the main reason he remained in Fresno as his fame grew. Schmoozing the press and meeting and greeting fans and bigwigs were nothing but necessary annoyances to him, something to be done with as quickly as possible. His brooding, standoffish behavior frustrated many of his admirers. His fearless style behind the wheel astonished and terrified them.

Simply put, he never slowed down. Vukovich got hooked on the thrill of living at the edge of catastrophe early in life and he stayed hooked. In the end, his obsessive love of speed led to his death at the peak of his career.

Born Vaso Vucerovich in 1918 in Alameda on San Francisco Bay, Vukovich grew up in the Depression, one of eight children of farming parents who immigrated from Serbia. On Vukovich's 14th birthday in 1932, his troubled father committed suicide, forcing the quiet, olive-skinned boy to quit school and go to work to help support the family. To relieve his stress, he started chasing jackrabbits across the countryside with his older brother Eli in a Model T Ford.

Bill won his first car race at 18 and moved quickly to the midget car circuit, barnstorming along the West Coast with Eli. Midgets were a nationwide craze in the 1930s and 1940s, especially in California. Vukovich raced in the Rose Bowl, the Los Angeles Coliseum and Gilmore Stadium, the midget mecca that was demolished in 1952 to make way for CBS Television City.

The drivers were bold and hungry, eager to move up quickly to faster, more powerful drives and bigger purses. They were also on the smallish side physically—Vukovich was 5-8, 155 pounds—because they had to fit into the colorful, 900-pound versions of Indy cars that raced on short, tight, dirt ovals.

In his first midget race in 1938, Vukovich flipped his car and broke his collarbone and several ribs. It was the first of innumerable injuries he suffered behind the wheel, including those that kept him from being drafted in World War II. Instead of serving in uniform, he maintained and repaired military vehicles at his garages in Fresno. After the war, in a bright red car he christened Old Ironsides, Vukovich won West Coast midget titles in 1946 and 1947. He captured the national crown in 1950.

By then he had his sights set on a bigger goal—the Indianapolis 500. First run in 1911, it had risen from humble beginnings to become the biggest motorsport show in America. In the 1950s, stock car racing was still in its infancy in the Southeast, looked on by most motorheads with a mixture of disdain and amusement. The Formula One Grand Prix circuit was largely confined to Europe. Indy was far and away the main event.

He arrived at the Brickyard in 1950, looking for a ride. He got one but failed to qualify for the race. In 1951, he earned a starting position and lasted 72 miles before exiting with an oil leak. The next year, driving for racing magnate Howard Keck, he led the race after 480 miles but scraped the wall and dropped out when a vital pin on his steering column broke.

On Memorial Day in 1953, in scorching heat that approached 130 degrees on the track, Vukovich started on the pole and won his first 500. He repeated as winner in 1954 from the 19th position. He won both races in Keck's Fuel Injection Special, each time without a relief driver. To deal with pain, exhaustion and heat, it was a common practice of the time for substitutes to spell main drivers for two or three periods of 15 to 20 minutes each during a race. In 1953, only five men drove at Indy without relief.

Vukovich had no use for relief drivers. He smoked and drank alcohol sparingly and ran or biked daily to stay in shape. It would be him and him alone behind the wheel for the duration of the race. No sharing. Given his prickly personality, that made perfect sense.

To the dismay of fans and promoters, he showed little interest in competing regularly on the national circuit. He raced infrequently and spent most of his time in Fresno. He grew up dirt poor, his father had deserted his family in the cruelest possible way, and in his early years on the track he had money waved in his face by slick-talking promoters only to have it evaporate when payday arrived. All of that instilled in him a strong need for steady employment. He once quipped that he ran a gas station for a living and only raced when he needed to earn some extra bucks.

Vukovich entered the 1955 race at Indianapolis with a chance to become the first man to win three times in a row. Howard Keck had dropped out of the business, and he drove for owner Lindsey Hopkins. Dressed in his usual T-shirt, cotton pants and bowling shoes, without gloves, he started from the fifth position on a damp, windy, overcast day. Like always he was supremely confident of victory, and he thrilled the crowd of 175,000 by weaving and surging to the head of the pack in a spectacular duel with archrival Jack McGrath.

Then fate intervened, and his luck ran out.

At the southeast turn on the 57th lap, he suddenly faced a tangle of three disabled cars spinning wildly across the pavement in front of him. He hit the gas and tried to weave quickly through the mess, but his car bounced off the rear tire of one of the others, then went airborne and cartwheeled over the outside wall. It clipped a utility pole and a safety patrol jeep before plowing into the ground upside down in an explosion of flame.

His skull and spine crushed, Vukovich died before he could be pulled from the smoldering wreckage. He was 36 years old.

Vukovich was one of 58 people to die in the Indy 500 through 2023. That number includes drivers, crew members, race officials and spectators killed during the race, practice laps or qualifying runs. The first fatality came in the inaugural race in 1911, when riding mechanic Sam Dickson was flung from his car into a wall. Riding mechanics sat behind drivers and massaged their hands, pumped oil and fuel, checked gauges and tire pressure and looked out for other cars. They were mandatory at Indy until 1923, then used on an optional basis before being abolished in 1938.

On June 4, 1955, an overflow crowd of 2,000 gathered in the red brick Free Evangelical Lutheran Church in Fresno to pay final respects to the town's most prominent citizen. After the service, Vukovich was buried in a bronze casket in Belmont Memorial Park next to his parents.

His son and grandson carried on in his name. Bill Jr., who was 11 when his father died, raced Indy cars for 12 years and was the 500 runner-up in 1973. Bill III earned rookie of the year honors at Indy in 1988 and then, at 27, followed his grandfather to a tragic end. On November 25, 1990, he crashed into a wall and died during a practice lap for a sprint race at Mesa Marin Speedway in Bakersfield, California.

## The Dakar Rally: Desert Storm
### *Off Road Racing 1988*

In 1975, a young French motorbike racer named Thierry Sabine journeyed to Africa to compete in a grueling event called the Abidjan-Nice Rally. When he lost his way along the off-road route in the forbidding terrain of the Tchigaï Plateau in Niger, he had a vision.

He foresaw an even more challenging race for cars, trucks and motorcycles, running somewhere between 18 and 23 days and covering 6,000 to 8,000 miles. It would kick off in Paris. From there drivers and crews would head south and ferry across the Mediterranean Sea to Algeria and Morocco. Then they would move through Niger, Mali, Mauritania and finally Senegal, finishing in the capital city of Dakar (DAK-are or duh-KARR).

Like the Tour de France and the Iditarod, the race would be divided into stages, with tent encampments set up each night, usually near airstrips so planes and helicopters could fly in food, vehicles parts, and other supplies. The teams with the fastest cumulative times in each vehicle class would be declared the winners.

Sabine worked quickly to turn his vision into reality. The first Paris to Dakar Rally in 1979 attracted 182 vehicles. Only 74 made it to the finish line. By 1984 the number of entries had grown to 427, and the rally was on its way to becoming the most extraordinary event in all of motorsports. It soon became known as the Dakar Rally, or simply the Dakar.

It wasn't popular in the U.S., which supplied a tiny number of competitors. No Americans even completed the race until 1996, when a seven-man Hummer team led by Ron Hall celebrated with other finishers on the beach in Dakar. But it was a rage in Japan and Europe, especially in France, the home nation of more than half the entries.

Professional factory teams like Peugeot, Citroën and Mitsubishi soon entered the fray and captured most of the prize money. But 80 percent of the drivers and crews each year were amateurs, known as privateers. Sabine concocted a motto that captured the essence of his creation well—*A challenge for those who go. A dream for those who stay behind.*

Even as it was invaded by swarms of swashbuckling motorheads, the compelling landscape remained the star of the Dakar. It was like the Iditarod in that respect. But instead of ice and snow and frozen tundra, the main feature was sand—soft, brilliantly yellow and blinding, and piled in dunes high enough to suck in and bury humans and vehicles. With the sand came dust and dirt. There were also plenty of ditches, boulders and rock fields, along with an occasional dry lake bed. One-hundred-degree heat in the daytime was the norm.

A second similarity was that the ordeal quickly winnowed out weaker entries. In a typical year, half or more of the sled dogs in the Iditarod break down with physical injuries and fail to finish the race. Likewise, the Dakar Rally route was littered with ravaged, broken machines taken down by the elements on the worst roads the mind could ever imagine. Some got fixed and moved on. Some didn't get fixed and remained forever in the blistering sun, where they were often stripped clean by scavengers.

But there were differences between the two events as well. The impoverished natives of northwest Africa didn't greet the contestants with the kind of affection that Alaskans shower on mushers and their dogs. Far from it. Each year they came out of their mud huts and arrived on foot or camels to line the route and watch warily as the spectacle unfolded. Some of the bolder ones begged the white men for cans of soda pop, scraps of food or T-shirts. Other than that they pretty much kept their distance.

There was also the ominous presence of radical Islamic terrorists, which forced revised routing on several occasions. The radicals did not take kindly to rich, decadent infidels from Europe throwing a giant, boisterous party on wheels on their home turf. Bloodshed was not unheard of. In 1991, a sniper in Mali shot and killed a supply truck driver.

In 2008, following terrorist threats in the Sahel region, the rally was cancelled. The next year, the entire show relocated to South America. There it would remain for 10 years, largely run in Argentina, Peru, Chile and Bolivia. The Dakar as originally conceived became a thing of the past.

The biggest difference of all between the two events was the death toll, what number crunchers call the mortality rate. Dogs perish in the Iditarod on a regular basis, but there hasn't been a human fatality since the race's inception in 1967. The same cannot be said for the Dakar. Starting with Patrice Dodin wiping out on his Yamaha bike in Niger in 1979, 76 people are believed to have died in the rally through 2023. The number includes 31 drivers and 45 journalists, spectators, bystanders and crew members.

The 1988 rally holds the grim distinction of being the deadliest ever. A record 603 vehicles started at Versailles Palace outside Paris—311 cars, 183 motorcycles and 109 trucks. Only 151 would arrive in Dakar 22 days later after completing the 8,000-mile route through six countries.

Along the way seven people died. On January 9, engineer Kees van Loevezijn from the Netherlands was thrown out of a truck when it hit a rocky sand dune near Djado, Niger, at 110 mph and somersaulted several times. He died instantly. On the same day co-driver Patrick Canado of France died when his Range Rover collided with a Mercedes-Benz near Arlit, Niger. On the 17th, Frenchman Jean Claude Hager crashed his BMV bike in the harsh outback of Mali and smashed his head into a boulder. He was life-flighted to Paris, where he died two days later.

Next came the spectators. On the 18th, a 10-year-old native girl named Baye Sabi was struck and killed by a Toyota Land Cruiser near Kita, Mali, when the driver was blinded by heavy dust. Three days later a mother and child in Mauritania were run over by a camera truck. And on the last day of the rally a man was killed by a vehicle in Dakar. There were also 50 injuries, including two drivers who were paralyzed.

The critics turned the heat up high. They'd been vocal from the beginning, but the events of 1988 emboldened them. The president of Senegal said that perhaps the time had come to pull the plug on the whole mess. In Côte d'Ivoire, the government newspaper called the rally "the last refuge of people nostalgic

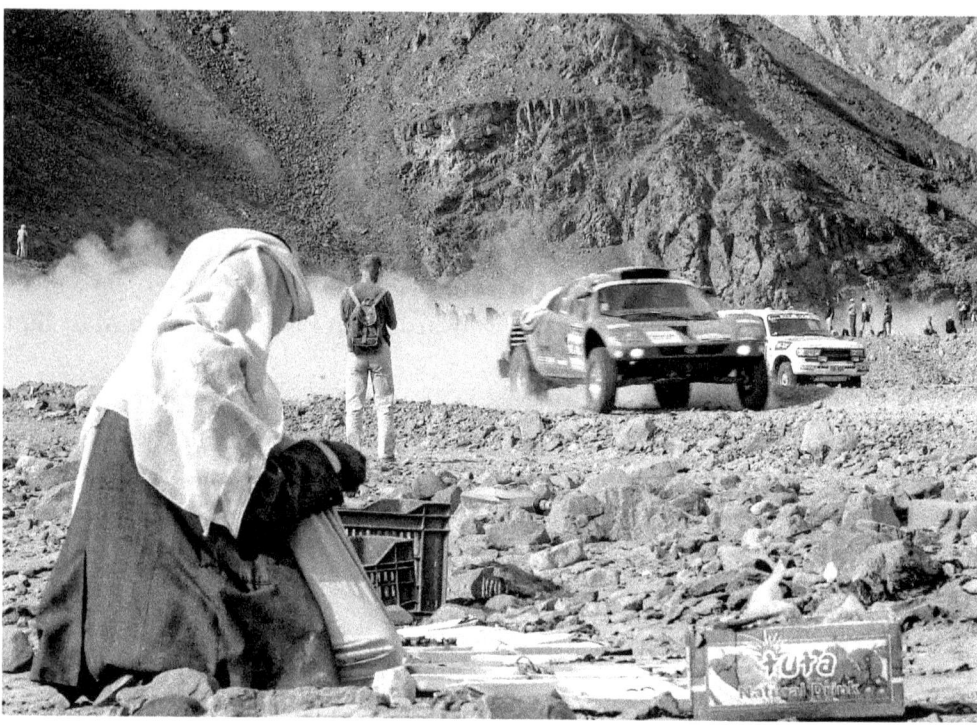

An Egyptian woman lays out her wares as a vehicle approaches her during the 2003 Dakar Rally in South Sinai, some 360 miles south of Cairo. The route of the event was moved that year from its traditional start and finish points in Paris and Dakar. Behind the wheel of the oncoming Mitsubishi is Jutta Kleinschmidt, who in 2001 became the only woman ever to win the grueling off-road race. She finished first in the car class (AP Images / Amr Nabil).

for the saga of Lawrence of Arabia."[1] PANA, the African news agency based in Dakar, wrote that the deaths of the African spectators were "insignificant for the organizers."[2]

Even the Vatican weighed in, describing the event as "the bloody race of irresponsibility" and a "vulgar display of power and wealth in places where men [sic] continue to die of hunger and thirst."[3]

Dakar survived the 1988 debacle and the ongoing chorus of disapproval. Today it may not be thriving, but it's surviving. In 2020, the rally left South America and returned to its spiritual home in the desert, this time in Saudi Arabia, with a route stretching from the beaches of the Red Sea to the sands of the Arabian Gulf in Damman.

As for death, it comes with the territory, no matter where on Earth that territory might be. Since relocating to Saudi Arabia, three motorcycle racers, a mechanic and a photographer have died.

Later in this chapter we'll visit the Isle of Man for a look at the freewheeling Tourist Trophy motorcycle races. I think you'll note a strong resemblance to Dakar.

## Ayrton Senna: Collision Course
*Formula One 1994*

Ayrton Senna presented two faces to the world. You could almost call him a Jekyll and Hyde personality.

When it came to racing, the three-time Formula One champion could be an arrogant bully. He demanded everything of himself. Like Bill Vukovich, he was obsessed with winning, and he had no use for anyone standing in his way. At times that included the men who designed and built his cars, his team owners, his pit crew, and many Grand Prix bureaucrats and honchos. He also disdained media types, who retaliated by churning out story after story spotlighting his nasty, cutthroat side.

But Senna reserved most of his animosity for fellow drivers, especially Nelson Piquet and archrival Alain Prost. Inflated egos and ugly confrontations run rampant on the F1 circuit, but Senna managed to stand out on both counts.

Moving at 170 mph at the Japanese Grand Prix in 1990, he purposely rammed Prost's car at the first corner of the first lap, sending both of them into the gravel trap, through the tire barrier and out of the race. Why? By denying his teammate a chance to continue, he assured himself of the point margin he needed to win the individual world championship.

He initially claimed that the collision was an accident. No one bought his story. A year later he finally fessed up, and the two members of the McLaren team eventually reached an uneasy truce. But the incident confirmed yet again what had been crystal clear since Senna's first F1 race in 1984 at the Brazilian Grand Prix in Rio de Janeiro. He was not in the game to make friends—and he didn't.

At the same time he loved his fans, and they loved him back. He was adored by millions, especially in his native Brazil. The hero worship was extreme, and he was considered the equal of soccer legend Pelé. There was something almost mystical about him, and his humbleness and staunch Catholic faith demanded respect. Senna was born into a wealthy family of land and factory owners, and he became astronomically rich himself, but he donated millions of dollars to charitable causes. He also remained fiercely loyal to the people who helped him early in his career.

Many call him the greatest F1 driver ever. The numbers present a strong case. Sixty-five starts on the pole, still third all-time. Forty-one wins, fifth all-time behind Lewis Hamilton (103), Michael Schumacher (91), Sebastian Vettel (53) and Alain Prost (51). World championships in 1988, 1990 and 1991. And he did it all in a career cut short way too soon at age 34, in the third race of his 11th F1 season.

The shattering end came in Imola, Italy, on May 1, 1994. At the San Marino Grand Prix in the Ferrari Autodrome, Senna was looking to win his first race for the Williams-Renault team after leaving McLaren-Honda in 1993. The mood in the pit lanes and paddock was somber that Sunday. Austrian Roland Ratzenberger had been killed the day before during a qualifying run, the first death on the F1 tour in 12 years.

Seconds after the start, two drivers collided in a wreck that injured a policeman and eight spectators. The field drove behind a safety car for five laps as debris were cleared. After the restart, as he approached a perilous 90-degree left turn in first place, Senna's car didn't turn and he plowed straight into a concrete barrier at 131 mph, after braking from 190 mph. The impact tore off the right front wheel. Chunks of metal flew back into the cockpit and one struck Senna full force in the head.

First responders pried him out of his seat and laid him flat on the blood-stained pavement. In an effort to induce breathing they performed a tracheotomy, placing a tube into his windpipe through an incision in the neck. It was a lost cause. Senna had suffered massive trauma at the base of his skull. He was transported via helicopter to a hospital in Bologna, where he was pronounced dead at 6:05 p.m.

Escorted by fighter jets, his coffin was flown home on a Varig Airlines plane not in the cargo hold but in the first-class cabin. The president of Brazil declared a three-day national mourning period, and the crowd that lined the streets of his hometown of Sao Paulo to view his funeral motorcade was estimated to be as large as three million. Alain Prost, Jackie Stewart and Emerson Fittipaldi were among the pallbearers at his service.

Under a legal duty to investigate the accident because it occurred at a sporting event, Italian prosecutors concluded that the wreck had been caused by a defective steering column that broke during the race. They were convinced it was both poorly designed and improperly installed. They filed manslaughter charges against Williams-Renault team chairman Frank Williams, technical manager Patrick Head and four others. The condition of the track was also cited as a factor in the crash.

It was an unprecedented situation that sent the F1 tour reeling. Here was the powerful hand of the law dragging the gritty details of their grand enterprise into a public courtroom for all the world to see and hear. The intrusion ripped into the very soul of a sport where mechanics, machines and technology play a role as vital as the drivers, if not more so. To blame a driver's death on a difficult but routine procedure like replacing a steering column was a warning shot across the bow. A finding of guilt would signal that business as usual would no longer be tolerated. It might well threaten the future of racing in Italy and perhaps even the rest of Europe.

So pronounced the doomsayers.

Those fears were never realized. After the acquittal of all defendants in the first trial in 1997, prosecutors pursued their case through appeals and retrials for seven more years. Patrick Head's eventual conviction on manslaughter charges was largely symbolic because it came after the statute of limitations had expired.

He paid no fines and was never imprisoned. The specific causes of the accident remain elusive after 35 years.

Ayrton Senna is buried in Cemitério do Morumbi in São Paulo. The epitaph on his gravestone reads, "Nothing can separate me from the love of God."

## Dale Earnhardt: Long Live the King
### NASCAR 2001

As the 21st century arrived, stock car racing in America was as hot as highway blacktop in August and getting hotter.

NASCAR had moved beyond its Appalachian roots in the North Carolina Piedmont with a vengeance. With a rapidly expanding fan base and a new multi-billion-dollar broadcast deal with Fox, NBC and Turner Broadcasting, it had morphed into a sport with the potential to become a bona fide equal to the Big Four—football, baseball, basketball and hockey.

Not everybody was happy with the change. There were purists who preferred the days when weekend warriors raced on dirt tracks and beaches in cars that were slightly souped-up versions of ones you could buy off a lot in your hometown. They liked their idols raw and unpolished, and they relished the thought of disputes between drivers being settled with fisticuffs on pit roads. But they couldn't turn back the clock. For the old school crowd, the choice was clear. Hop on the fancy, shiny new bus or get left behind in the dust.

Two thousand one shone all the brighter because Dale Earnhardt looked to be returning to prime form. It wasn't as if NASCAR's biggest star was mired in a deep slump. He'd finished fourth, fifth, eighth and seventh in the Winston Cup standings from 1996 through 1999, with six wins and $8.58 million in earnings. But for a man with 76 career wins and seven cup titles that was subpar, and it had been seven years since his last championship. With one more title he would surpass Richard Petty as the all-time leader.

In the late 1990s Earnhardt suffered one mishap after another on the track. A fractured sternum and broken left collarbone after hitting a wall at the Die Hard 500 at Talladega. A mysterious blackout at the Southern 500 at Darlington that doctors never fully explained. Second-degree burns on his face after a fiery rollover, again at the Die Hard. Surgery to remove a ruptured disc after a slide into a wall at the Cracker Barrel 500 at the Atlanta Motor Speedway.

The highlight of those years was his 1998 win at the Daytona 500. He had won 34 times at the fabled oval but that was his lone victory in NASCAR's most celebrated race.

As he prepared for the 2001 edition on February 18, the 49-year-old nicknamed the Intimidator for his aggressive personality on and off the track was playing hurt. His pain wasn't so intense that he was driving with one arm like he'd been doing a few years before. But it was there. He didn't obsess about it. A lot of other guys were playing hurt too. It was the way of their world.

So was the omnipresent possibility of death. Earnhardt didn't obsess about that either. There was a new contraption on the circuit called the HANS (head and neck support) device. It was a U-shaped carbon fiber brace supported by the shoulders that protected the head and neck from the force of collisions. A few drivers were getting fitted for one, but Earnhardt wanted nothing to do with what he called "a damn noose."[4] He was so old school that he still wore an open face helmet without a shield, which he insisted impaired his vision. He'd say no thank you to the HANS, keep his fingers crossed and take his chances.

His future looked bright. He finished strong in 2000, winning the Winston 500 at Talladega in October and placing second in the final cup standings to Bobby Labonte. And for the first time he was a car owner. One of the drivers for Dale Earnhardt Incorporated (DEI) was Michael Waltrip, the brother of Darrell. Another was his 26-year-old son Dale Junior, who'd had his breakout Winston Cup season the year before. People sensed that the Intimidator was excited and gratified to be competing alongside his own flesh and blood.

The race in front of a crowd of 150,000 and a national TV audience on Fox was a humdinger. There were 49 lead changes among 14 drivers over 200 laps. In his trademark #3 black Chevy Monte Carlo, Earnhardt started in the seventh position and led for 17 laps, always lurking near the front.

With 27 laps left, Tony Stewart's orange Pontiac was tapped from behind on the backstretch and went airborne, triggering a 20-car pileup that halted the race for 16 minutes as crews cleared away the wreckage. When the action resumed Earnhardt was in third place, running interference for Michael Waltrip and Dale Junior battling for the lead ahead of him. He was minutes away from seeing his first win at Daytona as an owner.

With one lap left, Earnhardt's Chevy wiggled slightly after tapping Sterling Marlin's Dodge near Turn 4. The Chevy veered toward the flat apron at the bottom of the track before shooting abruptly back up to the right. Ken Schrader's oncoming Pontiac slammed into Earnhardt's passenger side door and pushed him into the concrete wall. Both cars then slid slowly down the banking and stopped nose-to-door on the infield grass.

Most people in the grandstand were focused on the finish line and didn't see the crash. To those who did it hardly seemed like much at all. No rollovers, no flying tires, no shooting flames. Just some mild-looking contact between the front bumper and the wall.

But the crash was absolutely as bad as could be. It was the angle of the impact between car and wall—virtually head-on—that ended Earnhardt's life in a millisecond.

He had a broken left ankle, eight broken ribs, a fractured sternum, partially collapsed lungs and cuts on his scalp and chin. He might well have survived all

## 9. Motorsport Mishaps

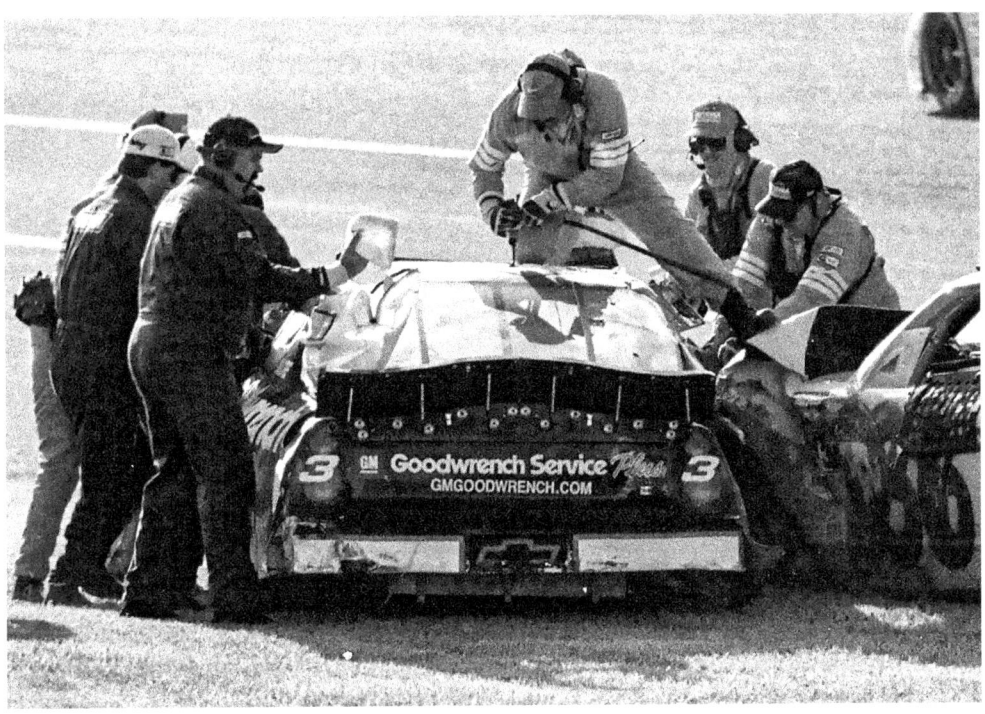

**Rescue workers try to extract Dale Earnhardt from his Number 3 Chevy Monte Carlo at the Daytona 500 on February 18, 2001. Their efforts were futile. The NASCAR legend with seven Winston Cup titles died on impact when his car slammed into a concrete retaining wall a few hundred yards from the finish line (AP Images / Greg Suvino).**

that. The fatal blow was a basilar skull fracture, caused by a violent whiplash that rips the brain stem loose from the spine. He died when he hit the concrete. It was the same type of injury that killed Bill Vukovich in 1955 at the Indy 500.

As Michael Waltrip rolled into Victory Lane after edging Dale Junior by 0.124 seconds, both were aware of the crash but didn't yet know who was involved. An hour later, Dale Junior walked into the trauma wing at Halifax Medical Center fearing the worst. When he saw Earnhardt's body, he knew right away that his father was gone. Doctors officially pronounced Earnhardt dead at 5:16 p.m.

There was immediate speculation about whether a HANS device would have saved his life. Some medical experts said yes, some said no. Only five of the 43 drivers that day wore one. In October, eight months after Earnhardt's death, NASCAR mandated its use by all drivers in it top three series.

The Intimidator's passing ripped the heart and soul out of the NASCAR community. It didn't help that drivers Adam Petty, Kenny Irwin, Jr., and Tony Roper had all been killed by basilar skull fractures in the previous eight months. But Earnhardt was the King. Losing him was the most devastating blow imaginable. It was like tennis losing Serena Williams or basketball losing LeBron James or golf losing Tiger Woods.

On February 22, Fox Sports Net broadcast live coverage of the invitation-only funeral at Charlotte Calvary Church. After the funeral thousands of fans flocked to Center Grove Lutheran Cemetery expecting to find Earnhardt's grave. But it was nowhere to be seen. Seeking to avoid what the family described as "an Elvis situation,"[5] they chose to bury him on their private estate in Mooresville, 25 miles north of Charlotte. The public is not permitted to visit the site.

Many people were upset that they chose to do things that way. But when all was said and done, it didn't matter much where Earnhardt was laid to rest. He was a legend in his own time, he is one today, and he'll be one tomorrow.

The King is dead. Long live the King.

## Jessi Combs: Speed Kills
*Speed Racing 2019*

Jessi Combs sped through her short life in a hurry, following a road not often taken by the so-called fairer sex. The urge to be bold and different and play with the boys ran in her blood.

Born and raised in the Black Hills of western South Dakota, she started driving sitting on her dad's lap in his truck. She was taking a cue from her great-grandmother Nina DeBow, a jazz pianist who worked and lived in the rowdy outlaw town of Deadwood and made a name for herself in the Roaring Twenties racing Stanley Steamers against all sorts of rough-and-tumble men.

After graduating from Stevens High School in Rapid City in 1998, Jessi launched a career as a metal fabricator, a field utterly dominated by males. Her courses at WyoTec, an auto tech school in Laramie, Wyoming, led to a job building a car from the ground up with a classmate to display at a trade show.

The gig was a way to get her foot in the door toward her real goal of becoming a professional race car driver. If you were a woman trying to break into that exclusive club, it was a big advantage to know more than most of the guys about how vehicles worked. And she did.

Combs achieved her goal in short order. Other than her brains and energy, the main factors in her quick rise were a lust for speed and adrenaline and heady skills behind the wheel. Her gorgeous blonde looks and spunky personality didn't hurt the cause. They also helped make her a TV star. It wasn't on her to-do list, but it happened anyway.

There's a saying in show business—*the camera loves her*. That was the case with Combs. She got lured in by the spell of the screen and hosted and guested on a bundle of shows—*Xtreme 4 × 4* on Spike TV, *Mythbusters, The List: 1,001 Car Things to Do Before You Die, All Girls Garage, Overhaulin,' Jay Leno's Garage*.

By 2013, she'd earned a shot at the ultimate prize of breaking the women's land speed record. Speed racing is among the riskiest endeavors in the sports world, with huge, complex machines moving at hundreds of miles per hour while facing a host of hostile forces including wind, rain, rough and ruptured surfaces, mechanical breakdowns and flying debris. Any of those alone or in the wrong combination at the wrong place at the wrong time can mean the end of the road for both car and driver.

Officially, the sexes compete on an equal basis. The International Automobile Federation (FIA) and other sanctioning bodies do not recognize separate records. But *The Guinness Book of World Records* does, giving women a measure of visibility and respect that they don't get from the overseers.

They have a long history in the sport, dating back to Dorothy Levitt's measured kilometer run at 96 mph in England in 1906. Aerobatics pilot Betty Skelton and drag racer and funny car pioneer Paula Murphy followed in her footsteps. By the time Combs arrived on the scene, the vehicles had evolved into sleek, dart-shaped cars with engines transplanted from jet airplanes.

Guinness recognized two marks for women—the absolute record of 512.710 mph set by Kitty O'Neil in a three-wheeled car in 1976 and the four-wheel record of 306.506 set by Lee Breedlove in 1965. She was the wife of land speed legend Craig Breedlove and she'd driven his car, *Spirit of America—Sonic I*. Three-wheeled cars were generally thought to be faster because they were lighter and faced less wind resistance. With a single axle there was also less friction along the undercarriage.

On October 9, 2013, Combs climbed into the *North American Eagle* at the Alvord Desert, a dry lake bed 12 miles long and seven miles wide in southeastern Oregon. Technically the *Eagle* was a 56-foot car, but it was actually more of a jet on wheels, built to break the existing men's land speed record of 763 mph set by Royal Air Force pilot Andy Green in *Thrust SSC* in 1997. The fuselage and cockpit were modeled after the Lockheed Starfighter, down to the original flight stick. There was no steering wheel. The wheels were solid billet aluminum, and at 52,000 HP, the engine was 375 times more powerful than the one in a Honda Civic.

The protocol for record attempts is standardized. There are two runs of about 10 miles each. The car accelerates as it approaches the measured mile—usually mile 4 to 5—and then decelerates as it moves toward the end of the course. The driver then turns around and makes the same run in the opposite direction and the two measured miles are averaged. The final number must exceed the existing speed mark by at least 1 percent to be certified as a new record.

Combs smashed Breedlove's mark with a run of 398.954 mph. Then as the reigning four-wheel record holder she won five titles, including the Ultra 4 King of the Hammers, an off-road desert race that included rock crawling. In 2016, driving a car called *The Other Eagle*, she eclipsed her own record with a run of 477.59, but because of timing issues the mark was not certified. She made another attempt in 2018 but had to abandon the run when high winds ripped a door off the car.

Those efforts set the stage for the final challenge of besting O'Neil's absolute record. Driving the four-wheeled *North American Eagle* like she had in 2013, Combs prepared to make history once again at the Alvord Desert. The *Eagle*'s enormous engine trumped any speed advantage a three-wheeler might offer.

The night before the attempt she had a heart-to-heart talk with her love and life partner Terry Madden. The dangers of her chosen profession were starting to weigh heavily on both of them. She was 39. She'd been racing for nearly 20 years. How long could she keep going before encountering a calamity? She and Madden decided that tomorrow would be her last hurrah.

That made what happened on August 27, 2019, all the more tragic. She completed her first run with a time of 515.346 mph. But after completing the second measured mile at a speed approaching 550 mph, the *Eagle* hit an object on the surface that caused the front wheel assembly to collapse. Unable to stop, the car rocketed beyond the lake bed, then exploded and burst into flames before finally lurching to a halt and disintegrating.

She died of blunt force trauma, probably when her head slammed against the instrument panel in the cockpit before the explosion and fire.

A year after her death, Guinness officially recognized her fatal run at 522.783 mph. It took dying to do it, but Jessi Combs had become the fastest woman ever on wheels.

## IMTT: Full Throttle
*Motorcycle 2022*

It was the last week of May in 2022, and the island was humming. After a two-year hiatus due to the scourge of Covid, the Isle of Man Tourist Trophy—the "TT"—was up and running again in all its not-so-righteous glory.

In the capital of Douglas and other port towns, some 35,000 visitors poured off ferries from England and Ireland. Nearly all of them were there simply to soak up the festive atmosphere, but the others wheeled off motorcycles of every conceivable size, color, weight and design. Only three to four hundred bikers ended up competing in the eight races that took place over the next two weeks. Most of them were privateers, unattached to the big factory teams like Haith Honda, PHR Performance, Milenco, and Ashcourt. Some fell out of contention after qualifying runs and even more were stymied by mechanical breakdowns.

The rest of the bikers were content to cut laps on their own time around the picturesque island in the Irish Sea aboard Kawasakis, Yamahas, Ducatis, Sennas, Triumphs, BMWs, Nortons and Sunbeams. There were even a small number of Harleys on hand, nearly all ridden by Americans. Just about everybody revved up on Mad Sunday, the day before races start, when the island's streets and highways were open to all comers.

## 9. Motorsport Mishaps

The TT takes place entirely in a dependency of the United Kingdom as big as the city of Tucson, Arizona, with a population the size of Sioux City, Iowa. The heart of it all is the Snaefell Mountain Course, a 37.73-mile loop around the center part of the island. It's the venue not only for TT races but also for the Manx Grand Prix for novice motor bikers held in August or September.

Bikers take off from the start line alone in 10-second intervals and complete the loop in anywhere from 17 to 22 minutes. The single lap record for the TT Senior Race is 16:42.778—an average speed of 135 mph. It was set by Peter Hickman in 2018 on a BMW.

The course is as different as can be from a NASCAR, Formula One or Indy-Car track. There are no nets or barriers to absorb shock, no gravel pits, and no runoff lanes. It includes 200 corners and consists entirely of public highways that are closed for the competition. But all of the features lining the winding mountain roads and narrow village streets remain as is—driveways, mail boxes, trash cans, fences, streetlights, yards and cow pastures.

There is no speed limit. The gutsier drivers can hit 170 mph on straightaways. Or is it 180? Can you say 190? For a long time it was a mystery because no one was measuring except the drivers themselves, reading their speedometers. And the tales grew taller at the end of the day as they tipped a few and moseyed up and down the bar. After the 21st century arrived datalogging devices were installed on bikes to provide accurate numbers. A handful of speeds above 200 mph have been recorded in practice runs.

The first race was held on the island in 1907 on a shorter course. The action moved to Snaefell in 1911 and has been there ever since. Before the Covid pause the event was cancelled during World War I (1915–1919) and World War II (1940–1946), and the 2001 edition was scratched because of an outbreak of hoof-and-mouth disease.

Two thousand twenty-two picked up where all its predecessors left off. It was as if the party lights never dimmed. Along with spectacular racing, revelry and high spirits came the other staple of the event that, with the Dakar Rally, is regarded as the most dangerous in the realm of motorsports.

That, of course, would be death. On June 1, Welsh biker Mark Purslow, 29, died after a crash at Ballagarey during a qualifying run. Three days later, side car driver Cesar Chanal met his end at a spot called Ago's Leap just a mile into the course in his TT debut. His passenger, Frenchman Olivier Lavorel, who was riding in the three-wheeled bike to help steer and control speed, barely survived. An unfortunate mix-up at the hospital had media reporting him and not Chanal as the fatality for three days. On June 6, Northern Irishman Davy Morgan died on the final lap of the Supersport Race for lighter, less powerful bikes. And on June 10, the father and son sidecar duo of Roger and Bradley Stockton, 56 and 21, died at Ago's Leap.

Five is quite a number, big enough to pop the eyeballs of sports fans who only casually follow the action. But it isn't a record for a single year on the Snaefell Mountain Course. That honor goes to 1993, when 11 riders died, followed by 1995 with 10 and 2007 with seven. From the first fatality in 1911 through 2022, the death count stands at 265 competitors. Seventeen spectators, bystanders and race officials have also died.

The toll includes three women. Marie Lambert, a side car passenger with her husband Richard driving, died after a smash-up in 1961. Brit Pam Cannell died in the Manx Grand Prix in 1997 and marshal April Bolster, an island native and one of 1,500 volunteer crew members, was struck and killed by a biker in 2005. The ongoing blood fest has spawned a grisly nickname for the Isle of Man—Isle of Manslaughter.

The carnage boggles the mind, and it has from the beginning. People have been clamoring for a ban on the TT since 1913, when pioneer feminists called suffragettes poured crushed glass up and down the course to protest what they saw as a grotesque display of male machismo. So why do the races survive? Improvements and modifications added through the years have made the course safer, even if those changes aren't reflected in the death count. That's a spur to go on. The TT is also a rainmaker for the government of the island and hundreds of merchants and small business owners.

But there's more to it than that. The main reason for the event's long life is the ethos of those who ride. Call it a mindset, an attitude, a point of view that guides their take on the long history of mayhem and the dangers they face themselves.

First and foremost, they know what they're getting into. Racing is entirely a matter of free will. Nobody is pointing a gun at anybody's head demanding that they participate.

Everybody who takes off from the start line knows that they could go home in a box that day. The odds of that happening are slim, but they're greater than zero. If riders haven't come to grips with that reality, they wouldn't be there in the first place. It likely won't be him or her transitioning to heaven. But sooner or later it will be someone else. Probably sooner.

That attitude extends to friends and loved ones too. The statement released by Mark Purslow's family after his death at Ago's Leap says it well. "If he was going to go, this is the way he would want to ... he would be telling us all to stop crying, have a laugh and a drink on him, and celebrate his achievements."[6]

There are other sports in which the attitude toward death is similar. Boxing and auto racing in all its many variations come immediately to mind. After further thought you might add bull riding and land and water speed racing. There are also the untold number of thoroughbred racehorses and sled dogs who perish each year. They're not aware of the fact that they might soon die. At least that's the conventional wisdom. But the human beings surrounding them certainly are.

What sets the TT apart from all the others is the element of glorification. Death is not merely expected and accepted. It's almost exalted. Meeting your maker on the highways of the Isle of Man seems like a badge of honor. It's as if the dead are joining some sort of select honorable circle.

So the races go on, confounding the critics who want to get rid of them. Hundreds of riders will continue to pour off ferries every spring with bikes in tow. The last year with no fatalities was 1982, so next year's races will likely bring tragedy, as will the races after that.

Here's one last question to ponder. Is the TT, in its essence, really a competition?

For the riders the answer is a resounding yes. But looking on from afar it's easy to view it all as an extended exercise in risk taking. Out on the island's roads, you don't see motorsport versions of Rory McElroy and Roger Federer and Usain Bolt. You see Caleb Moore backflipping his snowmobile on Buttermilk Mountain in Aspen. Sarah Burke laying out acrobatic moves inside a half pipe on her snowboard. Nick Mevoli powering down through the Atlantic Ocean in the Bahamas trying to become the deepest man on Earth.

And who is that way off in the distance? None other than Evel Knievel, the greatest stunt performer ever, hurtling over the Snake River Canyon in Idaho in his rocket-powered Skycycle.

Every spring on the Isle of Manslaughter, perhaps athletic skill is taking a back seat to pure daredevilry.

# 10

## Team Tragedy

### Spokane Indians: Such Hell
*Baseball 1946*

When a star falls alone in the sports world, it's heartbreaking. No matter how or why or when death comes calling, grief is sure to follow. But when an entire team faces catastrophe together, the blow can be overwhelming. The nightmare of so many lives lost at once triggers immeasurable sorrow not only in their home community but in wider society as well.

The Spokane Indians were one such team. In 1946 they were playing in their seventh season in the Class B Western International League. Most of the ballplayers were under 30. Nearly all were veterans of World War II, born and raised in Far Western states. Nine of the 18 were married.

Two had been to the majors for short stints. A few were talented enough to move up to A or AA ball, and three were serious big-league prospects. But for the rest, Spokane (spo-CAN) was as high as they were going to rise in the game, playing in small-town ballparks for a couple of hundred bucks a month for two or three or four seasons, unless they got banged up so badly they had to quit sooner.

On Sunday night, June 23, the Indians scored three runs in the bottom of the ninth to win a 10–9 grinder against the Salem Senators at Ferris Field in Spokane. The next morning, they boarded a 21-seat charter bus for a 320-mile journey to Bremerton on the far side of Puget Sound, directly west of Seattle.

There they'd play a series with the Bluejackets—single games Tuesday through Saturday and a doubleheader on Sunday. A seven-game series was outside the box for sure, but that was life in the "Willy Loop." The terrain was rugged, the roads were narrow and rutty, and the eight towns weren't packed in tightly on the map like they were in the minor leagues back East and down South. Vancouver in Canada was 413 miles away, Salem 400, Tacoma 294. Geography forced a different way of doing things.

At 11:30 the coach left Spokane and started to creak and crawl west at 35 mph under overcast skies. Pitchers Milt Candinha and Joe Faria were absent, making the trip with their wives in Faria's car. Around 3 p.m. driver Glen Berg, 24, pulled in for a pit stop in Ellensburg, and it was there that slugging third baseman Jack Lohrke got a message from the club office. Owner Sam Collins had asked police to track down the bus to deliver the news. Lohrke was being promoted. The San Diego Padres of the AAA Pacific Coast League needed him ASAP. He grabbed his suitcase, hitchhiked back to Spokane and prepared to head south.

It was the luckiest day of Lohrke's life. He went on to play five seasons with the New York Giants and two with the Phillies. Vic Picetti and Fred "Marty" Martinez, the other two prospects on the team, would perish in the nightmare that unfolded five hours later.

As the bus moved through the Cascade Mountains on U.S. Route 10, a drizzly rain persisted. Traffic picked up as they got closer to Seattle. The pavement was slick and wet as they drove through Snoqualmie Pass at the summit and began to ease down the steep, wooded western slope. As dusk arrived at 8, they were still 110 miles from Bremerton. That meant three more dreary hours in the bus, maybe longer if the traffic and rain kept up.

On a long, straight, treeless stretch of road, Berg put the pedal down to make some time. A black car appeared in the twilight in front of him, its headlights beaming bright in his eyes. It was on the wrong side of the yellow line, heading right at the bus.

In an instant, Berg faced a choice—crash into it head-on or pull over. He pulled over, rumbled along the shoulder, lurched back onto the pavement, then fell off again and slammed into the steel guardrails. Levi "Chief" McCormack knew what was about to happen. The Nez Perce Indian was the old man of the squad at 33 and he'd been around the block a few times.

He dove onto the floor, grabbed a footrest and hung on for dear life.

The bus sheared off 30 yards of heavy metal, then went over the cliff. There were no trees to break its fall. It smashed into a giant boulder and kept rolling. Sparks flashed. Flaming fuel spewed out of the ruptured gas tank. Shattered glass filled the cabin and everything in the overhead compartments flew out.

McCormack damaged his neck and vocal cords so severely that he could not speak for several hours after the accident. When he recovered his voice he described the scene to reporters from his hospital bed—"I've never heard such hell."[1]

After tumbling 350 feet down the slope, the bus came to rest upright on top of a giant log. The entire vehicle was aflame. A truck driver up ahead on Route 10 named Nelson Allen saw the bus go over in his rearview mirror. He ran back, tied a thick rope to a guardrail and dropped down the slope.

Two burning bodies were sprawled out near the twisted hulk of metal that minutes before had been a bus. He dragged them away and snuffed out the flames with his jacket, but they were already gone. Berg and several players were free of the wreckage, some walking around dazed, others passed out on the ground, most with cuts and broken bones and severe burns. The rest were still trapped inside, screaming for help, but the heat and flames were far too intense to render aid. Their screams soon stopped. What Allen remembered most vividly for the rest of his life was the silence that followed.

He wanted to secure the bodies and haul them up to the road himself. But the job was way too difficult for one man with a rope. After first responders and volunteers arrived, they had to wait hours for a mechanized trolley to arrive from Olympia to carry out the forbidding task. Two state troopers were injured during the recovery effort.

Six men were pronounced dead at the scene, including player-manager Mel Cole. One died en route to Harborview Hospital in Seattle and two more died there in the following days. Three of the victims had pregnant wives. Six players survived. The driver of the black car who forced the bus off the road and sped on was never apprehended.

Owner Sam Collins ignored his doctor's orders to stay at home and rest and worked around the clock to arrange funerals, transportation and financial aid for the bereaved. The baseball world responded quickly. MLB commissioner Happy Chandler sent $25,000 to the Spokane community relief fund established for the team. Casey Stengel, manager of the Oakland Acorns of the Pacific Coast League, arranged a benefit game in Spokane with the Seattle Rainiers that raised $21,326. Bob Hope bought 50 box seats, and Bing Crosby, who had attended Gonzaga University in Spokane, bought 250.

Main Street America pitched in as well. A bartender from New York City mailed in a dollar, a barber shop in New Castle, Indiana, mailed in two, and two softball teams in New Haven, Connecticut, sent $20.67.

The Indians rebooted their season on July 4. Several teams in the WIL had promised to donate players, but their offers never materialized. Play resumed with a gang of also-rans and outcasts who offered their services, including a Korean third baseman named Ping Ho. The Kings finished in seventh place with a record of 54–78.

In 1996, novelist Beth Mary Bollinger published *Until the End of the Ninth*, a fictionalized account of the tragedy. Outfielder Gus Hallbourg, the last living survivor, died in 2007 in Manteca, California, at age 87.

*Fatalities.* Mel Cole, 25, catcher-manager; Chris Hartje, 30, catcher; Bob James, 24, right fielder; Bob Kinnaman, 27, pitcher; George Lyden, 22, pitcher; Fred Martinez, 24, second baseman; Bob Patterson, 22, center fielder; Vic Picetti, 18, first baseman; and George Risk, 25, shortstop.

*Survivors.* Pete Barisoff, pitcher; Glen Berg, bus driver; Bob Geraghty, infielder; Gus Hallbourg, outfielder; Irv Konopka, catcher; Levi McCormack, left fielder; and Dick Powers, pitcher.

## Duluth Dukes: North Country Inferno
### *Baseball 1948*

Two years and a month after the Snoqualmie Pass plunge, tragedy struck the baseball world again.

On July 24, 1948, the team-owned bus carrying the Duluth Dukes cruised down Minnesota Highway 36 through Roseville, a Twin Cities suburb. On the sunny, cloudless Saturday morning, they were en route from Eau Claire, Wisconsin, to St. Cloud, Minnesota, for a game with the St. Cloud Rox. Behind the wheel was George Treadwell, 42, the player-manager of the Class C Northern League squad.

At 11:20 a.m. a dry ice truck approaching the crest of a hill lurched left of center on the rutty, skinny, two-lane road, directly into the path of the bus. Witnesses said later that it looked like the vehicle's heavy load had shifted suddenly to the rear, leaving the driver unable to steer. Treadwell swerved quickly and hard to the right. The truck slammed into the left side of the bus and sent it tumbling into a deep ditch, where it landed on its side and burst into flames.

Treadwell and truck driver James Grealish perished at the scene. So did three Dukes players—outfielder Gerald "Peanuts" Peterson, 23; pitcher Don Schuchman, 20; and outfielder Gil Krirdla, 19. Second baseman Steve Lazar, 23, died two days later. Thirteen other players were injured, most suffering severe burns.

Led by farmer Frank Kurkowski, who was plowing a nearby field, Good Samaritans pulled many victims from the mangled wreckage. A doctor who arrived on the scene took a canister of lipstick from a woman and triaged the injured, scrawling instructions for hospital staffers on the seared flesh of the players as they were loaded into ambulances.

Like the Spokane Indians, the Dukes valiantly continued to compete that summer with players provided by the Northern League and the St. Louis Cardinals, their major league club. A benefit campaign raised $82,000 for the families of the injured and deceased.

Only four of the surviving players continued in baseball, including Mel McGaha, who later managed the Cleveland Indians and Kansas City A's. Pitcher Don Gilmore served 12 years in the Ohio House of Representatives from 1989 through 2000. Catcher Bernard "Bernie" Gerl was the last survivor of the accident. He'd arrived at the hospital with a face looking like "burnt toast"[2] and lost 70 pounds during his 40-day stay. He died in Joliet, Illinois, on November 7, 2020, at age 94.

## Cal Poly Mustangs: Lost in the Fog
*College Football 1960*

The chartered plane had been sitting at the end of the runway for 20 minutes, hoping for the dense fog to clear up before taking off for the long trip west to California. All incoming and outgoing commercial flights at Toledo Express Airport were shut down on the night of October 29, 1960. Departure for the Arctic Pacific Airlines Curtiss C-46 Commando had already been delayed two hours.

The fog never lifted. Instead it got thicker. The decision to stay put or go was in the hands of the pilot and co-pilot. They chose to go. As the aircraft with 48 aboard roared down the runway at 10 p.m., visibility had reached zero.

Liftoff was rough and very loud. The plane was airborne for just 15 seconds when the left engine stalled and lost power. It fell back to the ground, cartwheeled madly, broke into two pieces and caught fire. As first responders converged the flames surged 300 feet into the darkness.

By morning hundreds of curiosity seekers were swarming the site with binoculars, cameras and grocery bags, many hoping to scoop up personal effects, clothing and scraps of metal as souvenirs. They were restrained from rummaging through the wreckage by police and members of the Civil Air Patrol. Authorities did not want a reprise of what happened in 1931, when Knute Rockne's plane went down in a Kansas wheat field and scavengers picked the unattended craft clean.

There were 26 survivors and 22 fatalities. The dead included 16 members of the football team from California State Polytechnic College at San Luis Obispo, known as Cal Poly. Life or death was largely a matter of where you were sitting. The passengers in the rear of the cabin catapulted out of the plane to safety. Those in front plunged down into the flames.

The school with an enrollment of 5,000 was located in a town of 18,000, 190 miles northwest up the coast from Los Angeles. It was all-male until 1961, the year after the crash, when the first females were admitted. Earlier that Saturday, the Mustangs had faced off against powerful Bowling Green at University Stadium 30 miles south of Toledo, losing 50–6.

Why in the world would a small college team from California make a 4,500-mile round trip in an airplane to play a football game? Because the situation demanded it. Cal Poly was a strong program, compiling a 67–29–1 record in the 1950s under coach LeRoy (Roy) Hughes. Their two most notable players in that decade were legend-to-be John Madden, a brawny tackle on both offense and defense, and Bobby Beathard, a quarterback-defensive back who went on to play in the NFL and serve as GM of the Redskins and Chargers. Many schools of equal size were dropping Cal Poly from their schedules to avoid ugly losses. The powerhouses of the West Coast like Stanford, USC and UCLA had no interest in playing them either.

Money was a constant concern. Every dollar counted. Staying afloat was a year-to-year challenge. Attendance at Mustang Stadium was low, and the appearance fees that opponents paid them to go on the road were usually more than the proceeds they could reap from a home game. Cal Poly had no choice but to accept their offers.

As for flying, it had become a routine practice in college football by 1960. But routine did not mean trouble-free. Based at Oakland International Airport, Arctic Pacific played fast and loose with the rules. Perhaps you had to when your fleet consisted of three old planes. The fatal flight was later found to be 2,000 pounds over the mandated weight limit. Pilot Donald Cresher had been cited by the FAA for several violations—no manifests, no logs, excessive hours in the cockpit, claiming to have a co-pilot aboard when he didn't. On the night of the tragedy he was flying without certification. The FAA had revoked it but permitted him to keep working pending an appeal. Cresher and co-pilot Howard Perovich both died in the crash.

Their last days on the job were busy. After dropping the Cal Poly team in Toledo they went to Youngstown, picked up the Youngstown State Penguins and flew them to New Haven for a game against Southern Connecticut College. Late on Saturday afternoon, they dropped the Penguins back home and then proceeded to Toledo to pick up the Mustangs. At no time during those two days was the Commando serviced.

Why did Cresher and Perovich decide to take off that night instead of waiting until the next morning? That's an enduring mystery.

Perhaps it all came back to money. An overnight stay would have required extra lodging and meal expenses for the Cal Poly team and staff. With a budget as tight as theirs, that mattered. Arctic Pacific also might have needed their plane back in Oakland as soon as possible for another assignment.

We don't know what conversations occurred inside the aircraft in the hours before the ill-fated takeoff. Were all parties in agreement that departing immediately was the best course of action? Or was their conflict on that point?

In 1970, a full decade after the crash, a federal appeals court in San Francisco ruled that the FAA controllers in the tower at Toledo Express had acted negligently by leaving the decision in the hands of the flight crew during such dangerous weather conditions. The court held that the controllers possessed the legal authority to bar the takeoff and should have done so.

On Thanksgiving Day 1961, Fresno State defeated Bowling Green 36–6 in the Mercy Bowl before a crowd of 33,145 in the Los Angeles Coliseum. Organized by Bob Hope and others, the one-time event raised $178,000 for the victims of the crash and their families.

Mustangs starting quarterback Ted Tollner was one of the lucky ones who lived. After boarding, he switched seats with wide receiver Curtis Hill, an NFL prospect who died. Tollner went on to serve as head coach at San Diego State from 1973 to 1980 and at USC from 1983 to 1986. He also worked in the NFL for 15 seasons as an assistant coach.

Fatalities. *Players.* Larry Austin; Rod Baughan; John Bell; Dean Carlson; Franklin Joe Copeland; Victor Hall; Guy Hennigan; Curtis Hill; Marshall J. Kulju; Jim Ledbetter; Lynn Lobaugh; Donald O'Meara; Raymond Parras; Wayne Sorenson; Bill Stewart; and Edward "Gary" Van Horn. *Manager.* Wendell Miner.

Survivors. *Players.* Donald Adams; Karl Bowser; Fred Brown; Bill Dauphin; James Fahey; Brent Jobe; Robert Johnson; Roger Kelly; Al Maranai; Richard McBride; General Owens, Jr.; Billy Ross; Roy Scialabba; Walter Shimek; Gil Stork;

Ted Tollner; Gerard Williams; and Russell Woods. *Coaches.* Sheldon Hardin; Roy Hughes, head coach; Howard O'Daniels; and Walt Williamson.

## USA Figure Skating: Total Eclipse
### *Figure Skating 1961*

In February 1961, as the United States figure skating team geared up for the world championships in Prague, Czechoslovakia, optimism was running high.

America had dominated the singles competition in the first decades of the Cold War era, producing five Olympic gold medalists—Richard "Dick" Button (1948, 1952), Tenley Albright (1956), Hayes Alan Jenkins (1956), Carol Heiss (1960) and David W. Jenkins, younger brother of Hayes Alan (1960). There was every reason to expect that level of excellence to continue. The 1961 team was young, spirited and very talented. The next American solo gold medalist would almost certainly be one of the athletes making the trip to Prague.

The candidate of the moment was Laurence "Laurie" Owen, 16, nicknamed the Winchester Pixie after her hairstyle and her hometown in Massachusetts eight miles north of Boston. She was sassy and spunky, with an air of charisma and command that riveted fans. You couldn't take your eyes off her. She'd just won the North American singles title in Philadelphia and was gracing the current cover of *Sports Illustrated* as "America's most exciting girl skater."[3]

Just before 10 on the morning of February 15, after an eight-hour journey across the Atlantic from Idlewild Airport in New York City, Sabena Airlines Flight 548 was preparing to land at Zaventem Airport, four miles northeast of Brussels, Belgium. The flight would proceed from there to Prague.

For reasons never determined, the cockpit lost radio contact with the control tower 20 minutes before the scheduled arrival. The crew was flying the giant silver and blue Boeing 707 on their own, with no help from the ground.

The first approach under bright blue skies was aborted because a small plane was idling on the runway. The pilots then violated protocol by attempting a second landing on an adjacent runway that was closed to all traffic.

The tower could see that they were struggling to control the aircraft. But there was no way to contact them to assist. Experts concluded later that the device designed to stabilize the tail had stopped functioning. From a height of 1,500 feet, the plane dropped rapidly in a near nose dive, lurched up violently at 300 feet, then plowed straight down through power lines into a marshy patch of land surrounded by farms. It exploded and caught fire on impact.

Theo de Later, 21, a worker in a nearby field, was killed by a chunk of flying aluminum shrapnel. All 61 passengers died, as did the crew of 11. The toll included 58 Americans. The crash was the first involving a Boeing 707 in regular service, which began in October 1958. It remains the deadliest air accident in Belgian history.

Initially there was eerie speculation that the event might somehow have been prompted by a total eclipse of the sun that was moving that morning across a wide swath of Europe, including Belgium. Observers quickly dismissed that theory because the darkness created by the moon completely covering the sun occurred 90 minutes before the crash. And it only lasted seven minutes.

But the term *total eclipse* was on point because for America's figure skating program the crash was exactly that. It was a colossal tragedy, almost inconceivable in its magnitude. All 18 team members died, along with six coaches, two judges, a referee, a team manager and six family members.

Nearly every sudden death in the sports world unleashes a flood of grief and shock. These deaths went

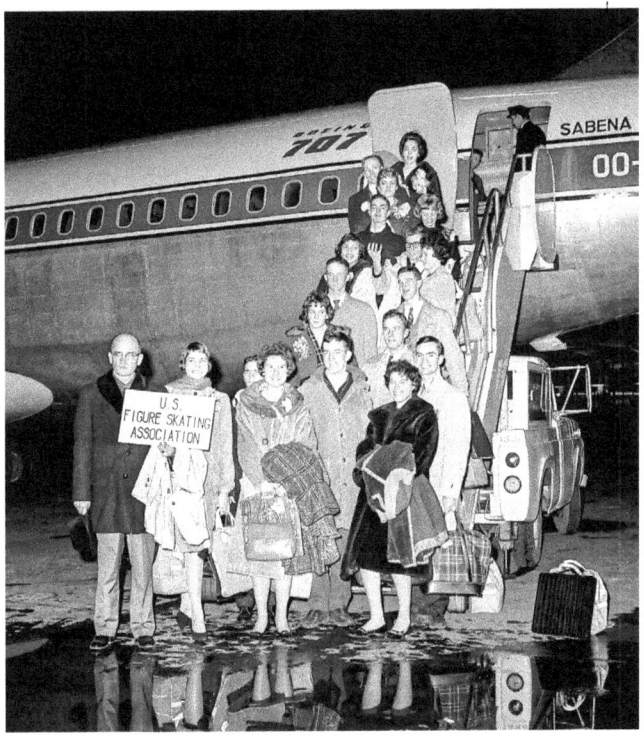

The U.S. figure skating team poses for a group photograph before boarding a Sabena Airlines Boeing 707 at Idlewild Airport in New York City on the night of February 14, 1961. All of them would perish 10 hours later when the flight crashed on approach to Zaventem Airport near Brussels, Belgium. On the far left is manager Deane McMinn, and next to him behind the sign is Laurence "Laurie" Owen, "America's most exciting girl skater" (AP Images / Matty Zimmerman).

above and beyond in that department. Nine of the skaters were teenagers. The oldest victim was 29. It was the sheer youthfulness of the victims that ripped human hearts to shreds. That and the fact that there were so many of them. There's a photograph of the ebullient team crowded together on the stairs in front of the 707 before they boarded Flight 548 at Idlewild. It's hard to look at it today and not feel a sickening sense of utter and total loss.

And then there were the telegraphs of condolence sent by the youngest man ever elected president, in office only 27 days. He and his magnetic wife were living symbols of hope, optimism and vigor, just like the team. No one could foresee that in 33 months he himself would be dead.

Days after the crash, supporters of the sport established the U.S. Figure Skating memorial fund. It has disbursed more than $20 million to support skaters' training and education costs.

The program rose from the ashes of Flight 548. The sun came out again and America reclaimed its elite standing in the world. Since that horrible February day the list of solo gold medalists has grown by eight—Peggy Fleming (1968), Dorothy Hamill (1976), Scott Hamilton (1984), Brian Boitano (1988), Kristi Yamaguchi (1992), Tara Lipinski (1998), Sarah Hughes (2002) and Evan Lysacek (2010).

Fatalities. *Skaters.* Roger Campbell, 19; Donna Lee Carrier, 20; Patricia Major Dineen, 24; Robert Dineen, 23; Ila Ray Hadley, 18; Ray Ellis Hadley, Jr., 17; Laurie Jean Hickox, 15; William Holmes Hickox, 19; Gregory Kelley, 16; Bradley Lord, 21; Rhode Lee Michelson, 17; Laurence Rochon "Laurie" Owen, 16; Maribel Yerxa Owen, 20; Larry Pierce, 24; Douglas Ramsay, 16; Dudley Shaw Richards, 29; Diane Carol "Dee Dee" Sherbloom, 18; and Stephanie "Steffi" Westerfeld, 17.

*Coaches.* Linda Hadley, mother of Ila Ray Hadley and Ray Ellis Hadley, Jr.; William Kipp; Daniel Ryan; Eduard "Edi" Scholdan; William Swallender; and Maribel Yerxa Vinson-Owen, mother of Laurie and Marabel Owen. *Judges.* Harold Hartshorne and Edward LeMaire. *Manager.* Deane McMinn. *Referee.* Walter S. Powell.

## Wichita State Shockers: Gold Flight
*College Football 1970*

It was a beautiful autumn day in the Rocky Mountains—60 degrees, sunny and cloudless, with a gentle breeze blowing up from the south.

At 1 p.m., a twin-engine Martin 404 airplane cruised westward across Colorado toward Loveland Pass and the Continental Divide. Aboard were football players, coaches, staffers and boosters from Wichita State University in Kansas. They were having a ball, laughing and swapping jokes, eating lunch and peering out the windows at the stunning landscape below. The "Gold Flight," reserved for team starters and VIPs, was enroute to Logan, Utah, for a game against the Utah State Aggies the next day. A second Martin 404, the "Black Flight" carrying second and third stringers and lower-level staffers, was also on its way there. Both planes had refueled in Denver.

As they prepared to leave Denver, Gold Flight pilot Danny Crocker and first officer Ronald Skipper decided on a whim to take the scenic route to Logan. They'd fly due west for 70 miles, then veer northwest over the most spectacular stretch of the Rockies. The Black Flight would follow the standard path, straight north out of Denver, then directly west to Logan.

Why was that standard? Because flying over high mountains can bring on many dangers—turbulence, updrafts, downdrafts and wind shear. The contour of the land can also play tricks on the eyes. You think you're in a safe place until all of a sudden you realize you're not.

That's what happened on the afternoon of October 2, 1970. Thirty minutes out of Denver, the scenic route turned very ugly.

## 10. Team Tragedy

Crocker and Skipper found themselves trapped in a narrow box canyon, flying too low and too slowly, with no chance to climb back to an altitude high enough to clear the tall mountains at the far end. They wanted to turn around and fly out of the canyon the same way they came in, and they made sharp turns to the left and right in a frantic effort to pull a quick 180. The plane began to vibrate loudly. Seconds later, it slammed into a wall of Mount Trelease, 10,750 feet above sea level, and fell into a dense cluster of pine trees.

Both wings were ripped off, but the fuselage was intact. Battered black and gold helmets and tattered shoes, shoulder pads and jerseys littered the ground. Many passengers dropped out of two holes in the side of the plane, most of them severely burned. The few who could walk scrambled down the mountain looking for help, which they found at a tunnel construction site. Some minutes later, the plane's two nearly full fuel tanks exploded.

Twenty-nine of the 40 people aboard perished at the scene. Two more died later at hospitals in Denver. One of the fatalities, defensive back Randy Kiesau, had switched planes during refueling to join the first stringers. The Black Flight arrived safely in Logan at 4 p.m., where the passengers learned of the crash, although details were sketchy for many hours.

The game with Utah State was cancelled, but the Shockers continued their season three weeks later at Arkansas. John Hoheisel, one of the survivors, drew a thunderous ovation from Razorback fans as he made his way to midfield on crutches for the pre-game coin toss.

In a hearing that began in Wichita 19 days after the accident, the NTSB pinned the blame squarely on Crocker, who died, and Skipper, who survived. Investigators determined that they had acted with utter recklessness and had no business taking the route they chose that afternoon. Skipper maintained for years that he and Crocker were scapegoated by a kangaroo court in front of a hometown crowd. He insisted that the real cause of the crash was failure of the right engine after it caught fire. The NTSB found no evidence to support his claim.

Visitors who make the climb up a steep, rugged trail can still see scraps of metal and chunks of the fuselage amidst fallen evergreens at the accident site. Just past mile marker 217 on westbound Interstate 70, a bronze plaque memorializes the victims.

As horrific as the crash of the Gold Flight was, it is to some extent forgotten today. That's largely because of what happened 43 days later in the heart of Appalachia.

Fatalities. *Players.* Marvin Brown; Don Christian; John Duren; Ron Johnson; Randy Kiesau; Mal Kimmel; Carl Krueger; Steve Moore; Tom Owen; Gene Robinson; Tom Shedden; Richard Stines; John Taylor; and Jack Vetter. *Coaches and Staff.* Floyd Farmer, ticket manager; Marty Harrison, head field manager; Bert Katzenmeyer, athletic director; Tom Reeves, head trainer; and Ben Wilson, head coach.

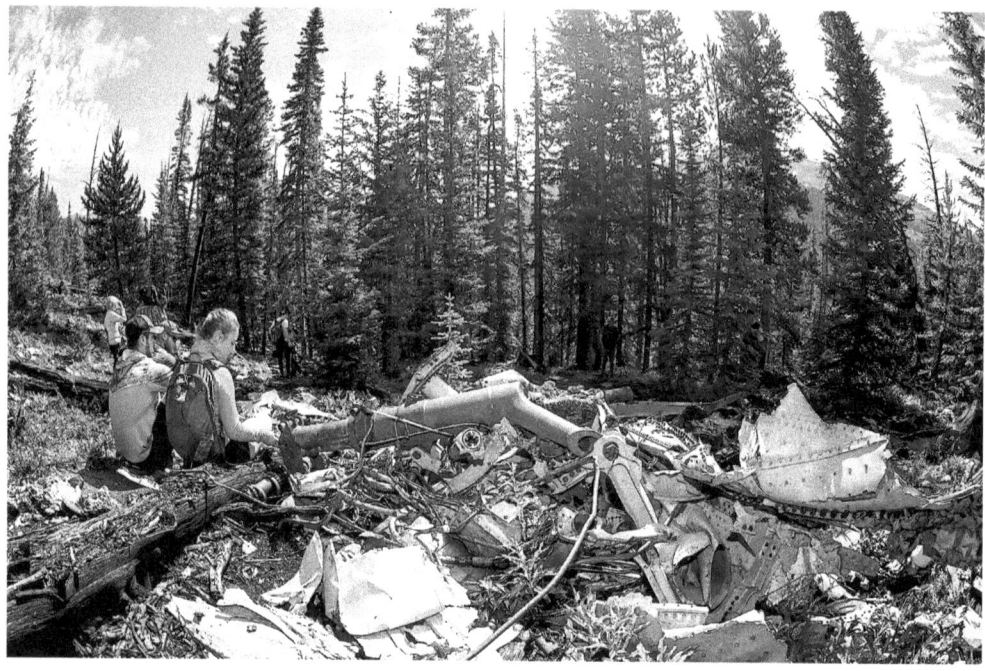

On July 27, 2020, visitors sit amidst the half-century-old wreckage of a twin-engine Martin 404 in the rugged terrain above Loveland Pass along Interstate 70 in Colorado. A crash into a dense cluster of pine trees on October 2, 1970, claimed the lives of 31 players, coaches, staffers and boosters of the Wichita State Shockers football team (AP Images / David Zalubowski).

Survivors. *Players*. Mike Bruce; John Hoheisel; Randy Jackson; Glen Kostall; David Lewis; Keith Morrison; Bob Renner; and Rich Stephens.

## Marshall Thundering Herd: The Worst
*College Football 1970*

As the Marshall University football team kicked off its 1970 season, the program was facing very hard times.

They had not had a winning season since 1964. The '67 and '68 campaigns were winless. The next year the NCAA placed the school on probation for more than 100 recruiting violations and alleged payments to players. Those misdeeds earned Marshall the heave-ho from the Mid–American Conference (MAC).

A load of players flew the coop, and the Thundering Herd opened the year with a depleted 40-man squad. On November 14, they played a road game in Greenville, North Carolina, losing 17–14 to the East Carolina Pirates. The defeat dropped their season record to 3–6. It looked as though the program might never climb out of the black hole they were in and regain some respect.

But something far worse than scandal and defeat on the field was just a few hours away.

## 10. Team Tragedy

After the game, the Herd traveling party boarded a chartered Southern Airways DC-9 in Kinston, North Carolina, for the 40-minute flight home to Huntington, West Virginia. It was their first air trip of the season. Southern was an established carrier with an excellent reputation for safety. Pilot Frank Abbott had logged more than 20,000 hours of cockpit time.

There was one ominous detail. The two men flying them home on Flight 932 were not the same ones who had flown them to Kinston the day before. Neither Abbott nor first officer Jerry Smith had ever landed at Tri-State Airport in Kenova, just outside of Huntington. Like many airports in the Appalachians, it sat on a tabletop plateau surrounded by hills and woods.

It was a nasty night for flying, rainy, windy and foggy. As the Ohio University Bobcats flew home after a game with Penn State, they battled the same storm. Just 15 days earlier, a small U.S. Army plane had crashed at Tri-State in similar conditions, killing three of the four aboard.

Abbott and Smith were attempting to land without the aid of precision instruments in the control tower. Tri-State did not have the state-of-the-art "Glide Float" system that best assists flight crews during adverse weather. Why not? Financing was an issue, but geography played the key role. Perched on an elevated plain, the airport was not surrounded by large tracts of flat, unoccupied land that were needed to install and operate the system.

As they approached Runway 11 from the west, everything seemed to be in order. The last communication between tower and crew 90 seconds before the crash was routine. At 7:42 p.m. the plane clipped a row of tall trees a mile west of the runway and smashed into a hillside. It then tumbled down into a thickly wooded ravine, exploded in flames and disintegrated.

Aboard were 37 players, eight coaches and athletic department staffers, 25 fans and boosters and a crew of five. All 75 died. Six injured players and a handful of players on the active squad did not make the trip. The bodies of six players were so badly mangled that they could not be identified. They are buried in adjacent graves in Spring Hill Cemetery overlooking the Marshall campus. The crash remains the deadliest tragedy in American sports history.

The accident left behind 29 orphans and traumatized the campus and the city of Huntington, which lost many of its most prominent citizens. The football program sank deeper into a black hole. In the 1970s they won only 22 games, the worst record in the nation. Some campaigned to drop the sport altogether.

But in the 1980s the Thundering Herd rallied from the depths. In 1984 the team had its first winning season in 20 years. They reached the Division I-AA playoffs in 1987 and 1988. In the 1990s, Marshall emerged as a real power, compiling a record of 114–25, a winning percentage of .820. They reached five I-AA title games and won two. The 1996 team finished 15–0. The next year Marshall moved up to Division I and rejoined the MAC. After many seasons in Conference USA, they now compete in the Sunbelt Conference.

Memorial Fountain was dedicated on the Marshall campus on November 12, 1972. Created by sculptor Harry Bertoia, the structure is in the shape of an upright flower, with water flowing out of 75 thin, intertwined steel strands at the top. A ceremony of remembrance is held every year on the anniversary of the crash.

*Fatalities.* Players. James Adams; Mark Andrews; Mike Blake; Dennis Blevins; Willie Bluford; Larry Brown; Tom Brown; Roger Childers; Stuart Cottrell; Rick Dardinger; David DeBord; Kevin Gilmore; Dave Griffith; Arthur Harris, Jr.; Bob Harris; Bob Hill; Joe Hood; Tom Howard; Marcelo Lajterman; Richard Lech; Barry Nash; Pat Norrell; James Robert Patterson; Scotty Reese; Jack Repasy; Larry Sanders; Al Saylor; Art Shannon; Ted Shoebridge; Allen Skeens; Jerry Stainback; Donald Tackett; Bob Van Horn; Roger Vanover; Fred Wilson; John Young; and Tom Zborill.

*Coaches and Staffers.* Deke Brackett, assistant coach; Al Carelli, Jr., assistant coach; Gary George, student assistant to Gary Morehouse; Charles E. Kautz, athletic director; Frank Loria, assistant coach; Gary Morehouse, sports information director; Jim "Shorty" Moss, assistant coach; Jeff Nathan, sports editor of the *Parthenon*, the Marshall student newspaper; Jim Schroer, trainer; and Rick Talley, head coach.

## Evansville Purple Aces: Basketball's Darkest Night
*Basketball 1977*

The raw, foggy afternoon of December 13, 1977, was turning to evening along the Ohio River in southwestern Indiana. The wet, dreary weather enveloping the city of Evansville was not going away.

Coaches, players and supporters of the University of Evansville basketball team were not sure when they would be able to board a chartered flight to Nashville, Tennessee. Their plane was late arriving at Dress Regional Airport, and takeoff had been delayed twice without explanation. Telephone calls were made to officials at Middle Tennessee State University in Murfreesboro, where the Purple Aces were scheduled to play the next night, to inform them of the status of Flight 216, operated by the National Jet Service of Indianapolis under the name Air Indiana.

Loaded to within 148 pounds of its 26,900-pound weight limit, the 30-year-old DC-3 finally left the ground at 7:20 p.m. Two minutes later, its engines whirring madly, the plane thudded to the ground on a mud-caked, wooded ridge near the eastern edge of the airport, just a few hundred yards from houses in the Melody Hills subdivision.

It exploded into flames. The fuselage was ripped open. Both wings had sheared off. The huge tail rested at the crest of the ridge as witnesses approached the wreckage and found bodies strewn across the ground.

Twenty-eight people aboard died at the scene from burns or the trauma of impact. The 29th victim was transported to Deaconess Hospital in Evansville, where he died later in the night. Early reports of survivors proved to be false. Eight of the 14 team members were freshmen, recruited by the school to help build a strong foundation for its first year in Division I competition after a long reign as a Division II superpower that included five national titles.

The only blessing of the night was that three assistant coaches—Ernon Simpson, Stafford Stephenson and Mark Sandy—had been on the road scouting future opponents and were not aboard the doomed craft.

As relatives of the victims were notified across Indiana, Ohio, Illinois, Pennsylvania, and North Carolina, rescue workers struggled at the crash site, fighting bad weather, confusion and a horde of curious onlookers. With no roads leading directly onto the ridge, bodies were placed in rubber bags and hauled by hand down a steep, stony embankment to a railroad track and a waiting Louisville and Nashville Railroad boxcar. An engine hauled the gruesome cargo, along with a caboose, to an emergency morgue in the gymnasium of the Evansville Community Center, where heaters had been turned off to prepare for the ordeal ahead.

Former Aces coach Arad McCutchan, just six months into retirement after 31 years at the helm, was called to the gym to help identify the players. He said later that it was the most painful and difficult task of his life.

The next morning, 1,500 students assembled in silence in the university chapel for eulogies and prayers. On December 18, 4,000 people paid final respects at a memorial service in Roberts Stadium, the Aces' home arena. The rest of the 1977–1978 season was cancelled after four games. Tragedy struck again 15 days later, when David Furr, an injured freshman who was sitting out the season with an ankle injury, died with his brother in an auto accident in Newton, Illinois.

Investigators seeking the cause of the crash found no evidence of engine malfunction. Attention then shifted to the immense load in the cargo hold, where imbalance or sudden shifting may have destabilized the plane and prevented it from gaining altitude. There was also a pilot-controlled rudder on one wing that had mistakenly remained locked after takeoff, making it more difficult to maintain control.

An illuminated fountain called the Weeping Basketball stands on the Evansville campus today as a memorial to those who died. The names of those lost are engraved on two stone slabs at the foot of the fountain.

Fatalities. *Players.* Warren Alston; Ray Comandella; Mike Duff; Kraig Heckendorn; Michael Joyner; Kevin Kingston; Barney Lewis; Stephen A. Miller; Keith Moon; Mark Siegel; Greg Smith; Bryan Taylor; John Ed Washington; and Marion A. "Tony" Winburn.

*Coaches and Staffers.* Jeff Bohnert, student manager; Bob Hudson, assistant athletic director; Mark Kirkpatrick, student manager; Mark Kneise, student manager; Greg Knipping, sports information director; and Bobby Watson, head coach.

## USA Boxing: KO'd by Fate
*Boxing 1980*

Most of the guys on the trip across the Atlantic were a few years north or south of 20. Walter Harris was the oldest at 27. Byron Payton, the youngest, was all of 16. They were just babies. That's what someone said after they were all gone. Of course they were more than babies, but you can see the point. They never had a shot at life.

As amateur members of the USA Boxing Team, they were still developing as fighters. All of them harbored Olympic ambitions. Light welterweight Lemuel Steeples from St. Louis, the best of the bunch, had his sights set on not just a gold medal but a pro career.

Fate snuffed out all their hopes and dreams on March 14, 1980. En route from New York City to Poland for a pair of dual meets in Kraków and Katowice, their Polish Airlines Ilyushin 62 ran into trouble with its landing gear approaching Warsaw Okęcie Airport. As pilots attempted to ease the craft down onto a foam-covered runway, excessive thrust caused a turbine disc in one of the engines to disintegrate. The plane lost altitude and shuddered violently, then exploded in mid-air and went down half a mile from the airport.

Most of the fuselage landed in a deep moat surrounding an army base that had been a fortress in the 19th century, sinking into 12 to 24 feet of water. A squad of frogmen worked for days to recover bodies. All 77 passengers and 10 crew members died, including 22 members of the USA Boxing traveling party.

They lost their lives by fate. Bobby Czyz was saved by fate. The New Jersey native who would become the light heavyweight champion in 1986 was planning to compete in Poland. But he was injured in a car accident a week before the flight and missed the trip. And Marvis Frazier, a 1979 AAU titlist, was saved by his old man, the heavyweight champion of the world from 1970 to 1973. Smokin' Joe had a profound fear of flying. He did not want his son setting foot in any airplane for any reason. He was the man of the house, and he ordered Marvis to remain stateside.

Two identical nine-foot metal sculptures commemorate the lives that were lost that Sunday. Titled *Down but Not Out, Lost but Not Forgotten*, they depict a fallen fighter struggling to get off the canvas. One stands outside the Museum of Sports and Tourism in Warsaw. The other is located at the U.S. Olympic and Paralympic training center in Colorado Springs, Colorado.

*Fatalities. Boxers.* Kelvin Anderson; Elliot Chavis; Gary Tyrone Clayton; Walter Harris; Byron Lindsay; Andre McCoy; Paul Palamino; Byron Payton; George Pimentel; Chuck Robinson; David Rodriguez; Lemuel Steeples; Jerome Stewart; and Lonnie Young.

*Coaches and Staff.* Joseph F. Bland, team manager; Colonel Bernard Callahan, referee-judge; Thomas "Sarge" Johnson, head coach; John Radison, referee-judge; Junior Robles, assistant coach; Steve Smigiel, interpreter; Delores Wesson, team assistant; and Doctor Ray Wesson, team physician.

# 11

## Red Highways

### Steve Prefontaine: Bell Lap
*Running 1975*

The gold MG convertible veered left of center on the narrow, winding road, jumping the shoulder, smashing a basalt embankment and flipping over in a field scattered with poison oak.

Pinned in the dirt beneath the sports car's bulk, surrounded by metal, glass, gasoline and blood, lay the driver Steve Prefontaine (pree-fawn-TAYNE), the greatest distance runner in America.

He'd run this very stretch of Skyline Boulevard outside of Eugene uncountable times. Just five hours before he'd won a 5K night race at Hayward Field on the University of Oregon campus, pulling away from close friend Frank Shorter in the stretch. It was a chilling omen that he wore a black singlet in a race for the first time in his career. Afterward he stopped at the Paddock Saloon and Grill on East Amazon Drive and then attended a private party for Finnish runners. He departed shortly after midnight, dropping his girlfriend Nancy Alleman at her car on campus before leaving Shorter at the home of runner Kenny Moore.

Ten minutes later Prefontaine was suffocating to death, his chest and stomach crushed by the wreckage. It was 12:39 a.m. on May 30, 1974. He was 24 years old.

With Pre, as he was called in the running world, it was never simply a matter of records broken and races won. Today more people remember his edgy, magnetic personality, his intensity in training and competition and a running style that Boston Marathon champion Jon Anderson called "always hard and straining and fierce."[1] Pre never did anything nice and easy, on the track or off. That is how he became a working-class hero and the pride of the Beaver State.

He grew up in the rugged fishing and lumbering town of Coos Bay, which he once described as a place where a man could get knocked on his ass for the offense of holding a beer stein the wrong way. The town had little use for a skinny, awkward boy who didn't even understand much English until he went to school because his mother Elfriede Sennholz spoke her native tongue in the family home. She met and married welder Raymond Prefontaine in Germany when he was stationed there with U.S. occupation forces after World War II.

The kid was a handful. His energy was boundless, and he was mad for sports. But he was short and weighed only 90 pounds, too small for the all–American holy trinity of football, basketball and baseball. At first, he resisted running because it seemed like drudgery. Then in eighth-grade gym class he discovered he was good at it. Big-time good, particularly in long runs of a mile or two or more.

He kept at it to prove his manhood and to resist the lure of switchblades, thieving gangs and life on the streets. At Marshfield High School he set a national record in the two-mile run. By the time he was a freshman on the renowned track team at Oregon he had appeared on the cover of *Sports Illustrated*.

For a runner he was short and squat at 5–9, 145. That didn't hold him back. He won 120 of the 153 races he entered in his career. In college he earned four NCAA three-mile crowns and three cross country titles. His dominance was astounding. The idea of limitations was foreign to his way of thinking. At the time of his death, he held American outdoor records in seven events—2K, 3K, two-mile, three-mile, 5K, six-mile and 10K. He also held indoor marks in the 3K and two-mile. His most painful setback came in the 5K final at the 1972 Olympics in Munich, where he faltered in the last 200 yards and finished fourth.

His most unabashed supporters were his boisterous fans in the stands, who came to be called Pre's People. After every win he liked to run two or three victory laps to commune with them and take in their wild chants and cheers. In every race he ran like a man with a score to settle with an unjust and uncaring world, possessed by an arrogance that both awed and repelled his rivals.

Off the track he lived with the same defiant abandon. He thumbed his nose at the AAU rules barring compensation for amateur athletes by becoming the first runner to take money for wearing and promoting Nike shoes. He attacked the AAU's mandatory event schedules that barred him from racing against elite international runners. His message to the powers that be was simple and direct. He wanted to be paid for his efforts. He wanted to be free to compete wherever, whenever and against whoever he wanted. And he wanted every other "amateur" athlete in America to be able to do the same.

He also ridiculed the facile patriotism of American sports fans. "People say I should be running for a gold medal for the good old red, white and blue," he said. "But it's not going to be that way. I'm the one who has made all the sacrifices. Those are my American records, not the country's."[2]

Prefontaine was not ashamed about his use of alcohol, and he made no effort to conceal it. He reveled in the taverns of Coos Bay and Eugene on a regular basis and occasionally bartended at the Paddock. One night after a poor showing in a race, he was tipping a few in a campus bar and lamenting the excess paunch in his belly. Another imbiber suggested that he might want to quit drinking beer. He replied that he would just as soon quit breathing.

So there was little surprise at the results of the BAC test taken on the morning he died—.16 percent, a level considered by Oregon law to impair driving skills significantly. He likely drank six or seven beers in the three or four hours before his death.

Questions have persisted for decades about the night of the accident. Was there a second vehicle involved? Did Prefontaine lurch left of center and smash the outcropping on his own or was he forced off the road? Was he drag racing with another driver? In fact, there was another MG on Skyline Boulevard that night, traveling very close to him. But the 20-year-old driver was cleared of wrongdoing after passing a polygraph test a week after the crash.

The police have stood by their story for half a century. Prefontaine was impaired and unbelted, he was driving way too fast for conditions, and he lost control of his vehicle on his own accord. No one else was involved.

After a funeral at Pirates Stadium in Coos Bay, Prefontaine was buried in Sunset Memorial Park. The next day, 4,000 people assembled at Hayward Field for a second service of memory. Frank Shorter, Oregon track coach Bill Bowerman and Kenny Moore delivered eulogies.

Three films portraying Pre's short life have been released—*Fire on the Track*, a 1995 documentary narrated by novelist Ken Kesey; *Prefontaine*, a 1997 Disney feature directed by Steve Jones with Jared Leto in the title role; and *Without Limits*, a 1998 Warner Brothers release directed by Robert Towne and starring Billy Crudup.

The most distinctive memorial to his life and legacy is Pre's Rock, located at the base of the roadside outcrop on Skyline Boulevard where he met his fate, a mile due east of Hayward Field. For many years before its formal dedication in 1997, runners and fans made pilgrimages to drop items at the foot of the engraved stone memorial, including race bibs, running shoes, singlets, medals, newspaper clippings, handwritten notes, flowers and photographs.

Now managed by Eugene Parks and Recreation, the makeshift, grassroots shrine arose with no civic or governmental involvement whatsoever. It was of the people, by the people, for the people. That makes it an appropriate tribute to the son of a welder and an immigrant, a little guy who dreamed big, worked hard and stood tall and proud in defiance of the system.

## Pelle Lindbergh: A Man and His Porsche
### *NHL 1985*

Pelle Lindbergh had plenty to be proud of. The Swedish-born hockey goalie earned a bronze medal with his country's team at the 1980 Olympics in Moscow. Just two years later, at 23, he was excelling for the Philadelphia Flyers. In the 1984–1985 season, he compiled a record of 40–17–7, won the Vezina Trophy as the NHL's best goalie and led the Flyers into the Stanley Cup finals.

But the one thing Lindbergh may have been most proud of was his car, a fire engine red Porsche 930 Turbo. He bought it for $52,000 and added $41,000 in customized alterations, including a radar detector and a speedometer that maxed out at 190 mph. He'd owned other pricey vehicles through the years, including a Corvette and a used Porsche 930. But the red-hot one was his abiding love. Sporting a set of blue and yellow Swedish license plates, it caught the eyes of everyone in the Moorings, a wooded, lakeside apartment complex in Marlton Evesham Township in south Jersey, where he lived with his fiancé Kerstin Pietzsch.

It turned heads on the roads of the region as well. Lindbergh fancied himself a stellar driver and aspired to race as a pro after his hockey career was over. He liked to drive fast. Who would own a Porsche 390 Turbo to take it easy in the right lane? He frightened the living daylights out many of his passengers, including Flyers GM Bobby Clarke. It sometimes seemed as if he *enjoyed* scaring them.

The young Swede's love affair with his gorgeous machine turned out to be the death of him.

On Saturday night, November 9, 1985, the Flyers defeated the Boston Bruins 5–3 at the Spectrum in Philadelphia, earning their 10th straight victory of the young season. Lindbergh did not play. Coach Mike Keenan put reserve goalie Bob Froese in the nets to give his starter some downtime.

After the game, Lindbergh was more than eager to join his teammates in a night of celebration. There was no practice on Sunday, the Flyers next game against the Edmonton Oilers wasn't until Thursday, and several of his friends from Sweden were in town and wanted to meet up.

He went to the Moorings first. On that particular night Kerstin did not want to join him, although she often did. Pelle's mother and brother-in-law were visiting, and she decided to stay home with them. So he headed out on the town alone.

After a stop at a place called Bennigan's, he arrived at the Coliseum After Dark at 2:40 Sunday morning. The Coliseum was a hopping after-hours watering hole, the destination of choice for cooks, servers, and dishwashers when their own shifts ended. It was located in Voorhees Township in the same complex as the Flyers practice facility. As he thundered into the parking lot, Voorhees police officer Ed Simpson nailed him for speeding. Simpson did not have his ticket book with him, so he let Lindbergh off with a warning.

Inside the place was packed to the gills. Eight bartenders worked the space. A half dozen Flyers mingled in the crowd. Lindbergh had never been perceived by his teammates to be an over-the-top drinker. Witnesses insisted later that they did not see him drink much and that he did not act or appear to be drunk at any time during the course of the evening. One described him as "more subdued than I had ever seen him."[3]

Appearances are often deceiving. You can be three sheets to the wind even if you don't look and act like it. Lindbergh was definitely drinking in the early morning hours of November 10. There is some disagreement about exactly how

## 11. Red Highways

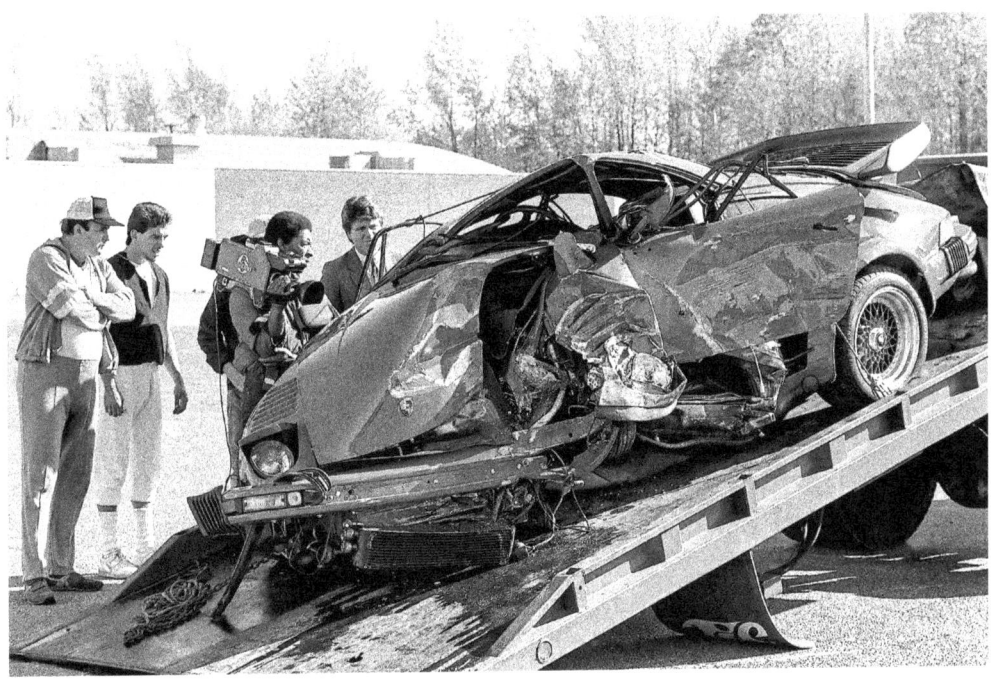

**Onlookers inspect Pelle Lindbergh's battered Porsche 930 Turbo as it is dropped at an auto repair shop in Stratford, New Jersey. Lindbergh died on November 12, 1985, two days after ramming the Porsche into a concrete wall at 80 mph following a night of heavy drinking. Two passengers survived (AP Images / G. Widman).**

much, where and when. Witnesses can also sugarcoat their memories after the fact to avoid speaking ill of the deceased.

As the Coliseum was closing at 5:30, Lindbergh went outside and revved up his pride and joy. With him were Ed Parvin, 28, and Kathyleen McNeal, 22, two friends who needed a lift home. None of the three fastened a seat belt. Lindbergh squealed out onto the street at a high rate of speed. A couple of blocks up the road he burned rubber as a light turned green.

At 5:41 a.m. Lindbergh failed to negotiate a hairpin curve at the corner of Somerdale Road and Ogg Avenue. Moving at 80 mph, he smashed into a low wall in front of an elementary school. Skid marks on the pavement indicated that he didn't brake until he was 10 to 20 feet away from it.

Parvin was in the passenger seat. McNeal was perched on the console between him and Lindbergh. Amazingly, given the force of the collision, they both survived and recovered from their injuries. Lindbergh was not as lucky. His body was plastered up tight against the steering wheel, and his brain, skull, legs and spinal cord were crushed. He had a pulse when paramedics arrived, then went into cardiac arrest as they struggled to extract him from the vehicle.

At John F. Kennedy Memorial Hospital in Stratford, his condition worsened. Kerstin Pietzsch was taken aback by the fact that he didn't really *look* too bad. That was a cruel illusion. He was soon declared brain dead and placed on life support. His father Sigge flew to Philadelphia to join his wife Anna Lissa, and they gave permission for many of his organs to be removed and donated. His heart was given to a 53-year-old father of three. Lindbergh died on November 12. He was 26 years old.

As they so often do when sports celebrities die, onlookers flocked to the crash site. Some scooped up tiny bits of twisted red fiberglass to keep as mementos. The next day school custodians painted the wall white to hide the damage inflicted by the impact. Folded up like an accordion, the Porsche was towed to an auto repair shop in Stratford, where it sat in the back of a flatbed truck partially covered with a blue tarp. A steady stream of the curious flowed through to gape at it through a chain link fence.

Several days later, Lindbergh's blood alcohol content was determined to be .24. The legal limit for drunkenness in New Jersey at the time was .10. A second test pegged his BAC at .17. The results indicated that he had consumed anywhere from eight to 12 standard units of alcohol in the four to five hours before the crash, probably beer, his beverage of choice.

Those startling numbers branded him in the eyes of many people as just another reckless, irresponsible drunk, much like they would in the case of Cleveland Indians pitcher Tim Crews after his boating accident in Florida eight years later. They refused to mourn Lindbergh's passing, and they were thankful that at least he had killed only himself and no one else.

Other people preferred to downplay the alcohol issue and instead remember the man they knew and loved. Several also regretted the fact that they hadn't done enough to try to get Lindbergh to control his rampant speeding and slow down.

On November 20, the remains of Per-Erik Lindbergh were buried at Skogskyrkogården ("The Woodlands Cemetery") in southern Stockholm. Four months after his death, fans selected him as the starting goalie on the NHL all-star team for the Prince of Wales Conference. He was the first player in a major sport to be awarded an all-star berth posthumously.

## Jackson State Tigers: Blue Bengal Curse?
*College Football 1988–1990*

Jackson State University does not have a prominent profile. Founded in 1877 as Natchez Seminary, the predominantly Black school in Mississippi's capital city earned a notorious place in history as the site of a student disturbance in 1970 in which police shot and killed two people. It happened just 11 days after the shootings at Kent State University in Ohio killed four.

Today, the school's major claim to fame is the Tigers football team. Known to their staunchest fans as the Blue Bengals, they've won 18 Southwestern Athletic Conference (SWAC) titles and claim four Black College national championships.

The program has sent nearly 100 players to the NFL, including four Hall of Famers—linebacker Robert Brazile, offensive tackle Jackie Slater, defensive back Lem Barney and running back Walter Payton. Among the rest are Wilbert Montgomery, Coy Bacon, Jimmy Smith, Harold Jackson and Willie and Gloster Richardson.

In 1988, the Blue Bengals started down the path to a far more disturbing type of prominence. The Grim Reaper arrived in their midst to rear his hideous head and would not go away.

On March 11, defensive back Antonio Rogers was killed in a one-car accident on his way to his home in Prichard, Alabama. The next year, on July 27, running back Earl Eatman died in a two-car wreck in his hometown of Hattiesburg, Mississippi.

At their core, the incidents weren't much different from thousands of others that play out on America's highways with mind numbing regularity. Young people cruising around in cars ending up in coffins and urns, taken off the playing field of life before their games have barely started. It has been ever thus. Excessive speed, for whatever reason, is almost always the root cause, and media accounts of the tragedies tend to blur together and recede to the back corners of the mind.

Until it happens in your town, your neighborhood, your school. To people you know and like and maybe even love. Then it's shattering.

The deaths shook the team, the campus and the Tigers faithful. But the worst was yet to come. Nine months later, on April 16, 1990, three players perished when a Ford Mustang lurched off the road at 2:25 a.m., rumbled 30 yards across a field and slammed into a tree outside Macon, Mississippi.

Linebacker Casey Connor, 19, was the driver. The passengers were defensive back Charles Ford, 20, and linebacker Michael Kimble, 22. They were returning from an Easter weekend in Memphis to Connor's home near Macon before heading back to campus to start spring quarter classes.

No alcohol or other drugs were found at the scene. Connor was on familiar turf, only six football fields or so away from his family's house. Police believe he fell asleep behind the wheel. Why? That is unknown. There were no survivors to offer their accounts of the events leading up to the crash. But the Mustang was destroyed, indicating a very high rate of speed at the instant of impact with the tree trunk.

A grief session for players organized by coach W.C. Gorden was not a quiet event. The screams and cries of anguish were loud and long. Soon the talk began. Were the Blue Bengals burdened with some kind of curse?

Five violent deaths in 25 months were hard to just shrug off. Were there forces at work within the program that spurred the recklessness and bad fortune? Those inclined to find a curse certainly had their reasons for thinking that way. But you could just as easily conclude that it was simply a case of abysmal bad luck in the high stakes game of Dying Young Poker, with the Tigers drawing a very poor hand.

Five years later, on June 3, 1995, two baseball players in a Cadillac Seville died in a shocking 100 mph rollover crash on I-220 in Jackson. It was a kind of grisly coda to the football carnage.

This time alcohol played a clear and convincing role. As first responders arrived the smell of it permeated the scene. Outfielder Henry Wallace III was the driver. Second baseman Willie James III was a passenger. They died along with Shone Taylor. James McAdory and LaMarcus Byrd, two other team members, were injured. Byrd walked away from the scene with minor injuries. He was the only one in the vehicle wearing a seat belt.

For once, it was nice to see the Grim Reaper lose a round.

## John Rodolph: Pure Soul
*Wheelchair Racing 1995*

John Rodolph was born in 1964 with spinal bifida, a congenital defect arising early in pregnancy in which the spinal cord is imperfectly closed so that part of it protrudes. The condition, which afflicts some 166,000 Americans, causes upheaval in the nervous system and can lead to severe challenges in life, among them the inability to walk. That was the case with him.

Rodolph was also born an athlete. The need to train, compete and push himself relentlessly was in his genes. So he took up wheelchair racing, a discipline open to amputees and those with spinal cord defects, cerebral palsy and other qualifying disabilities. He entered his first marathon in Hawaii at age 13, when the sport was no more than a bizarre novelty in the sports world.

In 1980 he pushed his first of five Boston Marathons. In his early days he didn't have much money so he raced in a thin, fold-up stainless-steel chair, a far cry from the state-of-the-art models that cost $5,000 and could reach speeds of up to 40 mph. That was kind of like a tennis player volleying with a ping pong racket or a sprinter settling into the starting blocks in a pair of flip flops.

He didn't care much for being patronized. He had zero interest in being the lead character in a golly-gee-whiz inspirational story designed to renew the world's lagging faith in the human species. The kind of feature you see at the tail end of the nightly news after all the murder, calamity and thievery has been reported. He wanted wheelchair racers to be respected for what they were—athletes, plain and simple. Let's all take off at the start and see who crosses the finish line first. No tears, please. And by all means, cancel the pity party.

After he got the equipment he needed, finishing first was something he did often. At the 1984 Paralympics in London, he won a gold as well as two silvers and a bronze in track events. The next year he set an American record of 4:21 at the Pepsi Invitational Mile and a world mark of 40:12 at the Gasparilla Distance

Classic 15K. After a decade out of racing he pushed another world record time of 18:55 in the *Deseret News* 10K in Salt Lake City, at an average speed of 19.7 mph. His new reason to get up in the morning was to earn a place on the American team for the 1996 Paralympics in Atlanta.

On October 1, 1995, he won the Duke City Marathon in Albuquerque. He'd convinced race officials to allow wheelchairs for the first time and organized the division himself.

Ten days later he was training on a bike path in Rio Rancho, near his hometown of Corrales, north of Albuquerque. As he waited for a traffic light to change, a dump truck blew through the red and plowed into a pickup truck in the middle of the intersection. They slid into Rodolph, sending him and both trucks hurtling into a rocky ravine.

The guy never had a chance. He died at the scene. John Rodolph was 31 years old.

## Judith Flannery: End of the Road
*Triathlon 1997*

On a spring morning, three cyclists pedaled west on River Road through Seneca Creek State Park in the verdant, rolling outer reaches of Montgomery County, Maryland. The White House lay 30 miles to the southeast.

They were just beyond the Bretton Woods golf course and heading toward Poolesville, the turnaround point on their regular 55-mile training loop. Two cyclists were abreast up front. The third rode 20 yards behind them. Traffic was sparse.

An oncoming car moving eastbound began swerving wildly on the two-lane road. As it approached the cyclists, it swerved across the double yellow line directly toward them. The two in the lead quickly turned out of its way, one veering to the left shoulder, one to the right. The white Hyundai Excel sped between them like a 2,000-pound bullet and struck the trailing cyclist's bike head-on before skidding to a stop 30 yards down the road. A hysterical teenage boy burst out of the driver's side door, screeching at the top of his lungs like a wounded animal.

Cary Bland and Joyce Gearhart were not injured. The victim lying dead on the pavement up ahead of her crumpled bike was their close friend, triathlete Judith Marie "Judy" Flannery, born Judith Sysko on Christmas Eve 1939 in Wilmington, Delaware. The force of the collision was so strong that she probably died within seconds. She was pronounced dead at the scene. It was 11 a.m., April 2, 1997.

The 57-year-old retired biochemist and mother of a son and four daughters was a legend in her own time, a mentor, role model and inspiration to hundreds of athletes. In 1978, at age 38, the woman who described herself as the original soccer mom began running marathons with her husband Dennis. Nine years later she started competing in triathlons, an event that combines consecutive legs of swimming, biking and running. In championship events the distances are a one-mile swim, a 25-mile bike ride and a 10-kilometer (6.214-mile) run.

Flannery held her own in the water, excelled in the run, and blew the field away when she got on her yellow and purple titanium bike. In a whimsical nod to her stout Catholic upbringing, her jock buddies nicknamed her Saint Judy, Our Lady of Perpetual Motion.

Her late bloomer status did nothing to hold her back. Truth be told, it was probably a plus. She was the kind of person who relished the challenge of making up for lost time. She won the first of six straight age group national titles in 1991. She captured the first of four world titles in 1992. At the time of her death, she was training for the 3,050-mile Race Across America, an ultra-endurance team event that stretched from Irvine, California, to Savannah, Georgia.

The tragedy was magnified when the sorry story of the Hyundai came to light. The driver was Timothy S. Rinehart, age 16, of Rockville, Maryland. He held neither a driver's license nor a learner's permit. In the passenger seat was his father, Ronald Milton Rinehart, 38, who'd been drinking alcohol while fishing on the morning of the accident. A teenage male riding in the back seat was not publicly identified because he was considered a witness.

Timothy S. Rinehart was convicted of reckless driving and driving on the wrong side of the road, but he served no jail time. Instead he was ordered to complete 300 hours of community service and attend school every day. He had dropped out after fifth grade.

After 11 hours of deliberation, a jury acquitted Ronald Milton Rinehart of manslaughter, vehicular homicide and driving under the influence but found him guilty of six lesser misdemeanor charges. During his trial he admitted that he and his son were wrestling for control of the steering wheel in the moments before the collision. But the prosecution could not prove conclusively that he ever had control of the vehicle, so he received what many people angrily dismissed as a slap on the wrist. Ronald Rinehart died in Frederick, Maryland, on March 12, 2008, at age 49.

Flannery's death was a bracing wake-up call for triathletes and cyclists everywhere. Many of her comrades probably shared the same thought—there but for the grace of God go I. Athletes who train along the highways do so at their peril. Bikers, skateboarders, walkers, runners and the wheelchair bound like John Rodolph can only do so much to protect themselves. Steel machines weighing whatever number of pounds and moving at however many miles per hour pose a constant and often terrifying threat.

Team Judith Flannery won the women's team division in the Race Across America. In 1998, the USA Women's Triathlon Committee established the Spirit of Judy Flannery Award in her memory.

## Dwayne Haskins: Running on Empty
*NFL 2022*

Not every star who falls on a highway is behind the wheel of a sexy sports car, like Steve Prefontaine in his MG or Pelle Lindbergh in his Porsche. Passengers die too, like Jackson State's Charles Ford, Michael Kimble, and Willie James III. John Rodolph met his end along a road in a wheelchair. Judith Flannery met hers on a bicycle.

Pedestrians can be victims as well. It happens about 20 times a day in America, mostly at night. That was the sad fate of Dwayne Haskins in the early morning hours of April 9, 2022.

The Pittsburgh Steelers quarterback was in South Florida for off-season training sessions with several teammates in Boca Raton. It was part of an effort to reboot a stalled career. There'd been a single brilliant campaign at Ohio State, when he threw for 50 touchdowns and 4,831 yards and led the Buckeyes to a 13–1 record. Then came two lackluster seasons with the Redskins, who released their former first-round pick in 2020, followed by a year on the Steelers bench. As 2022 approached he was vying with Mason Rudolph and Mitch Trubisky for the starting job.

After eating dinner with teammates on the evening of April 8, he went out with a friend or cousin later identified as Joey Smith[4] and drank heavily at a night club. At some point during the excursion they quarreled, laid angry hands on each other and went their separate ways.

Haskins later found himself stalled on the shoulder of I-595, an insanely busy 13-mile corridor that connects I-95 in Fort Lauderdale to the east with I-75 at the edge of the Everglades to the west. With him in his rented vehicle was an unidentified female.

They were out of gas. Haskins exited the car alone and went looking for a refill on foot. Gas can in hand, he wandered up and down on and off ramps and residential streets before stepping back onto the freeway.

He'd called his wife Kalabrya in Pittsburgh, told her what was happening and said he'd call her again when he got back to his car safely. They'd only been married for a year and 20 days. When she failed to hear from him, she called Broward County 911 and asked for a welfare check.

About 6:30 a.m., a nurse on her way to work reported a man dressed in all black stumbling along the interstate. About seven minutes later, the driver of an overloaded, old dump truck moving west in the pre-dawn darkness saw the same man out in front of him in the center lane, trying to wave him down. He may or may not have been speeding and he struck Haskins head-on. Seconds later he was grazed by another driver in an SUV trying to swerve out of his way.

He died at the scene of multiple blunt force injuries. Haskins was 24 years old.

On May 23, the Broward County medical examiner released his report on the incident. It was alarming. Two samples of Haskins' blood had alcohol readings of .20 and .24, well above Florida's legal limit of .08. His consumption level was right up there with Pelle Lindbergh's, if not higher.

Traces of the painkiller Ketamine were also found in his urine. Known as Special K and Super K on the street, it's a party drug that can be snorted in powdered form or swallowed as a pill. It's prized for its psychoactive and hallucinatory qualities. The death was ruled an accident, and the drivers who hit Haskins were absolved of all blame.

The man was hardly an innocent victim. His level of impairment was shockingly high. He displayed poor judgment by walking up and down an interstate in darkness. And running out of gas in the first place was not smart. The Haskins family has raised allegations of negligence against Joey Smith and three other individuals, the dump truck driver, the rental car company and the establishments that served Haskins alcohol in the hours before the accident.

The 7,465 pedestrian deaths documented by the NHTSA in 2021 was the highest total in four decades. Overall highway deaths in the same year numbered 42,915, a 16-year high and a 10.5 percent jump from 2020. Fatalities declined marginally in 2022. Experts blame the frightening spike on a surge in reckless driving, spurred largely by the Covid pandemic. It seems that more Americans than ever before are taking the wheel drunk, high, distracted—and angry. Or any combination of the above.

Services of memory for Dwayne Haskins, Jr., were held in Pennsylvania, in his native New Jersey and in Maryland, where he was a superstar at the Bullis School in Potomac. The location of his remains is unknown.

# 12

## The Savage God

### Rick Carter: No Goodbyes
*College Football 1986*

When he was growing up in Kettering, Ohio, in the 1950s, many people who knew Rick Carter had a nickname for him—God.

Carter was a three-sport captain at Fairmont High School in football, basketball and baseball. He was modest, kind, respectful and hard-working. He strived to be positive and uplifting in every aspect of his daily life. Above all, he never displayed anger.

It's the kind of behavior that *can* be off-putting. Mr. Perfect is not always Mr. Popular. But it wasn't that way with Carter. You wanted to be around him. His mere presence could lift your spirits. As for the ones who called him God, perhaps that was their way of ribbing the guy and maybe getting him to relax a little. He was laser-focused and more than a shade on the intense side.

He inherited his love of sports from his father Cloyd, the best friend he would ever have in life. Football was his favorite. He was small at 5–8, 150, but that didn't matter. He was big in everything else it took to compete and win. At Earlham College he started at quarterback for three years and became head coach at age 23. From there he went to Hanover College and the University of Dayton, where in 1980 he led the 14–0 Flyers to the Division III national title, earning him Coach of the Year honors. He downplayed that, saying it was really his staff who deserved the award.

His success brought him a ride aboard the private jet belonging to Edward Bennett Williams, the Washington super lawyer who owned big shares of the Redskins and Orioles and counseled Frank Sinatra, Hugh Hefner and Jimmy Hoffa. Williams was also chair of the board of trustees of the College of the Holy Cross, a Jesuit school with an enrollment of 2,250 in the old factory town of Worcester, Massachusetts. The jet picked up Carter in Dayton and flew him there for a meeting.

Holy Cross cherished its athletic programs. The Crusaders played in the Orange Bowl in 1946, won the NCAA basketball title in 1947 and took the baseball crown in 1952. Their track and field teams had excelled for decades. The school was looking for a new football coach and Carter was far and away their first choice. Really their only choice. He eagerly accepted the job, although it was just a steppingstone for him. Someday soon he wanted to take the reins of a powerhouse program. Ohio State or Michigan would be splendid. Notre Dame would be even better.

In 1983, after three winning seasons, he got an offer from North Carolina State of the ACC. It was a definite step up. But Williams and Holy Cross president the Rev. John Brooks refused to release him from his multi-year contract.

Carter accepted the decision like the loyal soldier he was. But inside he was bitter. Big-time football schools released coaches from their contracts on a regular basis. Nobody wanted to stand in the way of a man trying to advance himself in his profession. But Holy Cross didn't see it that way. The institution that thought the world of him now seemed to be holding him back.

Two years later, the school decided to go the way of the Ivy League and abolish athletic scholarships. As with other students, financial aid for athletes would now be based solely on need. Holy Cross planned to join the Colonial League, later renamed the Patriot League, a group of like-minded schools including Colgate, Bucknell and Lehigh. To Carter it was another slap in the face. Holy Cross was kicking him and the sport he loved to the curb.

Just before the start of the 1985 season, Cloyd Carter died of cancer a mere week after his diagnosis. Rick was shattered by the sudden loss. His father was the guiding light of his life. Then his mother Henrietta was diagnosed with cancer as well.

Autumn passed in a haze. Holy Cross finished at 4–6–1, Carter's third losing season in 20 years of coaching. His wife Deanna could see that he was suffering. Her husband, she later said, "was not in his right mind."[1] He was tired, unfocused and morose. He stopped eating and sleeping on a regular basis. He had trouble making even the simplest of decisions.

The illness that had frightened and bedeviled him nearly all his adult life was back, rearing its very ugly head again as he turned 42.

Carter was smart enough to know something was wrong with him. He'd been treated for depression once before in Massachusetts. He didn't want to create a stir in Worcester, so on January 24 he flew back home to seek treatment at Kettering Memorial Hospital. He visited his gravely ill mother, who was drifting in and out of a coma, and met with doctors who gave him antidepressant medication for the first time.

That in itself was a game changer. Forty years ago, society at large still viewed depression as a sign of weakness, a personal failing. The prevailing take on it was blunt.

Stop your sobbing, get over yourself, show some gumption and grit and move on with your life. It can't be *that* bad.

Carter himself probably agreed with that view to some extent. Only in the medical community was depression viewed as an illness that could be treated successfully with medication. Not that the meds always did their job. They were usually effective in rebalancing chemicals in the brain and controlling the symptoms of depression. But they were also known to trigger suicidal thoughts.

After four days Carter was deemed stable enough to be released. He arrived back in Massachusetts on Friday, the 31st. Things appeared to be on the upswing. The next day he left a film session with his coaches at 11 p.m. and drove to his home at 42 Townsend Drive in West Boylston, nine miles north of campus.

The call came into 9-1-1 at 8:41 Sunday morning. His older son had found his father hanging from a ceiling beam by a belt in the upstairs hallway of the house. He was DOA at Hollern Hospital, with the cause of death listed as "ligature compression of the neck."[2] That's a professional term for strangulation. Medical examiners ruled the death a suicide. Carter left no note.

He was survived by his wife Deanna; sons Nick, 21, and Andrew, 12; sister and brother-in-law Diane and Michael Brown; and his mother Henrietta, who died a week later. His 20-year record as a college coach was 137–58–7. He is buried in Forest Hill Cemetery in Piqua, Miami County, Ohio.

The mourning at Holy Cross was profound and deeply felt. On February 10, 2,500 people packed St. Joseph's Chapel on campus for a memorial service. Carter's casket was shrouded in white with a single red rose on top.

The elaborate, ceremonial display of grief was somewhat ironic, given the harsh Catholic strictures against suicide. Your life is the property of God, and if you destroy your own life, you are committing the mortal sin of asserting your will over the will of God. That was the orthodox view that had endured for centuries. A funeral Mass could not be held for anyone who died by suicide, and the person could not be buried in a Catholic cemetery.

By the 1980s, under the leadership of Pope John Paul II, those bans had eased. The church came to recognize that most who die by suicide are mentally ill. They experience anguish and despair to such an extreme degree that it prevents them from making clear, rational choices. To use Deanna Carter's phrase about her husband, they are not in their right minds.

The illness diminishes their responsibility for their actions, and for that reason the Catechism no longer views suicide as a mortal sin. That means it does not bar those who die of it from attaining eternal salvation. However, taking one's own life remains a "grave offense."[3]

Carter taught his players how to deal with loss as a family. With his painful, unexpected death, they were suddenly facing the greatest loss of all. The program rallied in spectacular fashion under new coach Mark Duffner, who had served as the team's defensive coordinator. In the next six years they compiled an eyepopping record of 60–5–1 and won five Colonial / Patriot League titles.

But along with the triumph there was an undercurrent of despair and anger. Terry Malone, who played under Carter and became an assistant coach at Holy

Cross, spoke for many when he said he'd always be hurt and resentful about what the man did. He couldn't fathom why Carter would leave the world forever without giving him and many others a chance to say goodbye. And he was upset that he would not be around to see Malone someday coach his own team.

Suicide can indeed leave a harsh, bitter legacy. Not every memory of the deceased is a happy one. Far from it, especially when, like Carter, they depart with no warning. In his provocative study of the subject published in 1971, A. Alvarez labeled suicide the Savage God. That's an apt description of a jarring act and the ferocious, disturbing forces that lead up to it.

## Jeff Alm: Very Close
### NFL 1993

The call came into Houston EMS at 2:32 on the morning of December 14, 1993.

The frantic caller was away from his cell phone, shouting to someone in the distance. "Sean, are you all right?" he screamed. He came back to his phone and tried to explain to the dispatcher exactly where he was on the interstate system.

"I had an accident on 59. 59 North at Loop 610, I think. My buddy ended up on 610."

"Are you northbound? North or south?"

The caller didn't respond and started sobbing. "Sean, are you all right?" he screamed again.[4]

Half a minute later, the dispatcher heard a booming gunshot. Fifteen seconds after that came a second shot. Ten seconds later came a third and finally a fourth. Then silence.

Arriving police found a huge, muscular young man sitting on the side of the elevated ramp, his back propped up against a guardrail, a cavernous, bloody wound inside his mouth. On the ground next to him was a Winchester pistol-grip shotgun. His cell phone rested on the top of a battered black Cadillac El Dorado.

Off the right shoulder, down a step grass embankment, a second corpse lay on a service road. When the vehicle slammed into the guardrail at 63 mph, he had catapulted out of the open front window, tumbled down the grass and come to rest on cold concrete. He probably died instantly. One of his cowboy boots, ripped off in the trauma, lay on the pavement 15 yards from his body.

The driver of the El Dorado was Jeff Alm, 25, a defensive tackle in his fourth season with the Houston Oilers. The unbelted, ejected passenger was Sean Lynch, also 25, Alm's best friend since their days together at Carl Sandburg High School in Orland Park, Illinois, in the outer suburbs of Chicagoland, 27 miles southwest of the Loop.

They were something of an odd couple. Alm was nearly 6'7" and weighed 270 pounds. Lynch was a foot shorter and more than a hundred pounds lighter. They met on the football practice field the summer before junior year when they were paired up for one-on-one drills.

Alm was the best player on the team. Lynch was a hardcore benchwarmer. But they took an instant liking to each other and became nearly inseparable. If you saw one of them coming down the hall toward you, you almost always saw the other. "They were very very very close," said Larry Lokanc, a football coach at Sandburg.[5]

Both were outsiders of sorts. That may have been what sparked the friendship.

Lynch was a transfer student from another school. Alm had arrived in Orland Park at age 11 by way of Rye, New York, and Marlboro, New Jersey, after his parents Betty and Larry divorced. His mother married roofer Bill Robson and took her two sons and daughter to live with him and his children in his hometown.

The bromance continued when Alm went to Notre Dame on a football scholarship in 1986 and Lynch started work as a manager at Jack Gibbons Garden, an old-school steakhouse in Oak Forest owned by his family for 70 years. He slapped a big Notre Dame sticker on the mirror behind the Jack Gibbons bar and attended many Irish home games in South Bend.

After seeing little playing time in his first two years, Alm blossomed into a nimble, formidable pass rusher on the 1988 national championship team. Following a sterling senior season, he was drafted by the Oilers in the second round of the 1990 draft, and Lynch came to Houston at least once every year to visit him. When he did, they went out on the town and partied hard. On their last night together they dined at the Old San Francisco Steakhouse on Westheimer Road.

Alm was not just one half of an odd couple. He himself seemed to be two different people. One was a polite, organized neatnik; a deep thinker; a meticulous record keeper and a mama's boy. He called her three or four times a week from Houston, often just to say hi. He also had a fear of heights. On a job one summer with his stepfather, he lasted less than an hour after he froze at the top of a ladder and couldn't muster the moxie to step onto the roof.

The other Alm was moody, feisty and prone to anger. He once exchanged blows with Spencer Tillman at an Oiler practice, and in 1991 he busted a guy's nose in a bar fight. He struck many as a pensive loner with a lot on his mind, living life on the edge and maybe even a shade or two beyond.

He was also fond of firearms. He owned numerous pieces and always carried one in the back seat of his vehicle. The shotgun he used on the freeway ramp to pump three bullets into the air and then a fourth into his mouth was a legal weapon. Oiler running back Lorenzo White, who spent hours rehabbing with Alm when they were both injured, recalls him rapping about a variety of "crazy things,"[6] especially death.

As the 1993 season began, Alm's usual testy state of mind was magnified by his ugly contract dispute with the Oilers. He'd rejected their offer of $2.3 million for three years, holding out for $3.0 million. It was a puzzling move for a player who had earned a total of $1.04 million in his first three seasons while starting only eight games. Management rudely countered with a one-year offer at $319,000, the lowest salary permissible under the NFL's collective bargaining agreement.

Alm went into a deep funk and held out for five games without pay, then rejoined the team. He played in only two games before fracturing his right leg. He was set to return to action against the Steelers on December 19.

It showed every sign of being a less than joyful homecoming. Under the guidance of head coach Jack Pardee and defensive coordinator Buddy Ryan, the Oilers were performing splendidly without him, winning five straight after a 1–4 start. And he had alienated the front office with his excessive salary demands. He realized that his days with the Oilers were very likely numbered.

His days in the NFL may well have been numbered too. After the tragedy, Larry Alm said that his son was fretful about a future after football. He had never held a real job outside the sport, and it worried him. Uncertainty loomed. What in the world was he going to do with his life now?

The accolades for Alm were numerous and heartfelt. But his death provoked anger as well. There was outrage when the BAC readings for Alm and Lynch were released to the public—Alm's was .143, Lynch's an astronomical 3.0. For a man of Lynch's size and weight that pointed to an eight-hour escapade featuring roughly 15 standard units of alcohol. Alm's blood also contained a medicinal amount of Fiorinal, a powerful painkiller used to treat tension headaches and inflamed muscles. Bad feelings also welled up in Orland Park, where Alm's hometown friends trashed news reports that he was violent and self-destructive and had a death wish.

There was bitterness in Alm's family too. His older sister Debbie O'Connor and her husband Mike each gave his casket a hard whack as it lay at the Schmaedeke Funeral Home in Worth, near Orland Park. The whacks were intended to deliver an angry, final message to the deceased. *Stop kidding yourself. You're no hero. You took the coward's way out. You committed the ultimate selfish act and inflicted horrible pain on your friends and family, pain we will feel every day for the rest of our lives. We're trying very hard to forgive you for what you did but we may not be able to.*

Perhaps the one thing you can say in Alm's defense is that his suicide looked to be triggered by overpowering guilt. Thanks to a driver's side air bag in the El Dorado, he walked away from the accident he caused with barely a scratch. His best friend died. Alm tried and convicted himself of doing something horribly wrong and decided there was only one appropriate punishment. He sentenced himself to death.

Sean Patrick Lynch is interred at Holy Sepulchre Cemetery in the village of Alsip in Cook County, Illinois. Jeffrey Lawrence Alm lies eight miles to the northwest in Fairmount-Willows Memorial Park.

# Erica Blasberg: Final Breath
*Golf 2010*

First responders found the corpse in an upstairs bedroom of the trim, tidy house in the trim, tidy community of Henderson, 15 miles southeast of downtown Las Vegas.

A dust cloth covered the young woman's head. Beneath the cloth was a plastic bag, secured tightly around the neck. It's a form of death called asphyxia by rebreathing. Deprived of fresh oxygen, she slowly but very surely suffocated on the exhaled carbon dioxide trapped inside the bag until she took her final breath.

Although suicide is no longer considered a crime in 48 states in America, we sometimes forget that it is an act with victims. The chief victim in this case was Erica Paige Blasberg, 25, a five-year veteran of the LPGA Tour. But there were others as well, including her parents Mel and Debbie Blasberg and the hundreds whose lives she touched in her brief time on Earth.

It was a bright sunny Sunday, May 9, 2010. Mother's Day. News of Blasberg's passing sent seismic shocks through three places—her hometown of Corona, 48 miles southeast of Los Angeles, the University of Arizona in Tucson, where she emerged as a collegiate superstar, and Mobile, Alabama, where LPGA Tour players were assembled for the Bell Micro Classic. Blasberg had planned to fly there from Las Vegas to play in the tournament herself. Her luggage and golf clubs were found packed in the trunk of her car.

It was a shattering end for a remarkable young woman who appeared to have the world by the tail. She was smart, beautiful and poised. Her work ethic was fierce. Her smile could drop your jaw. She had empathy, the ability to see life from other people's perspectives. She was financially secure and owned a two-story, three-bedroom house in Henderson that she bought in 2007.

Then there was golf. Oh yes, was there ever. Her father started her in on it when she was five, but she balked. Three years later he tried again, and she took to it. When Erica was 14, he started teaching at Eagle Glen Golf Club and things got serious. Never in his wildest dreams did Mel imagine that his prize pupil would be his own daughter.

At Corona High School she played on the boys' team and nearly always won. She captured 30 titles nationwide before she graduated. At Arizona she won six of 20 tournaments in two years and was the top-ranked college player in the nation as a freshman. She left after her sophomore year, spent time on the Futures Tour where she won her only pro title and joined the LPGA Tour in 2005.

Despite her astounding resume, success on the main stage proved hard to come by. She was only 20, facing life on the tour alone. Unlike most players, she didn't have a support group traveling with her. Mel and Debbie, who had split up during her senior year in high school, were back in Corona. And by all accounts she had only one close friend, fellow golfer Irene Cho. Her swing was nearly perfect.

Her distance and accuracy off the tee were consistent and her approach shots were solid. But her putting was very weak, especially from short distances. She finished her first season with earnings of just $52,522, tied for 109th on the money list.

The camera still loved her. So did her fans. She signed a contract with super agent Leigh Steinberg's firm and endorsement deals with Casio, Cleveland Golf and Puma Golf arrived in short order. That kept her bills paid as her slump on the course continued. From 2006 to 2009 she played in 66 events and managed only one top 10 finish. As the 2010 season began, she was relegated to limited status on the tour. That meant she had to play her way into tournaments in Monday qualifying rounds.

She gamely kept up a brave front. But all was not golden in the life of the beautiful All-American girl next door. It never had been.

The problems started with her dad. Mel was a stern, overbearing taskmaster. By his own admission he "force fed"[7] her both golf and his own personality, and he said he was happy to have done so because at the end of the day it was the best thing for her. They no doubt loved each other. But the relationship was abrasive and combative. Sometime near the end of 2009 they stopped talking to each other. It was not the first time.

Her relationships with guys were less troubling. They lined up to grab a spot next to her on the driving range. She didn't seek out the attention, but she got it anyway. Nor did she lack for boyfriends. Chase Callahan, one from high school, later became her agent, and through the years she had several beaus, some steady, some not.

Somewhere along the line she developed a thing for older men. At the posh Southern Highlands club in Las Vegas, she liked to crash the stag bar and send the wrinkly gray men into a tizzy. For several years she carried on an affair with John Broders, a wealthy, married man twice her age. Little has come to light about Broders. He is very much the mystery man of this story.

At least on the surface, it was his termination of their relationship near the end of 2009 that sent Blasberg into a death spiral. He was not willing to leave his wife for her. Heartbroken and devastated, she started hanging out with Doctor Thomas Hess, 43, also married, a family practitioner and the on-call physician at Southern Highlands. They met at the club when she asked him to look at a blister on her hand, thinking it might be infected.

The end came quickly after that.

On May 6 she played golf with Mel in Las Vegas. They'd patched up their rift and were speaking to each other again. Erica was focused and upbeat. Her funk seemed to be lifting. But that was a façade. Father and daughter talked about death that day, and her four-page suicide letter, which surfaced several months later, was dated May 6.

The next day she played golf with Hess at Southern Highlands before they went to a casino at the M Resort in Henderson to watch a hockey game. On May 8, Hess grew concerned about her state of mind, went to her house and poured two bottles of vodka down the kitchen sink. They watched TV and chipped some balls in the back yard. He went home at 9 p.m.

On May 9, Hess called her at her home 18 times, first in the early morning and then in the afternoon. She never picked up. He drove to her house, entered through an open sliding door in the back and discovered her body. He called 911 and left the scene in his Mercedes before responders arrived at 3 p.m.

A memorial service was held on May 19 at Eagle Glen Golf Club in Corona. Blasberg's silver coffin was rolled into a large ballroom in front of 250 mourners. Her tiny Yorkshire terrier Wynston was among them. The tears flowed freely, but there were laughs as well as people remembered her goofy humor and her affection for tabloids and the movie *The Hangover*, which she watched eight times. Blasberg is interred at Pacific View Memorial Park in Corona del Mar, on the ocean near Newport Beach.

At first Mel did not believe his daughter had killed herself. He was hellbent on making Hess the villain and demanded an explanation of what transpired between them in the days and nights leading up to May 9. None was forthcoming. Hess has since sworn on the life of his own daughter that the two of them never had sex and that they were nothing more than friends. At the time, Mel thought otherwise.

Many people believed he was lashing out at Hess to obscure his own culpability. He didn't give a damn what they thought. He launched a civil lawsuit against Hess, claiming that his breach of a physician's legal duty of care was the prime cause of Erica's death.

The process dragged on. The case did not go to trial until May of 2014, when an eight-person jury deliberated less than an hour before finding no liability. Mel Blasberg bitterly accepted the verdict but insisted that Nevada's statutes were skewed heavily in favor of medical professionals to the detriment of their patients.

Not that Hess was entirely blameless. After discovering the body and calling 911, he left the scene clutching some critical pieces of evidence. One was Blasberg's suicide letter. The contents became public in the early stages of the lawsuit.

He also made off with a package of Xanax, an anti-anxiety medication that Blasberg had purchased legally in Mexico a few weeks before while playing in a tournament there. A staggering number of other pills were found in her home—Tramadol and codeine for pain and a half dozen others to help her sleep, ease her migraines and suppress her cough. Medical examiner Doctor Alane Olson described the level of prescription meds in her system as toxic and called it a contributing factor in her death from asphyxia.

Nevada law bars public disclosure of the specific amounts of each drug. But there's no need to know the details. The picture is crystal clear. Blasberg was depressed and profoundly troubled, deep in the throes of a self-destructive

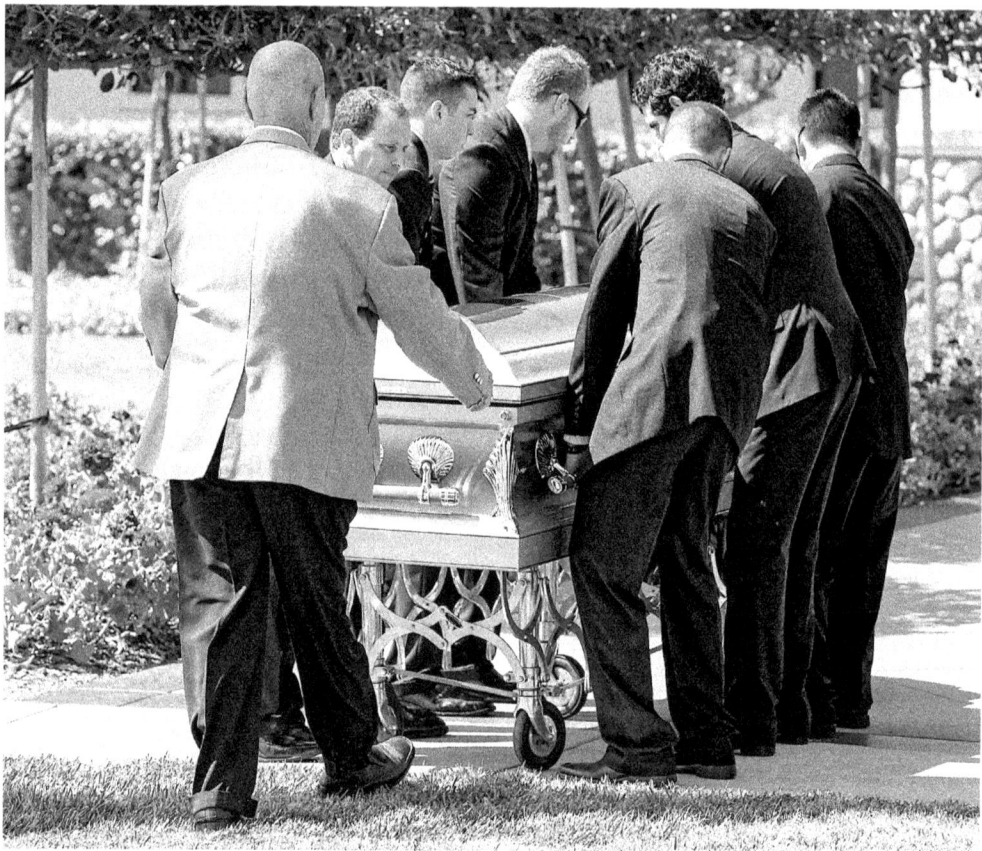

At the Eagle Glen Golf Club in Corona, California, pallbearers wheel Erica Blasberg's silver coffin into a ballroom for a memorial service on May 19, 2010. The troubled LPGA golfer died by suicide at her home in Henderson, Nevada, after enduring years of depression and prescription drug abuse (AP Images / Nick Ut).

lifestyle, swallowing way too many pills way too frequently. And let's not overlook the vodka that Hess poured down the drain. When it comes to substances that do a fine job of numbing pain, alcohol stands high on the list.

Did he prescribe any of her meds himself? That question has never been definitively answered. But the finger pointing in his direction continued.

Police arrested Hess on August 24 after discovering the letter and Xanax in the trunk of his Mercedes. He claimed that he removed them from the house to spare the Blasberg family additional anguish. For his actions that day, he was convicted on one count of obstruction of justice, sentenced to 40 hours of community service and placed on probation.

Fifteen years after the tragedy, the overarching question remains—why did it happen?

Blasberg's farewell letter, addressed to "Whoever," offers some hints. She knew she was "fucked up" in the head and she'd known it for many years. She considered herself incapable of living the life she led. She had the ability to behave normally but it was all a struggle and an act. Traveling on the LPGA Tour was "torture." She confessed to many failed suicide attempts. She was "sorry for all the people she was going to hurt" but they had to understand that she was "utterly miserable and had no other way to escape."[8]

For all the despair expressed in the language, no individuals are mentioned by name except her accountant in connection with her taxes. It leads you to believe that she shut people out. That comes through time and time again in the accounts of her life. She built walls around herself and shared her inner thoughts and emotions with absolutely no one. To a large degree, it seems as if she willed her situation on herself.

Why did she hate her life so much? What were the sources of her deep-rooted anguish? If she didn't want to be a golfer, what did she want to be? We will never find the answers to those questions. In spite of all we know about her life and death, Erica Blasberg remains largely an enigma.

The same can be said about all the other stars portrayed here. Each of their stories is incomplete. But even though the full truth remains elusive, there is one thing we know for sure. Every time one of these athletes died, the sports world lost a piece of its soul.

# Chapter Notes

## Chapter 1

1. John S. Watterson, "The Gridiron Crisis of 1905: Was It Really a Crisis?" *Journal of Sports Medicine*, Summer 2000, 293–297.
2. Aaron Gordon, "Did Football Cause 20 Deaths in 1905? Re-Investigating a Serial Killer," Deadspin, www.deadspin.com, January 22, 2014.
3. Christopher Klein, "How Teddy Roosevelt Saved Football," *History in the Headlines*, www.history.com, September 6, 2012.
4. Tale Runners, "Either I Win or I Die," www.talerunnerswordpress.com, November 4, 2019.
5. Curt Brown, "Sorrow, Past and Present, Masterton's Widow Hurt by Departure," *Minneapolis Star Tribune*, March 11, 1993, 7C.
6. George Puscas, "Hughes Died of Artery Disease," *Detroit Free Press*, October 26, 1971, 4A.
7. Bonnie Erbe, "Boxing Is Society's Worst Blood-Sport Throwback," Scripps Howard News Service in the *Columbus Dispatch*, July 2, 1997, 3C.
8. John Walters, "The Week in TV Sports," *Sports Illustrated*, April 7, 1997, 6.
9. Skip Mylenski, "A Rodeo Cowboy's Perfect Ride Ends in Death," *Chicago Tribune*, August 6, 1989, Section 3, 9.
10. Mylenski, "A Rodeo Cowboy's Perfect Ride Ends in Death," Section 3, 9.

## Chapter 2

1. Mark Hall, "5 Questions for Jim McKay," American Sportscasters Online, www.americansportscasters.com.
2. "Ballplayer's Parents File $462 Million Lawsuit," *New York Times*, December 24, 1981, 12.
3. "Player's Suicide Disputed," *New York Times*, September 3, 1981, 25.
4. Judith Cummings, "Inquiry on Jail Death of Black Athlete Widens Divisions in California Town," *New York Times*, November 2, 1981, 16.
5. Jack McCallum, "No Way to Die," *Sports Illustrated*, July 11, 1995, 27.
6. McCallum, "No Way to Die," 26.
7. Jeremy Wilson "Colombia Prepare for Biggest Ever World Cup Match on 20th Anniversary of Death," *The Telegraph*, www.telegraph.co.uk, July 2, 2014.
8. Pamela Mercer, "Outrage and Tears at Escobar Funeral," *New York Times*, July 4, 1994, 28.
9. Jane Ridley, "A Millionaire Murdered My Olympic Champion Brother," *New York Post*, www.nypost.com, November 12, 2015, 5.
10. Wright Thompson, "17 Days in November," ESPN, www.espn.com, August 20, 2012.
11. "Brother of Greg Halman Acquitted of Stabbing Seattle Mariner to Death," *The Guardian*, Associated Press, www.theguardian.com, August 20, 2012.

## Chapter 3

1. Sharon Kirkey, "The Dangerous Trance of Niagara Falls," *National Post*, www.nationalpost.com, February 20, 2018.
2. "Joe Delaney Headed for Chiefs Ring of Honor Sunday," Kansas City Chiefs, www.kcchiefs.com, September 23, 2004.
3. Jose Bermudez, "Speed Dream: Craig Arfons Remembered," *Sebring News-Sun*, July 13, 1994, 1A.
4. "Craig Arfons Killed When Jet Boat Flips," *Akron Beacon Journal*, July 10, 1989, 1.

## Chapter 4

1. Jerry Brondfield, *Rockne* (New York: Random House, 1976), 18.
2. Ivan Maisel, "Knute Rockne's Funeral and the Dawn of a New American Experience," ESPN, www.espn.com, April 4, 2019.
3. Mark Sabljak and Martin H. Greenberg, *Sports Babylon* (New York: Bell, 1988), 105.
4. Dick Brown, "Ruling: Munson 'Errors' Caused Crash," *Canton Repository*, April 17, 1980, 8.
5. Mike McCabe, "Detroiter Was Ideal Student and Athlete," *Detroit Free Press*, May 3, 1996, 7A.
6. "Tight Spot: Lessons from the Cory Lidle Accident," Aircraft Owners and Pilots Association (AOPA), www.aopa.org.

## Chapter 5

1. Gerald Eskenazi, "Nassau Grand Jury Exonerates Stewart," *New York Times*, June 9, 1970, 47.

2. Shirley Fischler, "Last Interview," *Hockey Illustrated*, November 1970, 21.
3. Brent Brookhouse, "Owen Hart's Legacy a Priority as Martha Hart's Wounds Have Healed, Though Her Distaste for WWE Has Not," CBS Sports, www.cbssports.com, May 18, 2020.
4. Brian Hedger, "Police Report Answers Some, Not All, Questions in Kivlenieks Fireworks Tragedy," *Columbus Dispatch*, December 2, 2021, 1C.

## Chapter 6

1. Tom Weir, "Hamilton Remembers Grinkov as 'Gentle Giant,'" *USA Today*, November 25, 1995, 3C.
2. Scott Powers and Tim Feran, "Bodybuilder's Death Puts Focus on Drugs," *Columbus Dispatch*, February 23, 1997, 1C.
3. Sam Farmer and Rene Lynch, "Vikings Say Stringer Had Diet Supplements," *Los Angeles Times*, www.latimes.com, November 17, 2001.
4. Philip Smith, "5 Drugs That Shaped Major League Baseball," Alternet, www.alternet.com, April 2, 2016, 2.
5. Mark Kreidler, "Baseball Finally Brings Amphetamines into the Light of Day," ESPN, www.espn.com, November 15, 2005, 2.

## Chapter 7

1. Christopher Clarey, "World Cup Skiing Star Dies After Crashing During Race," *New York Times*, January 30, 1994, Section 8, 9.
2. Clarey, "World Cup Skiing Star Dies After Crashing During Race," Section 8, 9.
3. Clarey, "World Cup Skiing Star Dies After Crashing During Race," Section 8, 1.
4. Peter Alfano, "Bench Jockeying: Lost Art in Baseball," *New York Times*, www.newyorktimes.com, August 15, 1983.
5. Richard Green, "Schott: A Day of Triumph and Tragedy," *Cincinnati Enquirer*, April 2, 1996, A4.
6. Rick Reilly, "Heaven Help Marge Schott: Cincinnati's Owner Is a Red Menace," *Sports Illustrated*, www.si.com, November 19, 2014.
7. Franz Lidz, "Well Off the Plate," *Sports Illustrated*, August 5, 1996, 78.
8. Sara Oliver, "Ice Cold Cruelty: The 8 Most Notorious Iditarod Mushers," PETA, www.peta.org, January 26, 2022.

## Chapter 8

1. "Jockey Dies as He Wins His First Race; Hayes Collapses After Passing the Winning Post," *New York Times*, June 5, 1923, 1.
2. Tom Pedulla, "The Imperial, Elegant Ruffian," https://www.americasbestracing.net, June 12, 1997.
3. Gene Smith, "Ruffian," *American Heritage*, September 1991, 53.
4. Smith, "Ruffian," 57.
5. Joseph Durso, "The End of a 'Gorgeous Beast,'" *New York Times*, July 8, 1975, 23.
6. Barry Horn, "Mary Bacon Ran Out of Rides," *Dallas Morning News*, September 29, 1991, C2.
7. "Report: Illegal Procedures Didn't Cause Deaths of Santa Anita Horses," NBC Los Angeles, www.nbclosangeles.com, March 10, 2020.

## Chapter 9

1. James Brooke, "Dangerous Paris-Dakar Race Is Endangered," *New York Times*, March 13, 1988, Section 1, 8.
2. Brooke, "Dangerous Paris-Dakar Race Is Endangered," Section 1,8.
3. Brooke, "Dangerous Paris-Dakar Race Is Endangered," Section 1,8.
4. Ryan McGee, "Dale Earnhardt's Death at the Daytona 500—Revisiting the Day of the Crash," ESPN, www.espn.com, February 11, 2021.
5. Rita DeMichael, "Dale Earnhardt's Grave Is Off-Limits, but You Can Still Honor the NASCAR Legend," Sportscasting, www.sportscasting.com, October 23, 2021.
6. Ben Hunt, "More Isle of Man TT Deaths Call for dangerous Race to Be Axed but Riders Know the Risks—the Decision Is Theirs," *Irish Sun*, www.thesun.ie, June 6, 2022.

## Chapter 10

1. "Death List in Flaming Bus Wreck Reaches 8," *New York Times*, July 26, 1946, 27.
2. Dave Deland, "Dukes' 1948 Tragedy Remains a Vivid Memory," *St. Cloud Times*, www.sctimes.com, July 23, 2015.
3. Kelyn Soong, "The Terrible Plane Crash That Devastated U.S. Figure Skating—and Still Shapes It Today," *Washington Post*, www.washingtonpost.com, February 20, 2018.

## Chapter 11

1. Kenny Moore, "A Final Drive to the Finish," *Sports Illustrated*, June 9, 1975, 23.
2. Neil Amdur, "Prefontaine, 24, Killed in Crash," *New York Times*, May 31, 1975, 21.
3. Marc Duvoisin, Al Morganti, and Tom Torok, "Lindbergh Was Heavily Intoxicated at Time of Crash, Blood Test Shows," *Philadelphia Inquirer*, November 12, 1985, 16A.
4. Justin Tasch, "Dwayne Haskins Drugged, Blackmailed and Robbed Before Death: Lawsuit," *New York Post*, www.nypost.com, April 10, 2023.

## Chapter 12

1. John W. German, "Rick Carter Was Sick Man, Treated for Depression," *Worcester Telegram*, February 24, 1986, 1A.

2. Ted Bunker, "Holy Cross' Rick Carter Dies at 42," *Worcester Telegram*, February 3, 1986, 1A.

3. Scott Alessi, "Is Suicide a Sin?" U.S. Catholic, www.uscatholic.org. October 2014, 12–17.

4. "Transcript of Jeff Alm's Phone Call to 911," *Houston Post*, December 23, 1993, A-1.

5. Robert Stanton and Richard Weiner, "Teammate's Death Stuns Oilers," *Houston Post*, December 15, 1993, A-1.

6. Doug Mitchell, "Oilers Try to Deal with Shock," *Houston Post*, December 15, 1993, C-1.

7. Alan Shipnuck, "The Mystery of Erica Blasberg," *Sports Illustrated*, www.si.com, December 13, 2010.

8. Mirjam Swanson, "Year Later: Family Haunted by Corona Golfer's Death," *Riverside Press-Enterprise*, www.pressenterprise.com, May 7, 2011.

# Bibliography

"Airliner with 48 Crashes at Airport; Football Team Aboard, 20 Are Killed." *Toledo Blade*, October 30, 1960: 1, 4–6.

Albom, Mitch. "Don't Blame Bearer for Lewis' Bad News." *Detroit Free Press*, November 21, 2008. www.mitchalbom.com.

Alessi, Scott. "Is Suicide a Sin?" U.S. Catholic, www.uscatholic.org, October 2014, 12–17.

Amdur, Neil. "Prefontaine, 24, Killed in Crash." *New York Times*, May 31, 1975, 21.

Anderson, Dave. "The Phone Stopped Ringing." *New York Times*, February 9, 1986, Section 5, 53.

Baker, Geoff. "Seattle Mariners Outfielder Greg Halman Killed." *Seattle Times*, www.seattletimes.com, November 22, 2011.

Barry, Scott. "Lucky Lohrke: 40 Years Ago, He Was Spared from Fatal Crash." *Seattle Times*, June 25, 1986, F1.

Bate, Beth. "Haughton 'Could Get Along with Anybody.'" *Yonkers Herald-Statesman*, July 16, 1986, E1, E6.

Beaven, Steve. *We Will Rise: A True Story of Tragedy and Resurrection in the American Heartland*. Seattle: Amazon, 2020.

Bechtel, Mark. "Crushing." *Sports Illustrated*, February 26, 2001, 37–43.

Beddoes, Richard, Stan Fischler, and Ira Gitler. *Hockey! The Story of the World's Fastest Sport*. New York: Macmillan, 1973.

*Berkshire Encyclopedia of Extreme Sports*. New Marlborough, MA: Berkshire, 2007.

Bermudez, Jose. "Speed Dream: Craig Arfons Remembered." *Sebring News-Sun*, July 13, 1994, 1A, 15A.

Binder, David. "Police Ordered 5 to Ambush Terrorists." *New York Times*, September 8, 1972, 1, 12.

Blood Alcohol Content (BAC) Calculator. American Addictions Center, www.alcohol.org.

Blunk, Frank M. "Auto Race Driver Killed Seeking Third Straight Victory at Indianapolis." *New York Times*, May 31, 1955, 1, 34.

Boating Accident Investigation Report. Florida Fish and Wildlife Conservation Commission, www.fws.gov, August 25, 2009.

Booker, Brakkton. "After Fatal Crash, Loved Ones Remember Racer Jessi Combs: 'She Was a Badass.'" National Public Radio, www.npr.org, August 29, 2019.

Boyer, Neal. "Man, 31, to Be Charged in Slaying of Baseball Player." *Gary Post-Tribune*, September 25, 1978, A1.

Bradley, John Ed. "Descent into the Maelstrom." *Sports Illustrated*, December 5, 1977, 121–127.

Branch, John. "The X Games, Driven by Risk, Have First Death." *New York Times*, www.nytimes.com, January 31, 2013.

Briqueiet, Kate. "Yankee Statue Destroyed—for the Metal." *New York Post*, www.nypost.com, February 23, 2014.

Britton, Bianca. "Frank Hayes: The Jockey Who Won a Race Despite Being Dead." CNN Sports, www.cnn.com, December 10, 2018.

Brondfield, Jerry. *Rockne*. New York: Random House, 1976.

Brooke, James. "Dangerous Paris-Dakar Race Is Endangered." *New York Times*, March 13, 1988, Section 1, 8.

Brookhouse, Brent. "Owen Hart's Legacy a Priority as Martha Hart's Wounds Have Healed, Though Her Distaste for WWE Has Not," CBS Sports, www.cbssports.com, May 18, 2020.

Brown, Gene, editor. *New York Times Encyclopedia of Sports*. New York: Arno Press, 1979.

Bunker, Ted. "Holy Cross' Rick Carter Dies at 42." *Worcester Telegram*, February 3, 1986, 1A.

"CAB Begins Inquiry in Crash at Airport Killing 16 Players, 6 Others on Football Plane." *Toledo Blade*, October 31, 1960, 1, 4–5.

Cady, Steve. "'Her' Favored to Beat 'Him' in Belmont Match Race Today." *New York Times*, July 6, 1975, 1, 9.

Caldwell, Suzanna. "Iditarod Dog Deaths Over the Last Decade." *Anchorage Daily News*, www.adn.com, March 15, 2017.

"Caleb Moore Dies One Week After Snowmobile Crash at Winter X Games." *Denver Post*, www.denverpost.com, January 31, 2013.

Callahan, Dorothy. *Ruffian*. Dubuque: Crestwood House, 1983.

Charlton, James, editor. *The Baseball Chronology*. New York: Macmillan, 1991.

Christine, Bill. "Bill Haughton Succumbs to Harness Race Injuries." *Los Angeles Times*, www.latimes.com, July 16, 1986.

Cilwick, Ted, and Monroe Dodd. "Chiefs Star Drowns in Rescue Effort." *Kansas City Times*, June 30, 1983, A1.

Clarey, Christopher. "World Cup Skiing Star Dies After Crashing During Race." *New York Times*, January 30, 1994, Section 8, 9.

Clark, Jim, and Diana Rossetti. "Crash Witness: 'No Hope.'" *Canton Repository*, August 3, 1979, 1, 6.

Clifford, Matthew. "Don Wilson: Houston's Fallen Star." Society for American Baseball Research, www.sabr.com.

Corzine, Nathan. *Team Chemistry: The History of Alcohol and Drugs in Major League Baseball*. Urbana: University of Illinois Press, 2016.

"Craig Arfons Killed When Jet Boat Flips." *Akron Beacon Journal*, July 10, 1989, A1, A4.

Crawford, Sarah. "Haughton Hero, NFL Star Joe Delaney Died 35 Years Ago." *Shreveport Times*, www.shreveporttimes.com, June 29, 2018.

Croft, Jay, and Matias Grez. "Details Emerge in 'Extremely Troubling' Slaying of Golf Champion Celia Barquín." CNN Sports, www.cnn.com, September 19, 2018.

Cummings, Judith. "Suit Over Football Player's Death in Coast Jail Settled." *New York Times*, www.nytimes.com, January 24, 1983.

Cutter, Robert, and Bob Fendell. *Encyclopedia of Auto Racing Greats*. Hoboken: Prentice Hall, 1973.

"Darkness and Light: Remembering Fabio Casartelli." *Rouleur* 18, no. 4, July 18, 2018, www.roleur.cc.

"Death and Discovery at 'Indy' Speedway." *Business Week*, June 4, 1955, 29–31.

DeLand, Dave. "Dukes' 1948 Tragedy Remains a Vivid Memory." *St. Cloud Times*, www.sctimes.com, July 23, 2015.

Demak, Richard. "Marfan Syndrome: A Silent Killer." *Sports Illustrated* Vault, February 17, 1986.

"'Difficult' Probe into Stewart Crash." MSNBC, www.msnbc.com, October 26, 1999.

Drape, Joe, and Corina Knoll. "Why So Many Horses Have Died at Santa Anita." *New York Times*, www.nytimes.com, June 26, 2019.

Drellich, Evan. "Mike Carp Carries Greg Halman with Him Everywhere," MassLive.com, May 16, 2013.

Duckworth, Mick. "Days of Future Past." *Cycle World*, September 1994, 67–80.

Dufresne, Chris. "Aloha to a Hero." *Los Angeles Times*, www.latimes.com, July 5, 1997.

Durso, Joseph. "The End of a 'Gorgeous Beast.'" *New York Times*, July 8, 1975, 23.

Duvoisin, Marc, Al Morganti, and Tom Torok. "Lindbergh Was Heavily Intoxicated at Time of Crash, Blood Test Shows." *Philadelphia Inquirer*, November 12, 1985, 15A, 16A.

"Eighth Snoqualmie Bus Victim Taken by Death." *Spokane Daily Chronicle*, June 25, 1946, 1–2.

"89 Years Later, Delahanty's Death Still a Mystery." *Washington Post*, September 22, 1992.

Eisenberg, John. "Jockey Weights Get Heavy Debate." *Baltimore Sun*, www.baltimoresun.com, March 11, 2003.

Elliott, Helene. "Sixtieth Anniversary of U.S. Figure Skating Crash Conjures Heartfelt Memories." *Los Angeles Times*, www.latimes.com, February 15, 2021.

Elmer-DeWitt, Philip. "Death on the Basketball Court." *Time*, March 19, 1990, 56.

Eskenazi, Gerald. "Nassau Grand Jury Exonerates Stewart." *New York Times*, June 9, 1970, 47.

———. "Police Link Sawchuck's Death to 'an Altercation.'" *New York Times*, June 2, 1970, 46.

———. "Pro Hockey Stunned by Death of Minnesota Player Hurt in Game." *New York Times*, January 15, 1968, 31.

Fallows, James. "The Cory Lidle Crash in New York City." *The Atlantic*, www.theatlantic.com, October 2006.

Falls, Joe. "Chuck Hughes Dies After Collapse During Game." *Detroit Free Press*, October 25, 1971, 1A, 8A.

Finnegan, William. "Can Horse Racing Survive?" *New Yorker*, www.newyorker.com, May 15, 2021.

Fotheringham, William. "Tour's Tragedy Still Resonates 10 Years On." *The Guardian*, www.guardian.com.uk, July 15, 2005.

Gasaway, John. *Miracles on the Hardwood*. New York: Twelve Books, 2012.

Gearan, John. "Rick Carter Was Sick Man, Treated for Depression." *Worcester Telegram*, February 24, 1986, 1A.

George, Thomas. "Pro Football: Heat Kills a Pro Football Player; N.F.L. Orders a Training Review." *New York Times*, August 2, 2001, A1.

Glick, Shiv. "Alabama Gang Loses Another; Tragic Story of Allisons Gets Another Chapter When Davey Allison, 32, Dies After Helicopter Crash." *Los Angeles Times*, www.latimes.com, July 14, 1993.

Gorman, Robert M., and David Weeks. *Death at the Ballpark*, 2d ed. Jefferson, NC: McFarland, 2015.

Gottfried, Mara H. "High School Hockey Coach Dies After Dispute Over Social Distancing Turned Violent at St. Paul Bar." *St. Paul Pioneer Press*, www.twincities.com, April 20, 2021.

Grady, Bill. "Baseball Star Slain; Man Held." *Chicago Tribune*, September 26, 1978, C3.

Green, Jerry. "Hughes Injured in Earlier Game." *Detroit News*, October 25, 1971, 1D, 2D.

Green, Richard. "Schott: A Day of Triumph and Tragedy." *Cincinnati Enquirer*, April 2, 1996, A4.

Greene, Dan. "The Owen Hart Tragedy Was the Moment We Came to See Wrestler as Human." *Sports Illustrated*, www.si.com, May 25, 2019.

Gustkey, Earl. "Twenty Years Later: The Cal Poly Survivors Can't Forget." *Los Angeles Times*, October 29, 1980, 1, 8–10.

Guthrow, Steven T. "Boating Accident Claims Two Cleveland Indians." *South Lake Press*, March 24, 1993, 1, 11.

Hackerman, Richard. "Today in Racing History: Mary Bacon." *The Racing Biz*, www.theracingbiz.com, June 24, 2014.

Hamilton, Maurice. "How Ayrton Senna's Death Rocked Motor Racing to Its Roots." ESPN, www.espn.com, April 30, 2020.

Hanley, Reid M. *Who's Who in Track and Field*. New York: Arlington House, 1973.

Harris, Chris. "Beloved Hockey Coach Is Killed in Bar Fight After Allegedly Confronting Man About Boorish Behavior." *People*, www.people.com, April 21, 2021.

Hart, Gene, with Buzz Ringe. "When the Clock Ran Out." *Philadelphia*, October 1990, 29–31.

Hedger, Brian. "He Had Dreams." *Columbus Dispatch*, July 18, 2021, 1C, 6C.

Hess, David. "Munson Errors Ruled Cause of Fatal Crash." *Akron Beacon Journal*, April 11, 1980, A1, A10.

Hinton, Ed. "How Much Can One Man Bear?" *Sports Illustrated*, February 10, 1997, 55–65.

Hobson, Geoff. "Knight, Reds 'crushed.'" *Cincinnati Enquirer*. April 2, 1996: D1, D5.

"Hockey: First Fatality." *Time*, January 26, 1968, 65.

Hotten, Jon. "Dying to Be Arnie." *The Observer*, www.observer, May 25, 2011.

_____. *Muscle: A Writer's Trip Through a Sport with No Boundaries*. London: Yellow Jersey Press, 2005.

Hovdey, Jay. "Ruffian Remembered." *Equus* 18 (December 1995), 27–32.

Hoynes, Paul, and James F. McCarty. "Boat Crash Kills Tribe's Olin." *Cleveland Plain Dealer*, March 23, 1993, 1-A, 7-A.

Hoyt, Alicia, and Jessika Toothman. "Do Horses With Broken Legs Have to Be Shot?" How Stuff Works, www.animals.howstuffworks.com, October 14, 2021.

Huff, Richard. "NASCAR Still Hasn't Fully Recovered from Dale Earnhardt's Death Ten Years Ago at Daytona 500." *New York Daily News*, www.nydailynews.com, February 17, 2011.

"In Memory." *Sports n' Spokes*, January/February 1996, 78.

"Israeli Team Had 18 Athletes and Coaches." *New York Times*, September 7, 1972, 1.

Jensen, Cheryl, and Christopher. "Survival of the Fittest." *Cleveland Plain Dealer*, February 4, 1996, 1-I, 6-I.

"Jessi Combs Named Fastest Woman on Earth." *Motorcycle Cruiser*, www.motorcyclecruiser.com, June 26, 2020.

Jhabvala, Nicki. "Dwayne Haskins Was Legally Drunk at Time of Death, Which Is Ruled an Accident." *Washington Post*, www.washingtonpost.com, May 23, 2022.

"Jockey Dies as He Wins His First Ride; Hayes Collapses Passing the Winning Post." *New York Times*, June 5, 1923, 1.

Jordan, Tom. *Pre: The Story of America's Greatest Running Legend, Steve Prefontaine*. Emmaus, PA: Rodale, 1977.

Kantrowitz, Barbara, and Anne Longley. "Beyond the Tears." *People*, March 25, 1996, 78–87.

Kardong, Don. "In Pre's Footsteps." *Runner's World*, May 1991, 52–57.

Klein, Christopher. "Crunch Time." *Boston Globe*, www.boston.com, November 21, 2010.

Lajoie, Ron, and Dene Creswell. "Tragedy Strikes Student Games." *Edmonton Journal*, July 16, 1983, 1A.

Landry, Chris. "NFL Deaths Blamed on anchoring Error." *Soundings*, www.soundingsonline.com, May 31, 2009.

Ledger, Kate. "Safety Did Not Come First." *Sports Illustrated*, www.vault.si.com, July 14, 1997.

Lidz, Frans. "38 Miles of Terror." *Sports Illustrated*, www.vault.si.com, September 8, 2003.

Lundberg, George D., M.D. "Blunt Force Violence in America—Shades of Gray and Red." *Journal of the American Medical Association* 275, No. 21 (June 5, 1996), 1684–1685.

MacPherson, Malcolm. *The Black Box: Cockpit Voice Recorder Accounts of Nineteen In-Flight Accidents*. New York: Quill, 1984.

Maisel, Ivan. "Knute Rockne's Funeral and the Dawn of a New American Experience." ESPN, ESPN.com, April 4, 2019.

Maraniss, David. *Path Lit by Lightning: The Life of Jim Thorpe*. New York: Macmillan, 2022.

The Marfan Foundation. www.marfan.org.

"Marfan syndrome." Mayo Clinic, www.mayoclinic.

"Masterton Dies of Head Injuries." *St. Paul Dispatch*, January 15, 1968, 10, 20.

McCallum, Jack. "Fair or Foul?" *Sports Illustrated*, March 20, 1995, 26–35.

McCallum, Jack, and Richard O'Brien. "A Teammate Remembered." *Sports Illustrated*, June 10, 1996, 27.

McCallum, John, and Paul Castner. *We Remember Rockne*. Huntington, IN: Our Sunday Visitor, 1975.

McGee, Ryan. "Dale Earnhardt's Death at the Daytona 500—Revisiting the Day of the Crash." ESPN, www.espn.com, February 11, 2021.

McMillen, Lauretta. "A beautiful fall day ... then an ominous sound." *Wichita Eagle*, September 30, 1990, 11A, 12A.

Meisel, Barry. "Alm Family Openly Deals with Nightmare." *Chicago Tribune*, www.chicagotribune.com, December 25, 1993.

Mell, Randall. "Blasberg's Father Still Struggling with Daughter's Suicide." *Golf Channel*, www.golfchannel.com, May 20, 2014.

Mercer, Pamela. "Colombian Who Made World Cup Error Is Slain." *New York Times*, July 3, 1994, 1, 13.

Michael, Brian. "The Strange Death of Ed Delahanty." Phillies Nation, www.philliesnation.com, November 25, 2022.

Minton, Eric. "John Rodolph: 1964–1995." *New Mobility*, December 1995, 24.

Mitani, Sam. "Granada-Dakar." *Road & Track*, May 1996, 108–114.

Mitchell, Doug. "Oilers Try to Deal with Shock." *Houston Post*, December 15, 1993, C-1, C-5.

Montague, James. "The Munich Massacre." CNN, www.cnn.com, September 5, 2012.

Montville, Leigh. "The Ghost Plane." *Sports Illustrated*, April 10, 2000, 104–120.

_____. "Love Story." *Sports Illustrated*, December 8, 1995, 33–57.

_____. "More Grief for Jackson State." *Sports Illustrated*, www.vault.si.com, April 30, 1990.

Moore, Colten, with Keith O'Brien. *Catching the Sky*. New York: Simon & Schuster, 2016.

Moore, Kenny. "A Final Drive to the Finish." *Sports Illustrated*, June 9, 1975, 22–23.

Moriarty, Tim. "Sawchuk and Stewart: A Tragic Odd Couple." *Newsday*, June 1, 1970, 35.

"Munich Massacre." Britannica, www.britannica.com, updated April 23, 2023.

Munnings, Frances. "The Death of Hank Gathers: A Legacy of Confusion." *The Physician and Sports Medicine* 18, no. 5 (May 1990), 97–102.

Mylenski, Skip. "A Rodeo Cowboy's Perfect Ride Ends in death." *Chicago Tribune*, August 6, 1989, Section 9: 1, 9.

Naughton, Jim. "Yankees' Thurman Munson Killed Piloting His Own Small Jet in Ohio." *New York Times*, August 3, 1979, A1, A15.

Neff, Craig. "Fatal Obsession." *Sports Illustrated*, February 5, 1996, 41–48.

Nicholson, Dave. "Arfons' Boat Went Airborne Like a Jet, Investigators Say." *Tampa Tribune*, July 11, 1989, 1B, 6B.

O'Brien, Jerry. "Baseball's Darkest Night." *Spokane Spokesman-Review*, June 24, 1956, 3–5.

"Odd Mishap Fells Tennis Official." *St. Petersburg Evening Independent*, September 12, 1983, 3-C.

O'Hagan, Simon. "The Life and Tragic Death of Ulli Maier." *The Independent*, www.independent.co.uk, February 6, 1994.

Okrent, Daniel, and Steve Wulf. *Baseball Anecdotes*. Oxford: Oxford University Press, 1989.

Oliver, Sara. "Ice Cold Cruelty: The 8 Most Notorious Iditarod Mushers." People for the Ethical Treatment of Animals (PETA), www.peta.org, January 26, 2022.

Olney, Ross. *Daredevils of the Speedway*. New York: Grosset & Dunlap, 1966.

Parker, Graham. "Andrés Escobar: A Matter of Life and Death." *Al Jazerra America*, www.aljazerra.com, July 2, 2014.

Parker, Wendy. "The Fatal Attraction of Death-Defying Extreme Sports." *Sports Biblio*, www.sports.biblio.com, January 18, 2016.

Paul, Tony. "Blue Jackets Goalie Matiss Kivlenieks Dies from Fireworks Explosion at Novi Holiday Party." *Detroit News*, www.detroitnews.com, July 5, 2021.

Pearlman, Jeff. "Fifth and Jackson." *ESPN Outside the Lines*, www.espn.com, September 18, 2008.

Pender, Matt. "Owen Hart's Death: What Really Happened, from Those There." *Pro Wrestling Stories*, www.prowrestlingstories.com, March 3, 2023.

Penner, Mike. "Summer of Tragedy." *Los Angeles Times*, www.latimes.com, September 3, 2001.

"Pilot Steadfast in Denying Fault: 'Someone Needed to Be blamed.'" *Wichita Eagle*, September 30, 1990, 12A.

Plummer, William, and Ken Baker. "Life Giver." *People*, April 21, 1997, 165–166.

Powers, Scott, and Tim Feran. "Bodybuilder's Death Puts Focus on Drugs." *Columbus Dispatch*, February 23, 1997, 1C, 2C.

Prasher, Shantanu. "The Untold Story of the Most Shocking Death in the History of Bodybuilding." *Mensxp*, www.mensxp.com, June 28, 2017.

Price, S.L. "Cut Off from the Herd." *Sports Illustrated*, August 15, 1997, 130–140.

_____. "Shadow of Shame." *Sports Illustrated*, May 23, 1994, 61–70.

Puente, Maria. "Du Pont's Sanity Argued in Trial." *USA Today*, January 28, 1997, 5A.

Rabinowitz, Bill. "Ex-OSU QB Haskins Killed in Florida." *Columbus Dispatch*, April 10, 2022, 1A, 4A.

_____. "Fireworks Experts Question Tragedy." *Columbus Dispatch*, July 9, 2021, 4C.

Red, Christian. "Ten Years Later, Pain Lingers After Payne Stewart's Tragic Crash Following U.S. Open Win." *New York Daily News*, www.nydailynews.com, October 26, 1999.

Reeve, Simon. *One Day in September*. New York: Arcade, 2000.

Rejebian, Michael. "3 on JSU's Football Team Die in Wreck." *Jackson [MS] Clarion-Ledger*, April 17, 1970, 1A, 7A.

Ren, Yuan. "China's Ultramarathon Tragedy Was a Fad Gone Bad." *Foreign Policy*, www.foreignpolicy.com, July 16, 2021.

"Report: Illegal Procedures Didn't Cause Deaths of Santa Anita Horses." NBC Los Angeles, www.nbclosangeles.com, March 10, 2020.

"Rethinking Drinking: Alcohol & Your Health." National Institutes of Health, www.niaa.nih.gov.

Richmond, Peter. "The Death of a Cowboy." *National Sports Daily*, July 22, 1990, 31–40.

Rosengren, John. "Rarely Told Reason Cited for Bill Masterton's Death Underlies Concussion Issue." ESPN, www.espn.com, March 3, 2016.

Rovin, Jeff, with Steve Burkow. *Sports Babylon*. New York: Signet, 1993.

Sabljak, Mark, and Martin H. Greenberg. *Sports Babylon*. New York: Bell, 1988.

Santos, Kendra. "Silver Screen Salutes Lane Frost." *Pro Rodeo Sports News* 3, February 9, 1994, 18–19, 34.

Schultz, Mark, with David Thomas. *Foxcatcher: The True Story of My Brother's Murder, John du Pont's Madness and the Quest for Olympic Gold*. New York: Dutton, 2014.

Schuyler, Nick, and Jeré Longman. *Not Without Hope*. New York: William Morrow, 2010.

Schwartz, Jane. *Ruffian: Burning from the Start*. New York: Ballantine Books, 1991.

Seibert, William, editor. *The Lincoln Library of Sports Champions.* Columbus, OH: Frontier Press, 1978.

Seifert, Kevin. "Korey Stringer's Death, 20 Years Later: The Lasting Impact and How the NFL Changed." ESPN, www.espn.com, July 30, 2021.

"75 on Football Team Plane Die in West Virginia Crash." *New York Times,* November 15, 1970, 1, 48.

Shaw, Bud. "A Moonless Evening, a Quiet Lake, a Tragedy: Recounting the 1993 Deaths of Indians Pitchers Steve Olin and Tim Crews." *Cleveland Plain Dealer,* www.cleveland.com, March 22, 2011.

Shepard, Alicia C. "The Journal's Reggie Lewis Bombshell." *American Journalism Review,* www.ajrarchive.org, May 1995.

Shipnuck, Alan. "The Mystery of Erica Blasberg." *Sports Illustrated,* vault.si.com, December 13, 2010.

Shpigel, Ben. "What to Know About CTE in Football." *New York Times,* www.nytimes.com, December 16, 2021.

Smith, Gene. "Ruffian." *American Heritage,* September 1993, 46–57.

Smith, Phillip. "5 Drugs That Shaped Major League Baseball." *Alter Net,* www.alternet.org, April 2, 2016.

Smith, Shelley. "A Bitter Legacy." *Sports Illustrated,* March 4, 1991, 62–66.

"Some Reflections on the Death of Lyman Bostock." *Gary Post-Tribune,* September 29, 1978, A6.

Soong, Kelyn. "The Terrible Plane Crash That Devastated U.S. Figure Skating—and Still Shapes It Today." *Washington Post,* www.washingtonpost.com, February 20, 2018.

Sowell, Mike. *July 2nd, 1903: The Mysterious Death of Hall-of-Famer Big Ed Delahanty.* New York: Macmillan, 1992.

_____. *The Pitch That Killed.* New York: Macmillan, 1989.

Spander, Art. "Who's to Blame for Gathers' Tragic Death." *Sporting News,* March 19, 1990, 5.

Starr, Mark. "Brave Heart, Broken Heart." *Newsweek.* December 4, 1995, 70–71.

Stathoplos, Demmie. "No One Does It Better." *Sports Illustrated,* vault.si.com, July 18, 1994.

Su, Alice. "He Was Deaf, Mute, a Champion Runner—and One of 21 Who Died in a Chinese Ultramarathon." *Los Angeles Times,* www.latimes.com, May 28, 2021.

Swanson, Mirjam. "Year Later: Family Haunted by Corona Golfer's Death." *Riverside Press-Enterprise,* www.pressenterrpise.com, May 6, 2011.

Takle, Abhisnek. "A Man of Contrasts: Remembering Ayrton Senna." *Economic Times,* www.economictimes.indiatimes.com, May 1, 2014.

Tasch, Justin. "Dwayne Haskins Drugged, Blackmailed and Robbed Before Death: Lawsuit." *New York Post,* www.nypost.com, April 10, 2023.

"Then All the Joy Turned to Sorrow." *Sports Illustrated,* vault.si.com, November 22, 1982.

Thevenot, Carri Geer. "Jury Finds in Favor of Doctor in Malpractice Suit Tied to Pro Golfer's Death." *Las Vegas Review-Journal,* www.reviewjournal.com, May 13, 2014.

"13 Football Players Die with 16 Others on Plane." *New York Times,* October 3, 1970, 1, 32.

Tomizawa, Roy. "U.S. Boxing Team Perishes in Air Crash." *The Olympians from 1964 to 2000,* www.olympians.com, March 16, 2016.

Townsend, Jon. "Andrés Escobar: When Football Kills." *These Football Times,* www.thesefootballtimes.com, August 27, 2015.

"Tragedy Strikes Indians." *Winter Haven News Chief,* March 23, 1993, 1A, 9A.

Twigg, Bob, Carol J. Castaneda, and Deborah Sharp. "Everglades Biggest Enemy of Recovery." *USA Today,* May 13, 1996, 3A.

"UE Basketball Team Dies in Plane Crash." *Evansville Courier,* December 14, 1977, 1, 5.

Verhovek, Sam Howe. "A Friend Dies, and Oiler Kills Himself." *New York Times,* December 15, 1993, B13, B17.

Vescey, George. "Sports of the Times: Remembering Flo Hyman." *New York Times,* www.nytimes.com, February 5, 1988.

_____. "Was a Medal So Important?" *New York Times,* July 31, 1983, V-1, V-8.

Wagner, George. "What to Know About the Investigation into Tyler Skaggs's Death." *New York Times,* www.nytimes.com, August 30, 2021.

Walsh, Katherine. "Cowboy Fatally Rammed by Bull at Rodeo." *Wyoming Eagle,* July 31, 1989, 1, 8.

Wathen, Pat. "DC-3 Struck Tress Near Byers' Home." *Evansville Courier,* December 17, 1977, 1, 2.

Webster, Jake. "Killer of Celia Barquín Arozamena Sentenced to Life Without Parole." *Iowa State Daily,* www.iowastatedaily.com, August 23, 2019.

*Wertheim vs. United States Tennis Association.* 150 A.D. 2d 157, NY App. Div., 1989.

Wiley, Ralph. "Knute Rockne Dies with Seven Others in Mail Plane Dive." *New York Times,* April 1, 1931: 24.

Wulf, Steve. "A Triumph of Will." *Time,* www.content.time.com, June 24, 2001.

"Yankees Pitcher Killed in Crash of Small Plane in Manhattan." CNN, www.cnn.com, October 11, 2006.

Young, Brock. *Famous Indianapolis Cars and Drivers.* New York: Harper & Brothers, 1960.

Young, Eugene. *With Rockne at Notre Dame.* New York: G.P. Putnam's Sons, 1951.

# Index

Numbers in **_bold italics_** indicate pages with illustrations

Abilene, TX  16
AC Milan (soccer club)  33
Adirondack Medical Center, NY  101
Ago's Leap, Isle of Man  161–162
Air Indiana (airline)  176
Akron, OH  50
Akron-Canton Regional Airport, OH  65
Alabama Gang (NASCAR)  68
Alaska Airlines  127
Albright, Tenley  170
Albuquerque, NM  187
alcohol use by athletes  48, 55, 66, 79, 111, 170, 180–181, 186
Algeria  150
*All Girls Garage* (TV show)  158
Alleman, Nancy  179
Allen, Nelson  165
Allison, Bobby  70
Allison, Clifford  70
Allison, Davey  68–70, **_69_**
Allison, Donnie  70
Allison, Elizabeth (Liz)  69
Allison, Judy  68
Alm, Jeff  48, 71, 194–196
Alpine tour (skiing)  116–117
Alvarez, A.  194
Alvidsen, John  26
Alvord Desert, OR  159–160
Amateur Athletic Union (AAU)  180
American Hockey League (AHL)  89
American Medical Association  21
American Pharoah (racehorse)  146
Ames, IA  41–42
amphetamines  10, 118, 144
anabolic steroids  104
Anchorage, AK  124–126
Anderson, Jeff  141
Anderson, Jerry D.  65
Anderson, Jon  179

Angel Stadium of Anaheim  111
Anti-Drug Abuse Act of 1986  97–98
antidepressant drugs  81, 192, 199–200
Arcadia, CA  144
Arctic Pacific Airlines  167–168
Ardan, Van  74
Arfons, Art  50
Arfons, Craig  50–52
Arfons, Walt  50–51
Argentina  151
Ariostea team (cycling)  118
Arizona Diamondbacks  109
Armstrong, Lance  144
Arnold Classic (bodybuilding)  105
Arozamena, Celia Barquín  41–44
arrhythmia  114
Aruba  39
Arum, Bob  18
Ascension Providence Hospital, MI  90
Ashland, OR  35
Aspen, CO  122–123
Aspen Valley Hospital, CO  123
aspiration pneumonia  125
aspirin  105
Astaire, Fred  140
atherosclerosis  16
Atoka, OK  24
Autin, Eraste  108

Bacon, Coy  185
Bacon, Johnny "Pug"  140
Bacon, Mary  140–142
Baer, Max  20
Baeza, Braulio  135
Baffert, Bob  146
Bahamas  123
Baiul, Oksana  103
Baldini, Ercole  118
Ballesteros, Seve  42

Baltic Sea  89
Baltimore Orioles  66
Balto (sled dog)  124
Bandera Downs, TX  142
Barney, Lem  184
*Baseball Almanac*  48
Basilica of the Sacred Heart, IN  64
Battuello, Patrick  144–145
Bazaar, KS  63
Beathard, Bobby  168
Beattie, Richie  125–126
Bechler, Steve  107
Belaire Apartments, NYC  76
Belcher, Jovan  8
Bell, Mike  137
Bell Micro Classic (LPGA)  197
Bellegarrigue, Stephanie  74
Belmont Memorial Park, CA  149
Belmont Park, NY  131–132, 134–137, 142
Bench, Johnny  67
Bennigan's (bar), NJ  182
Benscotter, Ben  75
Berg, Glen  164–165
Berger, David  27–29
Berkley, MI  81
Bertoia, Harry  176
beta-blockers  114
Bethea, Elvin  50
Bias, Len  94–98, **_97_**
Bird, Larry  99
Black Hills, SD  158
Black September (terrorist group)  28
Blair, Wren  15
Bland, Cary  187
Blasberg, Debbie  197
Blasberg, Erica  197–201, **_200_**
Blasberg, Mel  197–199
Bleakley, Will  58
blood alcohol concentration (BAC)  55, 180–181, 184, 190, 196
Bloomington Jefferson High School, MN  45–46

**213**

Blountville, TN 70
Blue, Vida 111
the Blue Blazer (pro wrestling) 87
Boca Raton, FL 189
Bodacious (bull) 24
Boeing 707 (aircraft) 170
Boitano, Brian 103, 172
Bolivia 151
Bollinger, Mary 166
Bologna, Italy 154
Bolster, April 162
Bonds, Barry 39, 112
Bonnett, David 68
Bonnett, Neil 68
Bonneville Salt Flats, UT 50
Bossier Parish, LA 50
Bostock, Lyman 29–30, 41
Boston Bruins 81
Boston Celtics 94, 98–99
Boston Marathon 186
Bowerman, Bill 181
Bowling Green State University, OH 168–169
Boyd, Dennis "Oil Can" 111
Brackett Field, CA 76
Bradenton, FL 52
Bradshaw, Terry 25
Brandeis University, MA 98
Brazile, Robert 185
Brazilian Grand Prix 153
Breeder's Cup (horse racing) 143, **145**
Breedlove, Craig 51, 159
Breedlove, Lee 159
Bremerton, WA 164–165
Bremigan, Nick 120
Brigmond, Perry 54
Brock, Lou 30
Broders, John 198
Brodeur, Martin 79
*Broken Harts* (book) 88
Brookline, MA 73
Brooklyn Dodgers 11
Brooks, Herb 44
Broughton's Rule (boxing) 21
Broward County, FL 189–190
Brown, Jerry Lee 31
Brown, Warren "Freckles" 26
Brussels, Belgium 170, 171
Buffalo, NY 48
Buffalo Bills 16–17
Buffalo Sabres 81
bull riding (scoring system) 24
bullfighting 127
Bullis School, MD 190
Burke, Sarah 123, 163
Buser, Martin 125
Bush, George H.W. 36, 50
Butcher, Susan 125
Butkus, Dick 16
Buttermilk Mountain, CO 122

Button, Richard "Dick" 170
Byrd, LaMarcus 186

Cadillac Seville (automobile) 186
Caesars Palace, NV 18–19
Cal Poly SLO Mustangs 167–170
Calder Trophy (NHL) 79
Calgary, AB 85, 88
California Angels 29–30
California Horse Racing Board 144
California State University, Long Beach 31
Callahan, Chase 198
Camp, Walter 7–8, 63
Campbell, Sir Donald 51
Canado, Patrick 151
Candinda, Milt 164
Cannell, Pam 162
Canseco, Jose 112
Canton, OH 67
Carey, Tim 56
Carl Sandburg High School, IL 194
Carraway Methodist Medical Center, AL 69
Carter, Cloyd 191
Carter, Deanna 192–193
Carter, Henrietta 192
Carter, Rick 191–194
Casartelli, Annalisa 118
Casartelli, Fabio 117–119
Cascade Mountains, WA 165
Cascardo, Pamela 33
Castro, Humberto 34
CBS Radio 64
CBS Television 135, 148
Cemetery of the Holy Rood, NY 140
Center Grove Lutheran Cemetery, NC 158
Central Park, NYC 124
Central Red Army Club (CSKA), Moscow 101–103
Cepeda, Francisco 118
Cessna Citation (aircraft) 65–66
Chamberlain, Wilt 92
Chanal, Cesar 161
Chandler, Happy 166
Chapman, Ray 11–13
Charlotte Calvary Church, NC 157
Charlotte Hornets 98
Cheyenne Frontier Days Rodeo, WY 25–26
Chicago Bears 16
*Chicago Tribune* 6
Chicago White Sox 13
Chile 151

China Sports Administration 130
Cho, Irene 197
chronic traumatic encephalopathy (CTE) 8
Cirrus SR 20 (aircraft) 75
Civil Air Patrol 168
Claiborne Farm, KY 134
Clarke, Bobby 182
Clearwater, FL 57, 60
Clermont, FL 53
Cleveland, OH 54
Cleveland Golf 198
Cleveland Indians 11, 52–55, 167
Cleveland Monsters 89
CNN 74
cocaine 95, 97, 99–100, 111
Cochran, Johnnie L. 31
cockfighting 127
codeine 199
Coldwater Golf Links, IA 41–44
Cole, Mel 166
Coliseum After Dark, NJ (bar) 182
College of the Holy Cross, MA 191–194
Collins, Sam 164–165
Colombia 33–35
Colonial League 192–193
Columbia University, NYC 27
Columbus Blue Jackets 89
Combs, Jessi 158–160
Comiskey Park 30
Conan Doyle, Sir Arthur 103
Conference USA 175
Connor, Casey 185
Continental Divide, CO 171
Cooper, Bruce 59
Cooper, Marquis 57–60, **59**
Coos Bay, OR 179, 181
Corendon Kinheim (baseball team) 40–41
Corona, CA 197
coronary artery disease 102
Corrales, NM 187
Côte d'Ivoire 151
Cottonwood Springs, KS 63
Covid pandemic 44–46, 89–90, 130, 161, 190
Cracker Barrel 500 (NASCAR) 155
Cresher Donald 169
Crews, Laurie 53
Crews, Tim 52–55, 184
Crimson (racehorse) 139
Critter's Creek, LA (water park) 49
Crocker, Danny 172
Crosby, Bing 143, 166
Crudup, Billy 181
Crump, Diane 140

# Index

Crump, Marva 115
Crusty Demons of Dirt Tour (ATV racing) 122
Culver, Karen 71
Culver, Rodney 70–*72*
Curtis C-46 Commando (aircraft) 167
Czyz, Bobby 178

Daiei, Inc. 93
*Daily Racing Form* 136
Dakar Rally 149–*152*
Dallas Cowboys 31
Damascus (racehorse) 134
Daniel Freeman Marina Hospital, CA 114
Dawn Valley Memorial Park, MN 46
*A Day at the Races* (film) 143
Daytona 500 (NASCAR) 69, 155–*157*
DC-3 (aircraft) 64
DC-9 (aircraft) 175–176
Deaconess Hospital, IN 177
Deadwood, SD 158
De Bow, Nina 158
Decker, Bernadette 6
de Gaulle, Charles 94
Delahanty, Ed 47–49, 111
Delaney, Carolyn 50
Delaney, Joe 49–50
de Later, Theo 170
Delaware Museum of Natural History 36
Denver, CO 172
depression (mental condition) 192–194
depressurization (aircrafts) 74–75
Des Moines, IA 42
*Deseret News* 10K (wheelchair racing) 187
Desert Spring Hospital, NV 19
Detroit Race Course, MI (horse racing) 140
Detroit Red Wings 79–81
Detroit Tigers 48
dexedrine 111
Diamond, Neil 67
Dickson, Sam 149
Dickson, Tyler 50
Die Hard 500 (NASCAR) 155
Discover Card Stars on Ice (figure skating) 102
Doctor Phillips Cemetery, FL 75
Dodin, Patrice 151
dogfighting 127
Dominick, Tony 66
Douglas, Isle of Man 160
*Down But Not Out, Lost But Not Forgotten* (sculpture) 178

downhill race (skiing) 115
Dress Regional Airport, IN 176
Driesell, Lefty 96
Drysdale, Don 13
Duffner, Mark 193
Duk Koo Kim 18–21, *19*
Duke City Marathon, NM 187
Duke Ellington Orchestra 136
Duke University, NC 119, 121
Dull, Dick 96
Duluth Dukes 166–167
Dunbar High School, MD 99
du Pont, John E. 35–38, 41
Durso, Joseph 137

Eagle Glen Golf Club, CA 197, 199, **200**
Earlham College, IN 191
Earnhardt, Dale 155–158, *157*
Earnhardt, Dale, Jr. 156–*157*
East Atlantic Beach, NY 80
East Carolina Pirates 174
East Liberty, OH 52
East River, NYC 77
Eatman, Earl 185
Eau Claire, WI 167
Edberg, Stefan 84
Edmonton, AB 22
Edmonton Oilers 182
Eglin Air Force Base, FL 73
*8 Seconds* (film) 26
Elliott, Bill 68
ephedra 105, 107
Erbe, Bonnie 21
Erie, PA 51
Escobar, Andrés 33–35
Escobar, Pablo 34
ESPN 48
*Esquire* 106
Eugene, OR 179–181
Evansville Purple Aces 176–177
Everglades 71–*72*
extreme fighting 21
Exxon 127

Fair Grounds Course, LA (horse racing) 141
Fairmount High School, OH 191
Fairmount-Willows Memorial Park, IL 196
Fairview Southdale Hospital, MN 14
Faria, Joe 164
Farmer, Red 68–*69*
Federal Amateur Hockey League 14
Federal Aviation Administration (FAA) 169
fentanyl 110

Fenway Park 39
Ferrari Autodrome, Italy 153
Ferris Field, WA 164
Fiorinal 196
*Fire on the Track* (film) 181
fireworks (regulations and injuries) 90–91
Fisk, Carlton 67
Fittipaldi, Emerson 154
Flannery, Judith 187–188
Fleisher, Gerry 31
Fleming, Peggy 172
Flight Schools International 67
Florida Gators 108
Flushing Hospital Medical Center, NY 84
Flynn, Errol 143
Fokker F-10 (aircraft) 61, 65
Foolish Pleasure (racehorse) 135–136
Ford, Charles 185
Ford, Chris 98
Ford Mustang (automobile) 185
Forest Hills Cemetery, MA 99, 193
Forest Lawn Memorial Park, CA 78
Formula One (auto racing) 153–155
Fort Erie, ON 48
Fort Lauderdale, FL 189
Fort Walton Beach, FL 73
Fort Worth, TX 142
Fox Broadcasting 155–157
Foxcatcher Training Facility, PA (wrestling) 36–37
Fraley, Robert 74
Frayling, James K. 131
Frazier, Joe 178
Frazier, Marvis 178
Frederick, MD 188
Free Evangelical Lutheran Church, CA 149
freediving 123, 163
Fresno, CA 147–149
Fresno State University, CA 169
Froese, Bob 182
Frost, Eloise 25
Frost, Lane 23–26
Furr, David 177

Gable, Clark 143
Gallón, Pedro David 34
Gallón, Santiago 34
Gamsu province, China 128–130
Garagiola, Joe 120
Garmisch-Partenkirchen, Germany 116
Gary, IN 29–30

Gasparilla Distance Classic 15K (wheelchair racing) 186–187
Gates of Heaven Cemetery, NY 121
Gathers, Hank 113–115
Gathers, Lucille 113, 115
Gaye, Marvin 141
Gearhart, Joyce 187
Gehrig, Lou 66
Gerl, Bernard "Bernie" 167
German, Domingo 13
Gersten Pavilion, CA 113, 115
Gifford, Frank 8
Gilmore, Don 167
Gilmore Stadium, CA 147
"Glide Float" system (aeronautics) 175
Gloversville, NY 139
the Godfather (pro wrestling) 87
Golden Age of Sports 62, 64–65
Gold's Gym 103
Gonzaga University, WA 166
Goodale, Pat 38
Goodwill Games 36
Gorbachev, Mikhail 101
Gordeeva, Ekaterina 100–103
Gorden, W.C. 185
Grand Junction, CO 123
Grant, Cary 143
Grealish, James 167
Green, Andy 159
Green, Richard 19, *21*
Green, Tim 50
Green, OH 52
Greenville, NC 174
Gregg, David 96
Gregg, Eric 121
greyhound racing 127
Griffey, Ken, Jr. 39
Griffith, Calvin 30
Griffith, Emile 20
Griggs, David 71
Grinkov, Daria 101
Grinkov, Sergei 100–103, *102*
Guanjuan, Huang 129
*Guinness Book of World Records* 132, 159–160
Gulf of Mexico 57–60, *59*
Gustavas Adolphus College, MN 45

Haarlem, the Netherlands 39
Hager, Jean Claude 151
Halifax Medical Center, NC 157
Hall, David 32
Hall, Ron 150
Hallion, Tom 120
Halman, Eddy 39
Halman, Greg 38–41

Halman, Jason 39–41
Hambletonian Stakes (harness racing) 138
Hamilton, Chris 73
Hamilton, Lewis 153
Hamilton, Scott 101, 103, 172
Hamlin, Damar 16
*The Hangover* (film) 199
Hanover College, IN 191
HANS device (NASCAR) 157
Happer, J.H. 63
Harborview Hospital, WA 166
Harkes, John 33
harness racing 138–140
Harris, Walter 178
Harris-Lewis, Donna 99
Hart, Bret 85, 87
Hart, Martha 85, 88
Hart, Owen 85–88, *87*
Hart, Stu 85
Hartford Civic Center, CT 103
Harvard University, MA 7
Haskins, Dwayne 189–190
Haskins, Kalabrya 189
Hattiesburg, MS 185
Haughton, Billy 138–140
Haughton, Dorothy Bischoff 138
Haughton, Peter 138
Haughton High School, LA 49
Hawkins Cemetery, LA 50
Hayes, Frank 131–134
Haynes, Richard "Racehorse" 83
Hayward Field, OR 179, 181
Head, Patrick 154
heart disease 16, 84, 93–94, 99–100, 102, 105, 114–115
heat stroke 107–108
Hedeman, Tuff 24–25
Heinbechner, Bruce 30
Heiss, Carol 170
helmet use: baseball 12–13; cycling 118–119; football 1; harness racing 139; hockey 14–15; NASCAR 156
Henderson, NV 197
Hennepin, Louis 47
Henry Ford Hospital, MI 16
hepatitis C 133
Herbie's on the Park, MN (restaurant) 44–46
Hernandez, Keith 111
Hess, Doctor Thomas 198–199
Hickman, Peter 161
Highland Cemetery, IN 64
Highland Memorial Gardens, AL 69
Highlands Regional Medical Center, FL 52
Hill, Curtis 169
Hill, Graham 70
Hoffa, Jimmy 191

Hoheisel, John 173
Holland, Harry Leon 50
Hollendorfer, Jerry 146
Hollern Hospital, MA 193
Holy Cross Crusaders 191–193
Holy Sepulchre Cemetery, IL 196
Holyoke, MA 92
Honeywell Corporation 14
Honolulu, HI 56
Hoover, Herbert 63
Hope, Bob 166, 169
Horseracing Integrity and Safety Act 146
Horseracing Wrongs 145
Hotten, Jon 103
Houk, Ralph 111
Houston, TX 82–83, 194–196
Houston Astros 82–83
Houston Oilers 194–196
Howe, Gordie 14, 81
Howe, Steve 111
Hueytown, AL 68
Hughes, Chuck 15–18, *17*, 81
Hughes, LeRoy (Roy) 168–169
Hughes, Sarah 172
Hughes, Sharon 16, 18
Hughes 369 HS (helicopter) 68–*69*
Huntington, WV 175
Hyattsville, MD 95
Hyman, Flo 92–94
Hyman, Michael 94
hypertrophic cardiomyopathy 100, 115

Ideral 114
Iditarod 124–128, *127*, 150
Idlewild Airport, NYC 170–171
Ilyushin 62 (aircraft) 62, 178
Immanuel and St. Joseph's Mayo Health System Hospital, MN 107
Imola, Italy 153
Indianapolis Colts 70
Indianapolis 500 148–149
Inglewood Park Cemetery, CA 30, 94
insulin 105
Intercollegiate Athletic Association 7
International Automobile Federation (FIA) 159
International Cycling Union (UCI) 119
International Railway Bridge, NY-ON 48
International Ski Federation (FIS) 117
International Swimming Hall of Fame, FL 36

## Index

International Volleyball Association 92
Interstate 70 173–*174*
Interstate 595 189
Iowa State University 41–43
Irvine, CA 188
Irwin, Kenny, Jr. 157
Isle of Man Tourist Trophy (IMTT) 152, 160–163

Jack Daniel's whiskey 127
Jack Trice Stadium, IA 41, *43*
Jackson, Harold 185
Jackson, Reggie 67
Jackson State University Tigers, MS 184–186
Jakes, Keith 17
James, LeBron 157
James, Willie III 186
Janney, Barbara 134, 137
Janney, Stuart, Jr. 134, 137
Japan 150
Japanese Grand Prix 153
*Jay Leno's Garage* (TV show) 158
Jenkins, David W. 170
Jenkins, Ferguson 111
Jenkins, Hayes Alan 170
Jenkins, Patricia 38
Jensen, Knud 10
Jing, Liang 129
Jockey Club 144
Jockey Guild 131
John F. Kennedy Memorial Hospital, NJ 183
John Smith Hospital, TX 142
Joliet, IL 167
Jones, Chipper 39
Jones, Steve 181
Jordan, Michael 95, 99
Justify (racehorse) 146

Kansas City A's 167
Kansas City Chiefs 49
Kansas City Municipal Airport, MO 61
Kapaa High School, HI 56
Kauai, HI 55–56
Kay, Eric 110
kayfabe (pro wrestling) 86
Keck, Howard 148–149
Keenan, Mike 182
Kelly, Red 15
Keming, Zhu 129
Kemper Arena, MO **87**–88
Kennedy, Edward 99
Kentucky Derby 146
Kesey, Ken 181
ketamine 190
Kettering, OH 191
Kettering Memorial Hospital, OH 192
Kidder, Margot 47

Kiesau, Randy 173
Kimble, Bo 113
Kimble, Michael 185
King, Billie Jean 135
King, Clyde 70
King Haakon (Norway) 63
Kinsman Aquatic Centre, AB 21
Kinston, NC 174
Kivilev, Andrey 119
Kivlenieks, Matīss 88–91
Kleinschmidt, Jetta 152
Kling, Michael 74
Knievel, Evel 163
Knight, Bob 95
Knight, Ray 120
Kojon Village Cemetery, Korea 21
Krirdla, Gil 19
Krum, TX
Ku Klux Klan 141
Kubeck, Candalyn 35
Kulwicki, Alan 70
Kurkowski, Frank 167
Kyle, Kellie 24

Labonte, Bobby 156
Ladies Professional Golf Association (LPGA) 197–198, 201
La Guardia Airport, NYC 76
Lake District, England 51
Lake Jackson, FL 51–52
Lake Nellie, FL 54
Lake Placid, NY 100
LaLanne, Jack 103
Lambert, Cody 25
Landover, MD 95
Landry, Greg 16
Laramie, WY 158
Larsen, Jonathan 94
Lasix 105, 133, 144
Latvia 89
Lauren, Lucien 135
Lavorel, Olivier 161
Lawrence Hospital, NY 139
Lawrence of Arabia 152
Lazar, Steve 167
Lázaro, Francisco 9–10, 19
Legace, Emmanuel "Manny" 89–90
Leland Memorial Hospital, MD 95
Leto, Jared 181
Let's Light the Way (racehorse) 142
Lewis, Reggie 98–100, 115
Lewmar, Inc. 88
Lexington, MA 84
Lidle, Cory 75–78, *77*
Lidle, Melanie 75, *77*
Lincoln, Abraham 94
Lincoln Memorial Cemetery, MD 95, 97

Lindbergh, Anna Lisa 184
Lindbergh, Charles 62, 64
Lindbergh, Pelle 55, 181–184, *183*
Lindbergh, Sigge 184
Lipinski, Tara 172
Little Brown Jug (harness racing) 138
Little Lake Nellie, FL 54
Lockheed Starfighter (aircraft) 159
Loevezijn, Kees van 151
Logan, UT 172
Lohrke, Jack "Lucky" 164
Lokanc, Larry 195
Lombardy, Italy 118
Long, Terry 95–96
Long Beach, NY 79
Longman, Jéré **59**
Los Angeles, CA 61, 63
Los Angeles Angels 40, 109–110
Los Angeles Coliseum 169
Los Angeles Dodgers 53
Los Angeles Kings 15
Louganis, Greg 22–23
Louisiana State University Tigers 114
Louisville and Nashville Railroad 177
Loveland Pass, CO 172, *174*
Loyola Marymount University, CA 113
Lutz, FL 58
Lynch, Edward 27
Lynch, Sean 194–196
Lynn, Lance 13
Lysacek, Evan 172

M Resort, NV 199
Ma Huang (herbal stimulant) 107
Maccabiah Games 28
Macon, MS 185
MacPhail, Larry 12
MacTavish, Craig 15
Madden, John 168
Madden, Terry 160
Madison Square Garden, NYC 20, 79, 89, 94, 103
Madonna del Ghisallo, Italy, 119
Maier, Melanie 117
Maier, Ulrike 116–118
Mali 150
Malone, Terry 193–194
Mancini, Ray "Boom Boom" 18–20, *19*
Mankato, MN 106
Manx Grand Prix (Isle of Man) 161, 162
Marfan, Antonine 93
Marfan syndrome 93–94

Marion du Pont Training Center, SC (racehorses) 134
Marlboro, NJ 195
Marlin, Sterling 156
Marlton Evesham Township, NJ 182
Marquis of Queensberry Rules (boxing) 21
Mars Retrograde (fireworks) 90
Marshall Thundering Herd 174–176
Marshall University Memorial Fountain, WV 176
Marshfield High School, OR 180
Martin, Billy 66, 121
Martin 404 (aircraft) 172
Martinez, Fred "Freddy" 165
Marx Brothers 143
MASO K Walsh (bull) 25
Masterton, Bill 13–15
Matsue, Japan 93
Maturna, Francisco 33–35
Mauritania 150
Mausoleum of Christian Heritage, CA 78
Mayfield Cemetery, OH 29
Mays, Carl 11–13
Mays, Willie 30
McAdory, James 186
McArthur, Ken 9
McBurney Y.M.C.A., NYC 27
McCormack, Levi "Chief" 165
McCourt, Owen (Bud) 14
McCutchan, Arad 177
McGaha, Mel 167
McGrath, Jack 149
McGwire, Mark 112
McHale, Kevin 99
McKay, Jim 29
McKenzie, Scott 133
McKinley, William 67
McLaren-Honda team (Formula One) 153
McMahon, Vince 86
McMinn, Deane *171*
McNeal, Kathyleen 183
McSherry, John 119–121
Meade, Nathan 22
Means, Jimmy 68
Medellín, Colombia 34
Medwick, Joe (Ducky) 12
Memorial Hospital, WY 25
Mercy Bowl, Los Angeles 169
Merrill, Charles 27
Merzlikins, Elvis 89
Mesa Marin Speedway, CA 149
Metropolitan Sports Arena, MN 14–15
Mevoli, Nick 123, 163
MGM Grand Arena, NV 24

Miami International Airport, FL 71
Michigan International Speedway 70
Mid-American Conference 174
Middle Tennessee State University 176
midget cars (auto racing) 147–148
Mijiashan Hill, China 128
Miley, Mike 30
Mina, ND 74
*Minneapolis Star-Tribune* 107
Minnesota Highway Thirty Six, 167
Minnesota North Stars 14
Minnesota State University 106
Minnesota Vikings 106–109
Minnesota Wild 44
Minsk, Russia 22
Mr. Olympia (bodybuilding) 104–105
Mitsubishi 150
mixed marital arts (MMA) 21
MLB player strike 75
Mobile, AL 197
Mohr, Charlie 21
Mongolian Groom (racehorse) *145*
Monroe, James 36
Monroe, Marilyn 47
Monroe, LA 49
Mont Ventoux, France 118
Montes, Fernando 54
Montgomery, Wilbert 185
Montgomery County, MD 187
Montreal Canadiens 14
Montreal Expos 112, 120
Moore, Caleb 121–124, 163
Moore, Colten 122, 124
Moore, Harold 5–8
Moore, Kenny 179–180
Mooresville, NC 158
Morgan, Davy 161
Morningside High School, CA 92
Morocco 150
Moss, Randy 107
Mount Hope Cemetery, MI 81
Mount Lawn Cemetery, PA 115
Mount Olivet Cemetery, OK 25
Mount Trelease, CO 173
MSNBC 74
Munich, West Germany 28–29, 105
Munson, Diana 67
Munson, Thurman 65–67
Muntean, Thais 23
Munzer, Andreas 103–106

Murcer, Bobby 67
Muscular Christianity 6
Museum of Sports and Tourism, Poland 178
Musson, Ron 51
myocarditis 115

Naismith, James 92
Nassau County, NY 80
Natchez Seminary, MS 184
National Collegiate Athletic Association (NCAA) 21, 174
National Highway Transportation Safety Administration (NHTSA) 190
National Jet Service 176
National Marfan Association 94
National Tennis Center, NYC 84
National Transportation Safety Board (NTSB) 67, 69, 76, 78, 173
Navarro, Chris 26
NBC 155
New Castle, IN 166
New England Baptist Hospital, MA 98
New Haven, CT 166, 169
New York Mets 13, 30
New York Presbyterian Hospital, NYC 80
New York Rangers 79–80
New York State Racing Association 135
New York Supreme Court 85
*New York Times* 59, 132, 137
New York University Violets 5
New York Yankees 13, 30, 65–67, 75–77
Newell, Pete 113
*Newsweek* 141
Newtown Square, PA 36
Nez Perce Indian tribe 165
Niagara Falls, NY-ON 47–49
Niagara River, NY 47–49
Niger 150–151
Nike 180
1964 Civil Rights Act 140
Nixon, Richard 29
Nome, AK 124–126
*North American Eagle* (jet-powered car) 159–160
North Carolina State University 58, 192
Northeastern University, MA 99
Northern League (baseball) 167
Northwestern Louisiana State University 49
*Not Without Hope* (book) 59

## Index

Notre Dame Fighting Irish 62–63, 70–72, 195–196
Novi, MI 89

Oakland Acorns, 166
Oakland A's 13
Oakland County, MI 89–90
Oakland International Airport, CA 168
Oakland Raiders 57
Oakland Seals 14
Oceanside, CA 62
O'Connor, Debbie 196
Ogdensburg, NY 7
Ohio Field, NYC 5, 7
Ohio House of Representatives 167
Ohio State Buckeyes 5, 189
Ohio University Bobcats 175
Ojeda, Bobby 53–55
Olin, Patty 54
Olin, Steve 52–55
Olson, Doctor Alane 199
Olympia, WA 166
O'Neal, Shaquille 114
O'Neil, Kitty 159
O'Neill, Tip 96
Orange Bowl 191
*Order of the Black Eagle* (film) 93
Orland Park, IL 194, 196
Orlando, FL 73
Orlando Regional Center, FL 53
Oshi (sled dog) 125–128, ***127***
Ostfriedhof Cemetery, Austria 117
Ouachita Parish, LA 49
*Overhaulin'* (TV show) 158
Owen, Laurence "Laurie" 170–***171***
oxycodone 110

Pacific Coast League (baseball) 165–166
Pacific View Memorial Park, CA 199
Pacino, Al 27
Pack, Austria 104
Paddock Saloon and Grill, OR 179–180
Page, Dorothy G. 124
Palo Alto, CA 35–36
Pan-American Games 36
PANA (African news agency) 152
Paralympic Games 129, 186–187
Paret, Benny (Kid) 20
Paris, France 150–151
Parish, Robert 99
Park City, UT 123
Parker, Dave 111

Parvin, Ed 183
Patriot League 192–193
Pavesi, Attilio 118
Payton, Byron 178
Payton, Walter 185
PCP (phencyclidine) 32
Pearson, David 68
Pebble Beach Golf Club, CA 75
pedestrian deaths in the U.S. 190
Peixoto, José Luis 10
Pelé 33, 153
Penn National Race Course (horse racing) 133
Penn State University, PA 175
pentathlon 36
People for the Ethical Treatment of Animals (PETA) 126–127, 143
Pepsi Invitational Miles (wheelchair racing) 186
Percocet 110
Perkins, Lancer Bernard 50
Perovich, Howard 169
Perry, Gaylord 13
Perry, Luke 26
Peru 151
Peterson, Gerald "Peanuts" 167
Petrenko, Viktor 103
Petty, Adam 157
Petty, Richard 155
Peugeot 150
Phelps, Michael 94
Philadelphia Eagles 16
Philadelphia Flyers 181–182
Philadelphia Phillies 48
Picetti, Vic 165
Pietzsch, Kerstin 182–183
Pineview Memorial Park, OH 109
Piniella, Lou 67
Piquet, Nelson 153
Pittsburgh Steelers 189
*Playboy* 141
Pocono International Speedway, PA 70
Polish Airlines 178
Polo Grounds, NYC 11
Poolesville, MD 187
Pope John Paul II 193
Pope Pius XXII 119
Porsche 930 Turbo (automobile) 182, ***183***
Portland, OR 54
Prague, Czechoslovakia 170
*Prefontaine* (film) 181
Prefontaine, Steve 55, 179–181
Pre's Rock, OR 181
Preservation Hall Jazz Band 136

Presidential Citizens Medal 50
Price, Lloyd 32
Prichard, AL 185
Prince of Wales Conference (NHL) 184
Princess Lili B (racehorse) 126
Princeton University, NJ 7
Professional Rodeo Cowboys Association (PRCA) 24
Progressive movement 6
Prost, Alain 153–154
PT X 3 (ice melting chemical) 117
Puente San Miguel, Spain 42
Puma Golf 198
*Pumping Iron* (film) 103
Purslow, Mark 161–162
Pyrenees Mountains, France 117

Queens' Park Mausoleum, AB 88

Race Across America (cycling) 188
*Rain-X Record Challenger* (jet-powered boat) 51–52
Raines, Tim 111
Ramos, Sugar 20
Ramsey County, MN 45
Ratzenberger, Roland 153
Rauris, Austria 116–117
Reagan, Ronald 50, 71, 98
Red Rock (bull) 24
Redington, Joe, Sr. 124
Reebok 94
Reed, William O. 137
Reese, Pee Wee 12
Reeve, Christopher 47
Reeves, Steve 103
Regions Hospital, MN 45
Rein, Bo 75
relief drivers (auto racing) 148
*Remember the Titans* (film) 107
Richard, Maurice 15
Richards, Collin Daniel 42–44
Richardson, Gloster 185
Richardson, Willie 185
Rickey, Branch 12
Riddles, Libby 125
riding mechanics (auto racing) 149
Riggs, Bobby 136
Rinehart, Ronald Milton 188
Rinehart, Timothy S. 188
*Ring* magazine 20
Rio Rancho, NM 187
Ripped Fuel (energy drink) 107–108
Rivera, Danielle 126

Riverfront Stadium, OH 16, 120
Roberts Stadium, IN 177
Robinson, Sugar Ray 20
Robinson R-22 (helicopter) 68
Rockne, Bonnie 64
Rockne, Knute 61–65, 168
*Rocky* (film) 26
Rodolph, John 186–187
Roe, Preacher 13
Rogers, Antonio 185
Rogers, Don 96
Rogers, Will 62–63
Romero, Randy 133
Romo, Sergio 13
Roosevelt, Theodore 6–7
Roper, Tony 157
Rose Bowl 33, 147
Roseville, MN 167
Royal Albert Hall, London 103
Rubin, Barbara Jo 140
Rudd, Ricky 68
Rudolph, Mason 189
Ruelas, Gabriel 20
Ruffian 134–137, 142
Ruiz, Chico 30
Ruth, Babe 62, 64, 121
Ryan, Mike 44–46
Ryder Cup 42, 73
Rye, NY 195

Sabena Airlines 170
Sabine, Thierry 149–150
SabreTech 72
St. Catherine's Church, HI 57
St. Cloud Rox 167
St. Francis Medical Center 50
St. Joseph's Chapel, MA 193
St. Louis Blues 14–15
St. Louis Cardinals 167
Saint Martin de Porres High School, MI 70
St. Mary Medical Center, IN 29
St. Mary's Hospital, CO 123
St. Nicholas of Tolentine Church, NY 121
Salem Senators 164
San Diego Chargers 70
San Jose Sharks 44
San Luis Obispo, CA 168
San Marino Grand Prix 153–154
Sanchez, Emmanuel Jose 133
Sandow, Eugen 103
Sandy, Mark 177
Santa Anita Park, CA 126, 142–146, *145*
Santa Monica, CA 109
São Paulo, Brazil 154–155
Sasso, Rosemary 80
Satterfield, Bob 71

Saudi Arabia 152
Savannah, GA 188
Sawchuk, Terry 48, 79–82
Scherzer, Max 13
Schmaedeke Funeral Home, IL 196
Schoedinger Funeral Home, OH 90
Schott, Marge 121
Schourek, Pete 120
Schrader, Ken 156
Schuchman, Dan 167
Schultz, Dave 35–38, *37*, 41, 86
Schultz, Nancy 36, 38
Schumacher, Michael 153
Schuyler, Nick 58
Schwarzenegger, Arnold 104–105
Schweighofer, Hubert 166–117
seat belt use 65, 139, 181, 183, 186
Seattle, WA 165
Seattle Mariners 40–41
Seattle Rainiers 166
Seattle Seahawks 31
Seattle Smashers 92
Seau, Junior 8
Sebring, FL 51–52
second impact syndrome (concussions) 14
Secretariat (racehorse) 135
Selinger, Arie 93
Seneca Creek State Park, MD 187
Senna, Ayrton 153–155
Seoul, Korea 18
"Serum Run," AK 124
Settles, Ron **31–33**
Shaker Heights, OH 27
Shalibashvili, Sergei 22–23
Shaw, Wilbur 70
Shelton, Lee (Stagger Lee) 32
Shinnick, Chris 56
Shore, Eddie 15
Shortall, Patrick A. 31
Shorter, Frank 179, 181
Sibley, Fred 51
Signal Hill, CA 31
silent heart attacks 102
Simpson, Ed 182
Simpson, Ernon 177
Simpson, O.J. 31
Simpson, Tom 118
Simsbury, CT 102
Sinatra, Frank 191
Sioux City, IA 161
Sitwell, Dame Edith 94
Six-Day War 28
Skaggs, Tyler 109–112, *111*
Skipper, Ronald 172
Skyline Boulevard, OR 181

Skyline Memorial Gardens, OR 55
Slater, Jackie 185
Slaughter, John B. 96
Smith, Corey 57–60, **59**
Smith, Davey Boy 87
Smith, Jimmy 185
Smith, Joey 189
Smith, Leonard 30
Smith, Robyn 140
Smith, Shannon 55–57
Snaefell Mountain Course (IMTT) 160–161
Snoqualmie Pass, WA 165
snowmobiles (X Games) 122
Solheim Cup (women's golf) 42
Sonny Key (racehorse) 139
Sosa, Sammy 112
South Sinai, Egypt *152*
Southern Connecticut College 169
Southern 500 (NASCAR) 155
Southern Highlands Club, NV 198
Southwestern Athletic Conference (SWAC) 184
Spears, Kenny 72
speciesism 126–127
speed racing records (measurement) 159–160
spinal bifida 186–187
spitballs (MLB) 12–13
Spokane Indians 164–166
*Sports Illustrated* 121, 176, 180
Spring Hill Cemetery, WV 175
Stabler, Ken 8
Stagg, Amos Alonzo 8
Stampede Wrestling Foundation 85–86
standing eight count (boxing) 21
Stanford University, CA 7, 37, 63
Stanger, Tyler 76–77
Stanley Cup 181
State Correctional Institution at Laurel Highlands, PA 38
statins 17, 82
Steeples, Lemuel 178
Steinberg, Leigh 198
Steinbrenner, George 66–67
Stello, Dick 120
Stengel, Casey 166
Stephenson, Stafford 177
Stewart, Jackie 154
Stewart, Payne 73–75
Stewart, Ron 80–81
Stewart, Tony 156
Stewart, Tracey Richardson 73
"sticky stuff" scandal (MLB) 13

# Index

Stockholm, Sweden 9
Stockton, Bradley 161
Stockton, Roger 161
*Story of Seabiscuit* (film) 143
Stratford, NJ 183–184
Street, Picabo 117
Stringer, Kelcie 107
Stringer, Korey 106–109, 112
Stronach, Brenda 144
Stronach, Frank 144
Stronach Group 142–143
suet 9
suicide 193–194, 196, 198, **200**–201
Suidegeest, Hanny 39–40
Summer Olympic Games 9, 10, 27–28, 36, 92–93, 118, 180
Sunbelt Conference 175
Sunjet Aviation 73
Sunset Hills Memorial Park, OH 67
Sunset Memorial Park, OR 181
Sunset Memorial Park, TX 17
Super Bowl 70
super giant slalom (skiing) 115
*Superman II* (film) 47
Suskind, Ron 100
Sweet Kiss (racehorse) 131–132

Tacoma Rainiers 40
Talladega Superspeedway, AL 68
Tampa General Hospital, FL 59
Taylor, Lee 51
Taylor, Shone 186
Team Judith Flannery (cycling) 188
Team Motorola (cycling) 118
Tel Aviv, Israel 28
Temple, Shirley 143
Teterboro Regional Airport, NJ 76
Texas Children's Hospital 83
Texas Rangers 109
Texas Western College 16
Thal, Austria 104
Thiros, Nick 30
*Thrust SSC* (jet-powered car) 159
*El Tiempo* (newspaper) 33
Tiger Stadium, MI 16
Tillman, Spencer 195
Toledo, OH 140
Toledo Express Airport 167–169
Tollner, Ted 169
Tom Collins Tour of World Champions (figure skating) 101

Tom Rolfe (racehorse) 134
Tour de France 117–119, 150
Towne, Robert 181
Tracy, Jim 120
Tracy, Spencer 143
Tramadol, 199
Transcontinental and Western Air (TWA) 61, 64
Treadwell, George 167
Tri-State Airport, WV 175
triathlon, 188
Tribble, Brian 95–96
Trubisky, Mitch 189
Truman Medical Center, MO 87
Trumbull County, OH 109
Tucson, AZ 161
Tulane University, LA 27
Turner, Curtis 70
Turner, Lana 143
Turner, Paul Corley 141
Turner Broadcasting 155

ultimate fighting 21
ultramarathons (running) 128–130
Union College, NY 5, 7
U.S. Coast Guard 59–60
U.S. Department of Commerce 61, 64
U.S. Hockey Hall of Fame 15
U.S. Olympic and Paralympic training center, CO 178
U.S. Open (golf) 75
U.S. Open (tennis) 84
U.S. Product Safety Commission 90
U.S. Tennis Association (USTA) 84–85
U.S. women's volleyball team 93
University of Alabama 197
University of Alberta 22
University of California at Irvine, 39
University of Cincinnati Hospital, OH 120
University of Dayton, OH 191
University of Denver, CO 13–14
University of Hawaii 56
University of Houston, TX 92
University of Maryland 94–96
University of Miami, FL 36
University of Nevada Las Vegas (UNLV) 115
University of Notre Dame, IN 62, 64
University of Oklahoma 35
University of Oregon 179–181
University of South Florida 58

University of Southern California 113–114
*Until the End of the Ninth* (novel) 166
Upper Arlington, OH 90
USA Boxing Team 178
USA Figure Skating Team 170–172, ***171***
USA Wrestling 36
Utah State University 172

Vagankovsky Cemetery, Russia 103
Valderrama, Carlos 33
Valencia, Adolfo 33
ValuJet Flight 592 71
Vancouver, BC 164
Vancouver Canucks 81
Vanderbilt, Alfred 140
Varig Airlines 153
Vasin, Vladimir 23
Vásquez, Jacinto 135–137
the Vatican 152
Versailles Palace, France 151
Vertical Blue Competition (free diving) 123
Vettel, Sebastian 153
Vezina Trophy (NHL) 79, 182
Vianelli, Pierfranco 118
*Vogue* 141
von Appen, Fred 56
**Vukovich, Bill** 147–149, 153, 157
Vukovich, Bill, Jr. 149
Vukovich, Bill III 149
Vukovich, Eli 147

Waipahee, HI 55
Wallace, Henry III 186
Wallace, Rusty 68
*Wall Street Journal* 100
Walsh, Christy 63
Waltham-Weston Hospital, MA 98
Waltrip, Michael 156
Warby, Ken 51–52
Warhol, Andy 27
Warsaw Okecie Airport, Poland 178
Washington, Denzel 107
*Washington Post* 104
Washington Redskins 168, 189
Washington Senators 48
Waters, Andre 8
Weaver, Earl 30
Weeping Basketball Memorial, IN 177
weight reduction: football 107–108; horse racing 132–134
Weiner, Benjamin 80
Wells Fargo Bank 127

**Wertheim, Richard** 84–85
West Boylston, MA 193
West Coast Conference 114
West Covina, CA 78
Westchester County Medical Center, NY 139
Western Air Express 62
Western International League (baseball) 164
Westerveld Cemetery, the Netherlands 41
Westhead, Paul 113
West Virginia 127
Weyer, Lee 120
Wheeler County, TX 123
Whisler, Ryan 45–46
White, Barry 141
White, Lorenzo 195
White, Rondell 120
Whiteley, Frank, Jr. 134–137
**Wichita State Shockers** 172–*174*
Wiggins, Alan 111
William Jewett College, MO 49
Williams, Edward Bennett 191–192
Williams, Frank 154
Williams, Serena 157
Williams-Renault team (Formula One) 153–154
Wilmarth, Dick 124
Wilmington, DE 187
Wilson, Bernice 82–83
**Wilson, Don** 48, 82–83
Wimbledon 84
Winchester, MA 170
Winnipeg, MB 13, 79
Winston Cup (NASCAR) 68, 155, 157
Winter Haven, FL 53–54
Winter Olympics 101–102, 116, 181
*Without Limits* (film) 181
Woodland Hills, CA 109
Woodland Memorial Park, FL 55
Woodland Park Cemetery South, FL 72
Woodlands Cemetery, Sweden 184
Woodrus, Robert, Jr. 71
Woods, Tiger 157
Woodstock, GA 71
Woolpert, Phil 113
Worcester, MA 191, 193
World Boxing Association (WBA) 18
World Cup (soccer) 33
World Series 11, 66
World University Games 22
World War I 161
World War II 111, 148, 161
World Wrestling Federation (WWF) 86, 88
Wrigley Field 39
Wylie, Paul 101

X Games 122–124
Xanax 199
Xcel Energy Center, MN 44
*Xtreme 4´4* (TV show) 158

Yagman, Stephen 32
Yale University, CT 7
Yamaguchi, Kristi 172
**Yellow River Stone Forest, China** 128–130
Yeltsin, Boris 102
Yonkers Raceway, NY 139
Yoranov, Valentine 38
Youl, Simon 84
Youngstown, OH 18
Youngstown State Penguins 169

Zanin, Mario 118
Zaventem Airport, Belgium 170–*171*
Zerlantes, Becky 20
ZG-Mobil team (cycling) 118
Ziegfeld, Florenz 103
Zoueva, Marina 101

www.ingramcontent.com/pod-product-compliance
Ingram Content Group UK Ltd.
Pitfield, Milton Keynes, MK11 3LW, UK
UKHW051905160525
458631UK00018B/180